Studies in Computational Intelligence

Volume 946

Series Editor

Janusz Kacprzyk, Polish Academy of Sciences, Warsaw, Poland

The series "Studies in Computational Intelligence" (SCI) publishes new developments and advances in the various areas of computational intelligence—quickly and with a high quality. The intent is to cover the theory, applications, and design methods of computational intelligence, as embedded in the fields of engineering, computer science, physics and life sciences, as well as the methodologies behind them. The series contains monographs, lecture notes and edited volumes in computational intelligence spanning the areas of neural networks, connectionist systems, genetic algorithms, evolutionary computation, artificial intelligence, cellular automata, self-organizing systems, soft computing, fuzzy systems, and hybrid intelligent systems. Of particular value to both the contributors and the readership are the short publication timeframe and the world-wide distribution, which enable both wide and rapid dissemination of research output.

Indexed by SCOPUS, DBLP, WTI Frankfurt eG, zbMATH, SCImago.

All books published in the series are submitted for consideration in Web of Science.

More information about this series at http://www.springer.com/series/7092

Zbigniew W. Ras · Alicja Wieczorkowska ·
Shusaku Tsumoto
Editors

Recommender Systems for Medicine and Music

Springer

Editors
Zbigniew W. Ras
Department of Computer Science
University of North Carolina
at Charlotte
Charlotte, NC, USA

Polish-Japanese Academy
of Information Technology
Warsaw, Poland

Alicja Wieczorkowska
Department of Multimedia
Polish-Japanese Academy
of Information Technology
Warsaw, Poland

Shusaku Tsumoto
Department of Medical Informatics
Faculty of Medicine
Shimane University
Izumo, Japan

ISSN 1860-949X ISSN 1860-9503 (electronic)
Studies in Computational Intelligence
ISBN 978-3-030-66448-0 ISBN 978-3-030-66450-3 (eBook)
https://doi.org/10.1007/978-3-030-66450-3

This Springer imprint is published by the registered company Springer Nature Switzerland AG
The registered company address is: Gewerbestrasse 11, 6330 Cham, Switzerland

Preface

We know that music has a large effect on us in general. It can make us smile when we are feeling stressed. The sound of music can cause our hearts to beat in healthier ways. It helps people regain inner peace and is the voice that binds us together. The positive relationship between music and medicine is widely known. Music has become an important tool for medical therapy. Sound healing therapy uses aspects of music to improve physical and emotional health and well-being. The person being treated partakes in the experience with a trained practitioner. Music therapy may involve listening to music, singing along to music, meditating, and playing an instrument. Evidence suggests that music therapy is beneficial for all individuals, both physically and mentally, but especially in aging societies.

Many papers on music therapy have been published, possibly because medical doctors have to deal with various kinds of chronic diseases, including cancers, in which music therapy helps to improve the symptoms. A recent study conducted at Johns Hopkins University found that Parkinson's patients singing weekly improved their quality of life, voice strength, and clarity. Music can have an impressive impact on people with Alzheimer's disease since it may reduce agitation and improve behavioral issues that are common in its middle-stages. There are papers reviewing the state of the art in applying music therapy to treat Alzheimer's disease [1,2]. Music provides a way to connect, even after verbal communication has become difficult. Listening to music may improve heart rate, respiratory rate, and blood pressure in people with heart disease. Music can be used to treat cancer, tinnitus, psychiatric disorders, and visually impaired patients.

Health intelligent systems have become indispensable tools in decision-making processes in the healthcare sector. Their main objective is to ensure the availability of valuable information at the right time by ensuring information quality, trustworthiness, authentication, and privacy concerns. As people use social networks to understand their health condition, the health recommender system is very important to derive outcomes such as recommending diagnoses and clinical pathway-based treatment methods taking into consideration the patient's health profile.

Part I of the book contains six contributions covering the area of recommender systems and their applications in healthcare.

The Chapter "Recommendation Systems in Healthcare", written by Madlen Ivanova and Zbigniew W. Raś, gives an overview of recommender systems and their classification which is based on filtering techniques. There are five common techniques—collaborative filtering, content-based, knowledge-based, group recommender systems, and hybrid. Each one is presented with examples covering the healthcare domain. Collaborative filtering recommendation can be further split into six subcategories—model-based, memory-based, clustering based, matrix and tensor factorization, deep learning, and hybrid method.

The Chapter "Recommender Systems in Healthcare: A Socio-Technical Systems Approach", written by Mila Kwiatkowska, describes healthcare as a socio-technical system that comprises interacting human and technical agents. Thus, any change to the system, such as an introduction of Recommender System based (RS-based) tools or methods, requires careful consideration of the technical and social aspects. The chapter presents the main issues which should be considered in the deployment of RS-based tools and techniques in healthcare: (1) adherence to the medical regulations for medical software, (2) compliance with the medical data privacy, (3) improvement of transparency and trustworthiness of recommendations, (4) analysis of short-term and long-term ethical issues, and (5) patient empowerment, doctor–patient relationship, and human aspects.

The Chapter "Computer Methods for Localization of the Subthalamic Nucleus During Deep Brain Stimulation Surgeries for Treatment of Parkinson Disease" concerns Parkinson's Disease (PD) and it is written by Konrad A. Ciecierski. In the neurosurgical treatment of PD, the goal is the precise placement of the stimulating electrode within the Subthalamic Nucleus (STN). As STN does not significantly differ from adjacent structures on images provided by the CT or MRI, these standard techniques of medical imaging can provide only the approximate localization of the STN. Its final localization is pinpointed during the surgery. The author shows how this localization can be found with very high precision using knowledge discovery techniques.

The Chapter "Stutter Detection and Remediation in Speech" concerns stuttered speech and it is written by Ayman Hajja and Pierre Arbajian. Authors provide a review of the most relevant literature on stutter detection and remediation, and then present a two-phase machine learning system capable of identifying stutter segments in a speech. It has been shown that the system is able to reduce stutter speech disfluency in speech recordings by removing undesired segments. Then the authors expand their discussion on this topic to include and elaborate the description of a web-platform developed by them. The motivation for the development of such a web-platform was to provide researchers with the ability to effectively collect pre-labeled audio information for further analysis.

The Chapter "Personalizing Patients to Enable Shared Decision Making", written by Mamoun T. Mardini, Amal Hashky, and Zbigniew W. Raś, presents an evidence-based platform that aims to facilitate the communication between patients and clinicians. The platform is tailored towards the hospital readmission problem. It was achieved by mining the Healthcare Cost and Utilization Project (H-CUP) dataset. Authors use machine learning techniques to build models that predict the readmissions, their number, and mortality for newly admitted patients. They also built a graph named procedure graph to visualize the primary procedures during the treatment course. The procedure graph is personalized to the patient's medical characteristics by applying rough clustering technique.

The last chapter in this section, written by Jeremy Beauchamp, Razvan Bunescu, and Cindy Marling, concerns people with type 1 diabetes. They must keep their Blood Glucose Levels (BGLs) as close to normal as possible. Insulin dosages and carbohydrate consumption are important considerations in managing BGLs. Since the 1960s, models have been developed to forecast blood glucose levels based on the history of BGLs, insulin dosages, carbohydrate intake, and other physiological and lifestyle factors. Such predictions can be used to alert people on unsafe BGLs or to control insulin flow in an artificial pancreas. In past work, the authors introduced an LSTM-based approach to blood glucose level prediction aimed at "what-if" scenarios, in which people could enter foods they might eat or insulin amounts they might take and then see the effect on future BGLs. Building on these neural models for "what-if" predictions, in this work authors derive a novel LSTM-based architecture that can be trained to make either insulin or carbohydrate recommendations to ensure that future BGLs attain a desired level. Experimental evaluations using data from the OhioT1DM dataset show that the neural architecture substantially outperforms the baselines. The promising results suggest that this novel approach could potentially be of practical use to people with type 1 diabetes for self-management of BGLs.

The Part II of the book contains five contributions covering the area of recommender systems in the music domain.

The Chapter "Music Recommendation Systems: A Survey", written by Mariusz Kleć and Alicja Wieczorkowska, presents an overview of music recommendation systems, supported by a comprehensive list of references. Authors pay special attention to user-centric systems which personalize their output by tracking the context of the user, including the user's emotions and personality. Authors emphasize the importance of social media, the usability of user interfaces, and the application of deep learning techniques in the recent developments in music recommendation systems. They also outline inspirations for future research in the field.

The Chapter "Repeated Listens in the Music Discovery Process" concerns the Long-Tail Problem (LTP) and it is written by Brian Manolovitz and Mitsunori Ogihara, Due to the nature of recommender systems, the most popular music is the easiest to recommend, but it is often the least interesting for the listeners. This is known as the long-tail problem for recommender systems. Authors propose to incorporate repetition in the music discovery process as a potential solution to LTP. Their studies showed that repetition of novel songs increases memory and liking of them as long as those songs remain novel. The psychological background for this phenomenon was extracted from various studies on music familiarity with respect to musical qualities and emotional and neurological responses.

The Chapter "What Songs We Listen to Together: Automatic Music Selection for Groups" concerns group recommender systems and is written by Jun'ichi Suzuki and Tetsuro Kitahara. Authors introduce several systems that aim at group music recommendation. The first one called MusicFX was developed by McCarthy and Anagnost. It was probably the earliest system that aims at group music selection and it was supposed to be used in fitness centers. The second one is called Flytrap—it automatically constructs a soundtrack that tries to please everyone in the room. The next one is called GroupFun which is a web application, implemented as a Facebook plug-in, that helps a group of friends to agree on a common music playlist. Finally, the authors present their Android application that tries to select songs that potentially please most of the people present in the same place under the assumption that they know each other well. The aim of this application is to automatically select and play the background music in which all members' musical preferences are equally reflected.

The Chapter "Body Data for Music Information Retrieval Tasks", written by Tejaswinee Kelkar, concerns a range of multimodal and cross modal music retrieval methods that help bring the ideas for music retrieval and music information retrieval, to incorporate data from the body. Treating sound-tracings as annotation material provides a new way of thinking about music analysis and studies on segmentation and phrasing. The author shows that people demonstrate a remarkable amount of consistency in their spatial and motor representations of music and sonic objects. Experiments akin to these could inform our understanding of musical phrasing, and the differences in people's phrasing boundaries in various contexts. This could help us build a more sophisticated understanding of music perception and create interesting interfaces for music retrieval.

The last chapter of this section is written by Jacek Grekow and it concerns the problem of searching different performances of the same composition. It mostly pertains to classical music, where the compositions of the greatest old masters, such as J. S. Bach, W. A. Mozart, L. v. Beethoven, R. Schumann, or F. Chopin, have many interpretations played by known and less known performers. Just as human speech has its emotional content, the same composition, based on one musical notation, can be performed differently with each performance differing in the emotional content. This chapter presents a content-based recommender system, which looks for similar performances in terms of emotional content of the same composition.

The Part III of the book contains three contributions covering the area of recommender systems focused on applications of music to healthcare.

The Chapter "Music and Healthcare Recommendation Systems" of this section is written by Mariusz Kleć and Alicja Wieczorkowska and it starts with an overview of healthcare recommender systems, supported by a comprehensive list of references. Next, the authors give a brief review of systems that recommend music for health purposes. Since systems that recommend music to treat medical problems are not commonly used yet, authors focus on studies that explore the influence of music on human health in general. They also outline the inspirations for the future development of music recommendation systems used for medical purposes.

The Chapter "Emotion-Based Music Recommender System for Tinnitus Patients (EMOTIN)" is written by Katarzyna Tarnowska and it describes a clinical decision support system for tinnitus diagnosis and music-based tinnitus therapy. This system utilizes a user-friendly graphical interface to enter patient- and visit-related data and to display the system's inference of diagnosis and effective treatment options. The rule engine is implemented using the Java Expert System Shell (JESS) framework. The system utilizes a pattern-matching algorithm to provide a diagnosis for a new patient based on a pre-coded set of decision rules. These decision rules encoded into the system are extracted from clinical datasets. Each decision rule assigns the tinnitus retraining therapy category based on the characteristics of a patient, such as initial interview and audiometry. The treatment recommendations are inferred from action rules extracted from clinical datasets first and then encoded into the knowledge base.

In the Chapter "A Model of Typhlo Music Therapy in Educational and Rehabilitation Work with Visually Impaired Persons", written by Pawel Cylulko and Joanna Gladyszewska-Cylulko, the authors present the specifics of a support intervention for visually impaired persons, carried out according to their model of typhlo music therapy. The model is mainly based on the sightless approach to experiencing music, the healing potential of music, and above all, the rehabilitative and therapeutic dimension of the human–music relationship. This model plays an important role in stimulating the individual development of persons with a disability, improving the impaired body functions, and in optimal adaptation to everyday functioning without sight or with serious visual impairment.

Music therapists and physicians already demonstrated the value of music in treating all diseases from Alzheimer's disease to chronic pain and substance abuse problems. Still, many questions remain to be answered. For instance, we need to know if specific sounds or tempos affect the heart regardless of the listener's musical preferences. Finding a relaxing melody that slows the heart rate, reduces blood pressure, and improves blood flow would make it easier to offer music therapy.

We are very grateful to all authors who contributed chapters to this book. Also, we hope that readers will find it interesting and useful.

Charlotte, NC, US
Warsaw, Poland
Shimane, Japan
September 2020

Zbigniew W. Ras
Alicja A. Wieczorkowska
Shusaku Tsumoto

References

Garcia-Casares N, Moreno-Leiva RM, Garcia-Arnes JA., Efecto de la musicoterapia como terapia no farmacologica en la enfermedad de Alzheimer. Revision sistematica [Music therapy as a non-pharmacological treatment in Alzheimer's disease. A systematic review]. Rev Neurol. 2017 Dec 16;65(12):529-538. Spanish. PMID: 29235615.

Leggieri M, Thaut MH, Fornazzari L, Schweizer TA, Barfett J, Munoz DG, Fischer CE., Music Intervention Approaches for Alzheimer's Disease: A Review of the Literature. Front Neurosci. 2019 Mar 12;13:132. doi: 10.3389/fnins.2019.00132. PMID: 30930728; PMCID: PMC6424022.

Acknowledgements

The editors of this volume are grateful to Aileen Benedict, Ph.D. student in CS Department at UNC-Charlotte, for converting two chapters of this book from word to latex format.

Contents

Contributors

Pierre Arbajian UNC Charlotte, Charlotte, NC, USA

Jeremy Beauchamp Ohio University, Athens, OH, USA

Razvan Bunescu University of North Carolina at Charlotte, Charlotte, NC, USA

Konrad A. Ciecierski Research and Academic Computer Network, Warszawa, Poland

Pawel Cylulko Karol Lipinski Academy of Music in Wroclaw, Wroclaw, Poland

Joanna Gladyszewska-Cylulko Institute of Pedagogy, University of Wroclaw, Wroclaw, Poland

Jacek Grekow Faculty of Computer Science, Bialystok University of Technology, Bialystok, Poland

Ayman Hajja College of Charleston, Charleston, SC, USA

Amal Hashky Georgia Institute of Technology, School of Computer Science, Atlanta, GA, USA

Madlen Ivanova Department of Computer Science, University of North Carolina, Charlotte, N.C., USA

Tejaswinee Kelkar Oslo, Norway

Tetsuro Kitahara Nihon University, Setagaya-ku, Tokyo, Japan

Mariusz Kleć Polish-Japanese Academy of Informtion Technology, Warsaw, Poland

Mila Kwiatkowska The Department of Computing Science, Thompson Rivers University, Kamloops, British Columbia, Canada

Brian Manolovitz University of Miami, Coral Gables, FL, USA

Mamoun T. Mardini College of Medicine, Dept. of Aging and Geriatric Research, University of Florida, Gainesville, FL, USA

Cindy Marling Ohio University, Athens, OH, USA

Mitsunori Ogihara University of Miami, Coral Gables, FL, USA

Zbigniew W. Raś Department of Computer Science, University of North Carolina, Charlotte, N.C., USA;
Polish-Japanese Academy of Information Technology, Warsaw, Poland

Jun'ichi Suzuki Nihon University, Setagaya-ku, Tokyo, Japan

Katarzyna A. Tarnowska San Jose State University, One Washington Square, San Jose, CA, USA

Alicja Wieczorkowska Polish-Japanese Academy of Informtion Technology, Warsaw, Poland

Recommendation Systems in Healthcare

Madlen Ivanova and Zbigniew W. Raś

Abstract Recommender systems are a subclass of information filtering systems which is broadly used to find the right products or services for the right consumers. In the era of 'Big Data', recommender systems are of great importance as they are used to solve the information overload in many areas of people's lives (e-commerce/e-shopping, e-library, movies, TV programs, prescriptions, health recommendations, news, cooking, and more). In their simplest form, recommender systems create a personalized list of predictions that are ranked based on the user's history, preference, solution/domain constraints, and other factors.

1 Introduction to Recommender Systems

Recommender systems are a subclass of information filtering systems which is broadly used to find the right products or services for the right consumers. In the era of 'Big Data', recommender systems are of great importance as they are used to solve the information overload in many areas of people's lives (e-commerce/e-shopping, e-library, movies, TV programs, prescriptions, health recommendations, news, cooking, and more). In their simplest form, recommender systems create a personalized list of predictions that are ranked based on the user's history, preference, solution/domain constraints, and other factors. What really matters for the customers today is their value experience as much as the actual products and services. They have proven their usefulness in the commercial market by improving the customers' decision-making process and satisfaction in the everyday life, as well as improving the customer retention and increasing the revenue for the service/product providers.

M. Ivanova (✉)
Department of Computer Science, University of North Carolina, Charlotte, N.C. 28223, USA
e-mail: mivanov1@uncc.edu

Z. W. Raś
Department of Computer Science, University of North Carolina, Charlotte, N.C. 28223, USA
e-mail: ras@uncc.edu

Polish-Japanese Academy of Information Technology, 02-008 Warsaw, Poland

Z. W. Ras et al. (eds.), *Recommender Systems for Medicine and Music*,
Studies in Computational Intelligence 946,
https://doi.org/10.1007/978-3-030-66450-3_1

2 Recommender System Classification

To bring out valuable insights from the massive amount of data with speed and precision, recommender systems rely on various data mining techniques for information retrieval [9]. The one criterion that is used to classify them is the filtering technique. There are five common techniques—Collaborative Filtering, Content-Based, Knowledge-based, Group recommender systems, and Hybrid [17]. The Recommender System classification could be broken down even more by the implementation approach and other specific to the filtering model characteristics. Additionally, there are external metadata characteristics that could be applied to each of the filtering models to further improve the accuracy of the system.

2.1 Collaborative Filtering

Collaborative Filtering is a technique used to make automatic predictions about the preference of a user derived by analyzing the preferences of other users that have similar interests. The underlined characteristic of this type of filtering is that if a person A has the same preference as person B, therefore, person A will be more likely to like another service/product that person B likes comparing to a random customer. In the e-commerce industry, for instance, based on products viewed and bought online, the system will recommend products to customers that are bought/viewed by people with similar taste. These product predictions will be specific to the individual customer, but the information used for the prediction will be filtered based on the online behavior of many users. Collaborative filtering recommendation is often based on trust and emotion [20, 30]. It can further split into six main categories—model-based, memory-based, clustering based, matrix and tensor factorization, deep learning, and hybrid method. Depending on the objective, the models could be also user-based and item-based.

2.1.1 Memory-Based Collaborative Filtering

The memory-based models are based on computing the correlation metrics of the user's rating and other behavioral metrics to recommend or predict the next item or set of items that users could be interested in. To compute the distance correlation, there are many statistical techniques that are widely used such as Euclidean distance, Jaccard distance, Pearson correlation coefficient, cosine similarity, adjusted cosine similarity, Manhattan distance, and others. There are two main approaches in memory-based filtering—user-based and item-based. The memory-based approach uses the entire data set to compute the correlations that makes it computationally expensive and unscalable in cases where we have massive datasets.

The item-based approach relies on the customer rating for the items viewed/bought. The rating could be determined not only from the implicit feedback of the users, but also the explicit. The target user's rating is used to compute the item similarity of the set of items the user has already rated and then select the most similar items to be recommended. This method does not perform well in cases where there are many items but comparatively few ratings.

The user-based collaborative filtering approach calculates similarity in opinion/interest between pairs of users and then use their item rating to recommend items that are new to the user at hand. Low-rank matrix approximation is one of the widely used methods for Collaborative Filtering due to high accuracy [26]. To be effective, this approach needs sufficient data on each user so it can be used to create the customer profile for the user-to-user similarity calculation.

2.1.2 Model-Based Collaborative Filtering

Comparing to the memory-based approach, the model-based one usually does not use the entire dataset to compute the predictions, but it uses a training set for predicting the future ratings. For recommending an item, a model first analyzes the user-item matrix. Next, it identifies the relationship among the items, and then it compares these relations with top-N recommendations list. After a model is constructed, predictions could be computed very fast. Model-based collaborative filtering methods usually achieve less accurate predictions than memory-based methods on dense data sets where a large fraction of user-item values are available in the training set but perform better on sparse data sets.

The emerging healthcare websites and online medical databases impose a new challenge for medical service recommendation. Model-based filtering is a popular technique used in the healthcare domain. In [31], it is used to better understand the interactions among different genes within the biological system. Results show clear advantages for the model-based over the model-free filtering techniques.

2.1.3 Clustering Based Collaborative Filtering

This method implies the usage of various clustering techniques to cluster the users and the items based on similar preferences and similar attributes correspondingly by using distance-based methods [23]. Neighborhood methods are centered on computing the relationships between users or, alternatively, between items. The user-based approach evaluates the user's neighborhood to determine what items users with the same interest in that neighborhood might be interested in.

An example of a clustering-based collaborative filtering in the healthcare domain is the application in the Clinical Decision Support System (CDSS) that helps with personalizing the diagnosis and treatment decisions [18]. The neighborhood-based Collaborative Filtering methods are used to exploit high-dimensional clinical data. The system is utilizing an exclusively data-driven approach, extended by a set of evidence-based contraindication rules. Patients having similar therapy characteristics and history can be analyzed to make a prediction for the therapy outcome. Trust plays a key role to leverage the acceptance and applicability of such systems. This Recommender System leverages the data-driven approach to increase trust and reduce the risk of the proposed system.

2.1.4 Matrix and Tensor Factorization-Based Collaborative Filtering

Some of the most successful implementations of latent factor models are based on matrix factorization [25, 30]. Recommender systems mainly base their suggestions on rating data of two entities (users and items), which are placed in a matrix with one representing the users and the other representing items of interest. Generally, matrix factorization characterizes both items and users by vectors of factors inferred from item rating patterns [26]. The overall interest of the item characteristics of a specific user is derived by computing the dot product of the given user interests based on corresponding factors related to the items and the actual item characteristics [37]. High correspondence between item and user factors leads to a better recommendation.

An example of matrix factorization in healthcare is the professionalized doctor recommendation system named iDoctor [49]. The system incorporates hybrid matrix factorization to propose a topic model-based approach to discover user preference distribution and doctor feature distribution to provide more accurate and personalized medical recommendations.

Tensor factorization has emerged as a powerful method to address the challenges of high dimensionality regarding disease development and comorbidity in healthcare. Patients suffering from one chronic disease have an elevated risk to get other diseases during aging as chronic diseases have a high likelihood to co-occur. In [49], two-tensor factorization-based methods are used to incorporate the clinical and sequential factors to reveal the latent patterns of co-occurring chronic diseases. The proposed predictive models could be used to inform proactive health management programs for patients at risk from different chronic conditions at discharge.

2.1.5 Deep Learning-Based Collaborative Filtering

Deep learning is a special type of model-based filtering methods that have proven to be powerful tools that complement traditional machine learning and allow the learning of nonlinear relationships between events, users, and products. Multilayer Perceptron (MLP), Convolutional Neural Network (CNN), Adversarial Networks (AN), Auto-Encoder (AE), Restricted Boltzmann Machine (RBM), Recurrent Neural Network (RNN), and its special case—Long Short Term Memory networks (LSTM) are the main components of the deep learning method [32, 48]. Due to their architectural structure, these methods integrate diverse data sets across heterogeneous data types. They are not simply based on classification accuracy, but provide greater generalization given the focus on representation learning.

The use of deep learning models for clinical applications has great potential to transform traditional healthcare service delivery. For instance, processing medical data with multilayer neural networks has increased the predictive power for several specific applications in different clinical domains. Many applications are using image processing to spot health problems on X-rays [36], Histology, Ultrasound, Magnetic Resonance Imaging, Computed Tomography, and other types of clinical imaging modalities [34]. For instance, as MRI is very sensitive to even small levels of subject motion during the scan, so it can produce artifacts in the final magnetic resonance (MR) image, which may result in misdiagnosis. To solve that, the Generative Adversarial Network (GAN) based MRI reconstruction method is presented in [45] that cleans the motion artifacts. Some other application areas which achieved human-level performance are ophthalmology [19], clinical pathology [7], and dermatology [16]. Deep learning uses efficient methods to do the diagnosis and to identify abnormalities, becoming a crucial component in the classification process of a health recommender system for diagnosis prediction.

2.1.6 Hybrid Collaborative Filtering

The hybrid collaborative filtering approach combines the user and item similarity techniques to improve the model performance as individually each collaborative filtering type of model has weaknesses, but in combination, they outperform the individual models. For instance, in [41], the authors introduce a Collaborative Filtering Neural network architecture (CFN) which computes a non-linear matrix factorization from sparse rating inputs and side information. The research shows that CFN outperforms the state of the art and benefits from side information.

2.2 Content-Based Recommender Systems

Content-based filtering is another type of filtering that is widely used to create recommendations based on item similarity. This system is heavily based on information retrieval and information filtering techniques where the weights are based on the item features and their utility for the individual users. Usually, the process involves creating a content-based profile for each user. Then the item importance weights are computed using one of many statistical techniques applied to the individually rated content vectors of the user profile.

These techniques could be as simple as using the average values of the rated item vector to more sophisticated such as using machine learning techniques (Bayesian classifiers, clustering, decision trees, neural networks/deep learning, etc.) to compute the likelihood of a user buying an item or liking a service. As this type of recommendation filtering is specific to the user, the advantages are that the model does not need a similarity index between users and can capture better user's specific interests as he/she might be interested in cases where user is interested in items that very few other users are interested in.

An example of a content-based filtering in healthcare is the content-based recommender system presented in [38] that links health care consumers to reputable health educational websites from MedlinePlus for a given health video from YouTube. The recommender system demonstrates the feasibility of using a semantic content-based recommender system to enrich YouTube health videos, where the recommendation relevancy is measured using information retrieval metrics such as precision and normalized discounted cumulative gain. Another example of a content-based filtering in healthcare is the paper written by Min Yen Wu which presents a deep architecture for depression detection using posting, behavior, and living environment data [47].

2.3 Knowledge-Based Recommender Systems

The knowledge-based recommender systems are based on explicit knowledge about the product, service, or recommendation criteria in a specific context. These types of systems are usually used in cases where the collaborative filtering or context-based filtering are not sufficient as there are domain knowledge expertise that needs to be considered.

The system makes use of the user profile and recommends items based on the user's need and user's implicit/explicit feedback. There are many ways to build such a system and its knowledge base using that feedback. For instance, the recommender system could walk the user down a discrimination tree of product features to build the knowledge base or use quantitative decision support tools for this task. The user profile definition process is usually partially automated as it involves both user-system interaction and the user's past behavior. The system also could rely on previous cases, then the recommendations are generated matching the new case with one that is stored in the knowledge base. The measures used to calculate the similarity between the items and the user profiles are based on the type of input (structured, unstructured data).

There are many applications in the healthcare environment that rely on domain specific knowledge. For instance, in [27], there have been implemented two popular knowledge-based techniques: case-based reasoning and rule-based reasoning. The paper discusses the development of a wellness recommender system that helps users to find suitable personalized wellness therapy treatments based on their individual needs. The system solves individual wellness problems for users by applying solutions from similar cases in the past by combining both case-based and rule-based reasoning in a hybrid approach. Case-based reasoning has been used for antibiotics therapy advice [39], electronic patient record system [10], and wellness therapy. The cycle consists of four main stages: retrieving previous cases from the case database, reusing a previous case to recommend a solution, revising a previous solution to match the current problem, and retaining new cases after a solution has been successfully found [39]. The rule-based reasoning, on the other hand, uses "if-then-else" rule statements. The engine looks for patterns in the rules matching to these in the data and the process is getting more complex over time as the number of rules increases [1].

During deep brain stimulation (DBS) treatment of Parkinson's disease, the target of the surgery is the subthalamic nucleus (STN). As STN is small and poorly visible on a computerized tomography (CT) scan or MRI, multi-electrode micro recording systems are used during DBS surgery for its better localization. Papers [11–14] present five different analytical methods, that can be used to construct an autonomic system assisting neurosurgeons in precise localization of the STN nucleus. Such autonomic knowledge-based recommender systems are currently used in Warsaw, Poland during surgical treatment for Parkinson's disease.

Tinnitus Retraining Therapy (TRT) is a complex treatment process which generates a high volume of matrix data over time: some attributes have relatively stable values while others may be subject to change as the doctors are tuning the treatment parameters while symptoms of patients are altering. Understanding the relationships between and patterns among treatment factors helps to optimize the treatment process. Based on the medical matrix data and knowledge, papers [24, 42–44] present a flexible temporal feature retrieval systems based on grouping the patients of similar visiting frequencies with connection to an action rules engine, which consists of four modules: a data grouping device, a temporal feature extraction engine, a decision tree classification device, and an action rules generation device. The system belongs to knowledge-based and group recommender systems.

Authors in [5, 6] present two different systems, whose purpose is to remedy a disfluent speech by automatically detecting blocked speech utterances and removing disfluent speech segments. Such systems are helpful to speakers who wish to make their speech easier, more convenient, and better understood. Remediation of disfluent speeches also reduces the need for a speech re-recording. For the first system, the dataset for training classifiers consists of speech and speaker metadata, and prequalified speech segments signal statistics. In the second approach, two classifiers were trained similarly, but with different datasets. The classifiers were capable to perform general speech scoring functions very well by analyzing a wide range of speech segments. Both systems belong to the knowledge-based recommender systems class.

2.4 Group Recommender Systems

The foundational concept of a group recommender system is that instead of user personalized recommendation, the system recommends services/items to a group of users based on the aggregated individual preference [15, 43, 44].

Group recommendation can be implemented using recommendation paradigms for individual users by using some of the filtering methods described in this chapter such as collaborative filtering, content-based filtering, knowledge-based filtering, and hybrid filtering. For instance, in [33], the authors have proposed a new approach to group recommender system using collaborative filtering technique where they have combined the features of both item-item and user-user collaborative filtering techniques to aggregate user preferences and make efficient group recommendation by creating homogeneous groups. Independent of the way, preferences are derived from individual group members, a key part of the group recommendation is determined by aggregating these preferences in one way or another [8].

Group recommender systems are applied in different ways in the healthcare domain. One is as an augmentation of the single user model to enhance the performance. An example of such a system is the HER system in [28], where social network groups of interests are used to enhance the Electronic Healthcare record system performance. On the other hand, it could be used as an additional recommender layer in more complex recommender systems in the instances where healthcare providers need recommendations on both patient group and individual levels. For instance, in [40], the group recommender system is used in a personal medical information recommendation system within the iManageCancer EU research project. The project has the objective to provide a cancer specific self-management platform designed according to the needs of patient groups, while in parallel focusing on the well-being of the cancer patient. The system aims to predict and detect in early stages events during the cancer therapy, and at the same time account for the psycho-emotional health of the patients and patients' individual goals. The platform is centered in a Personal Health Record which not only regularly monitors the psycho-emotional state of the patient, but also periodically captures the everyday life experiences of the cancer patient with respect to the therapy's unwanted side effects.

Distortions of the velopharyngeal closure, resulting in speech hypernasality, may cause speech disorders in children. The gathered geographic and medical data by the Children's Memorial Health Institute in Warsaw (Poland) also include general information on the patient's condition if it can be of importance, e.g., cerebral palsy, neurology, or myopathy. In [22], a decision support system for hypernasality treatment is presented. It discovers action rules recommending optimal personalized treatments to be followed by children with certain speech disorders to move them into less severe categories of hypernasality. The presented system belongs to the class of knowledge-based & group recommender systems.

2.5 *Hybrid Recommender Systems*

The main motivation behind the development of hybrid recommender systems is the opportunity to achieve a better accuracy as the hybrid approach is proven to perform better than the individual types of filtering approaches. The most popular hybrid approaches are those which use a heuristic combination of both collaborative filtering and content-based filtering, where the approach overcomes the major drawbacks of content-based and collaborative-based system such as cold-start problem, sparsity problem, gray-sheep problem, etc. Additionally, hybrid algorithms use item attributes and the ratings of all users. This type of system fuses multiple data sources, usually with static and nonadjustable weightings, to deliver recommendations [35].

The hybrid type of filtering is highly effective in combining the benefits of different recommender systems and have a broader application in the healthcare domain. In [46], an adaptive hybrid doctor-recommender system is proposed to address the problem of finding the right doctor for a patient. To tackle that problem, the researchers have combined different recommendation approaches: content-based, collaborative, and demographic filtering where the algorithm used a hierarchical structure to assign weights to identified doctor related attributes. The algorithm uses effectively an Analytical Hierarchical Process (APH) to translate the attributes and their relative importance into a nominal empirical model. The APH model is further used to recommend doctors to patients.

Papers [2–4, 21, 29] present novel algorithms used by a recommender system for reducing the number of readmissions by applying the concept of personalization and actionable patterns. First, all possible procedure paths (course of treatments) for a given medical procedure are extracted. Then, patients are clustered according to the similarities in their diagnoses with a goal to increase the predictability of the next procedure. Finally, the system provides recommendations (actionable knowledge) to the physicians to put patients on a treatment path that would result in an optimal reduction of the number of readmissions on the average case. The presented recommender system is collaborative, knowledge-based, and hybrid.

When comparing recommender systems with the search engines and other information retrieval systems, distinguishing criteria have been individualized, interesting, and useful. This should be the main objective of recommender systems.

References

1. Ali, R., Afzal, M., et al.: Multimodal hybrid reasoning methodology for personalized wellbeing services. Comput. Biol. Med. **69**, 10–28 (2016). Elsevier
2. Al-Mardini, M., Raś, Z.M.: A supervised model for predicting the risk of mortality and hospital readmissions for newly admitted patients. In: Foundations of Intelligent Systems, Proceedings of ISMIS'17 in Warsaw, Poland, LNAI, vol. 10352, pp. 29–36. Springer (2017)
3. Al-Mardini, M., Hajja, A., Raś, Z.W.: Reduction of readmissions to hospitals based on actionable knowledge discovery and personalization. In: Beyond Databases Architectures and Structures-BDAS, et al.: Conference Proceedings, Communications in Computer and Information Science, vol. 613, pp. 39–55. Springer (2016)
4. Al-Mardini, M., Hajja, A., Raś, Z.W. et. al.: Predicting the primary medical procedure through clustering of patients' diagnoses. In: New Frontiers in Mining Complex Patterns, LNAI, vol. 10312, pp. 117–131. Springer (2017)
5. Arbajian, P., Hajja, A., Raś, Z.W., Wieczorkowska, A.: Effect of speech segment samples selection in stutter block detection and remediation. J. Intell. Inform. Syst. **53**(2), 241–264 (2019). Springer
6. Arbajian, P., Hajja, A., Raś, Z.W., Wieczorkowska, A.: Segment-removal based stuttered speech remediation. In New Frontiers in Mining Complex Patterns, Post-Proceedings of NFMCP 2017, ECML/PKDD Workshop in Skopje, Macedonia, LNAI, vol. 10785, pp. 16-34. Springer (2018)
7. Bejnordi, B.E., et al.: Diagnostic assessment of deep learning algorithms for detection of lymph node metastases in women with breast cancer. Jama **318**(22), 2199–2210 (2017)

8. Bhattacharya, B., Burhanuddin, I., Sancheti, A., Satya, K.: Intent-Aware Contextual Recommendation System, IEEE International Conference on Data Mining Workshops (ICDMW), pp. 1–8. LA, New Orleans (2017)
9. Bobadilla, J., et al.: Recommender systems survey. Knowl. Based Syst. **46**, 109–132 (2013)
10. Branden, M., Wiratunga, N., Burton, D., Craw, S.: Integrating case-based reasoning with an electronic patient record system. Artif. Intell. Med. **51**(2), 117–123 (2011)
11. Ciecierski, K., Raś, Z.W., Przybyszewski, A.: Selection of the optimal electrode in Parkinson's disease DBS treatment, Foundations of Intelligent Systems, Proceedings of ISMIS 2011 Symposium, LNAI, vol. 6804, pp. 554-564. Springer (2011)
12. Ciecierski, K., Raś, Z.W., Przybyszewski, A.W.: Intraoperative Decision Making with Rough Set Rules for STN DBS in Parkinson Disease, Proceedings of the International Conference on Brain Informatics and Health, in Warsaw, Poland, LNCS, vol. 8609, pp. 323–334. Springer, (2014)
13. Ciecierski, K., Raś, Z.W., Przybyszewski, A.: Foundations of automatic system for intrasurgical localization of Subthalamic Nucleus in Parkinson patients. Web Intell. Agent Syst. Int. J. **12**(1), 63–82 (2014). IOS Press
14. Ciecierski, K., Raś, Z.W., Przybyszewski, A.: Foundations of recommender system for STN localization during DBS surgery in Parkinson's patients. Foundations of Intelligent Systems, Proceedings of ISMIS 2012 Symposium, LNAI, vol. 7661, pp. 234–243. Springer (2012)
15. Dara, S., Chowdary, C.R., Kumar, C.: A survey on group recommender systems. J. Intell. Inf. Syst. **54**, 271–295 (2020). Springer
16. Esteva, A., et al.: Dermatologist-level classification of skin cancer with deep neural networks. Nature **542**(7639), 115 (2017)
17. Felfernig, A. et al.: An overview of recommender systems in the internet of things. J. Intell. Inf. Syst. **52**(2), 285–309 (2019). Springer
18. Grasser, F., et al.: Neighborhood-based Collaborative Filtering for Therapy Decision Support, Proceedings of the Second International Workshop on Health Recommender Systems, ACM RecSys 2017. Como, Italy (2017)
19. Gulshan, V., et al.: Development and validation of a deep learning algorithm for detection of diabetic retinopathy in retinal fundus photographs. Jama **316**(22), 2402–2410 (2016)
20. Guo, L., et al.: Collaborative filtering recommendation based on trust and emotion. J. Intell. Inf. Syst. **53**, 113–135 (2019). Springer
21. Hajja, A., Touati, H., Raś, Z.W., Studnicki, J., Wieczorkowska, A.: Predicting negative side effects of surgeries through clustering. In: New Frontiers in Mining Complex Patterns, Post-proceedings of NFMCP, : ECML/PKDD Workshop, Nancy, France, LNAI, vol. 8983, pp. 41–55. Springer (2014)
22. Hajja, A., Wieczorkowska, A., Raś, Z.W., Gubrynowicz, R.: Pair-based object-driven action rules. In: New Frontiers in Mining Complex Patterns, NFMCP, : ECML/PKDD Workshop, LNAI 7765, pp. 79–93 . Springer (2012)
23. Kim, T.-H., et al.: Improving prediction quality in collaborative filtering based on clustering. Proceedings of IEEE/WIC/ACM International Conference on WI and IAT, Sydney, NSW, Australia (2008)
24. Kohli, D., Raś, Z.W. et. al.: From music to emotions and tinnitus treatment, initial study. Foundations of Intelligent Systems, Proceedings of ISMIS 2012 Symposium, LNAI, vol. 7661, pp. 244–253. Springer (2012)
25. Koren, Y., Bell, R., Volinsky, C.: Matrix factorization techniques for recommender systems. Computer **42**(8), 30–37 (2009)
26. Lee, J., Kim, S., Lebanon, G., Singer, Y.: Local low-rank matrix approximation. In: Proceedings of 30th International Conference on Machine Learning (ICML '13), pp. 82–90 (2013)
27. Lim, T.-P., Husain, W., Zakaria, N.: Recommender system for personalized wellness therapy. Int. J. Adv. Comput. Sci. Appl. (IJACSA) **4**(9) (2013). http://dx.doi.org/10.14569/IJACSA.2013.040909
28. Lopez-Nores, M. et. al.: Enhancing recommender systems with access to electronic health records and groups of interest in social networks. In: 2011 Seventh International Conference on Signal Image Technology & Internet-Based Systems, Dijon, pp. 105–110 (2011)

29. Mardini, M.T., Raś, Z.W.: Extraction of actionable knowledge to reduce hospital readmissions through patients personalization. Inf. Sci. J. **485**, 1–17 (2019). Elsevier
30. Nobahari, V., Jalali, M.: ISoTrustSeq: a social recommender system based on implicit interest, trust and sequential behaviors of users using matrix factorization. J. Intell. Inf. Syst. **52**, 239–268 (2019). Springer
31. Nounou, M.N., Nounou, H.N., Mansouri, M.: Model-based and model-free filtering of genomic data. In: Network Modeling Analysis in Health Informatics and Bioinformatics volume 2, pp. 109–121 (2013). Springer
32. Priyadarshini, R., Barik, R., Dubey, H., DeepFog: Fog computing-based deep neural architecture for prediction of stress types, diabetes and hypertension attacks. Computation **6**(4) (2018)
33. Pujahari, A., Padmanabhan, V.: Group Recommender systems: combining user-user and item-item collaborative filtering techniques. In: 2015 International Conference on Information Technology (ICIT), Bhubaneswar, pp. 148–152 (2015)
34. Qayyum, A., et al.: Secure and Robust Machine Learning for Healthcare: A Survey. https://arxiv.org/abs/2001.08103 (2020)
35. Rahdari, B., Tsai, C., Brusilovsky, P.: Expanding Controllability of Hybrid Recommender Systems: From Positive to Negative Relevance, FLAIRS'19 Proceedings. Fl, Sarasota (2019)
36. Rajpurkar, P. et al.: Chexnet: Radiologist level pneumonia detection on chest x-rays with deep learning. Cornell University. https://arxiv.org/abs/1711.05225 (2017)
37. Salakhutdinov, R., Mnih, A.: Probabilistic matrix factorization. In Advances in Neural Information Processing Systems (NIPS '08), pp. 1257–1264 (2008)
38. Sanchez Bocanegra, C.L., Sevillano Ramos, J.L., Rizo, C. et al.: Health RecSys: a semantic content-based recommender system to complement health videos. BMC Med. Inf. Decis. Mak **17**(63). https://doi.org/10.1186/s12911-017-0431-7 (2017)
39. Schmidt, R., Gierl, L.: Case-based reasoning for antibiotics therapy advice: an investigation of retrieval algorithms and prototypes. Artif. Intell. Med. **23**(2), 171–186 (2001)
40. Stratigi, M., Kondylakis, H., Stefanidis, K.: Fairness in group recommendations in the health domain. In: 2017 IEEE 33rd International Conference on Data Engineering (ICDE), Proceedings, pp. 1481–1488 (2017)
41. Strub, F., et. al.: Hybrid Collaborative Filtering with Neural Networks. https://hal.archives-ouvertes.fr/hal-01281794v1/document (2016)
42. Tarnowska, K.A., Raś, Z.W., Jastreboff, P.J.: Decision Support System for Diagnosis and Treatment of Hearing Disorders, The Case of Tinnitus, Studies in Computational Intelligence, vol. 685 (2017). Springer
43. Tarnowska, K.A., Raś, Z.W., Jastreboff, P.J.: Mining for actionable knowledge in tinnitus datasets. In: Thriving Rough Sets, Studies in Computational Intelligence, vol. 708, Chapter 18, pp. 367–396. Springer (2017)
44. Thompson, P., Zhang, X., Jiang, W., Raś, Z.W.: From mining tinnitus database to tinnitus decision-support system, initial study. In: Proceedings of IEEE/WIC/ACM International Conference on Intelligent Agent Technology (IAT 2007), IEEE Computer Society, San Jose, Calif., 203–206 (2007)
45. Usman, M., et al.: Retrospective motion correction in multi shot MRI using generative adversarial network. Sci. Rep. **10**(1), 1–11 (2020)
46. Waqar, M., Majeed, N. et. al.: An adaptive doctor-recommender system, Behaviour & Information Technology, vol. 38, Taylor & Francis, pp. 959-973 (2019)
47. Wu, M.Y., et al.: A deep architecture for depression detection using posting, behavior, and living environment data. J. Intell. Inf. Syst. **54**, 225–244 (2020)
48. Yuan, W., et al.: Socialized healthcare service recommendation using deep learning. Neural Comput. Appl. **30**, 2071–2082 (2018)
49. Zhang, Y., et al.: iDoctor: personalized and professionalized medical recommendations based on hybrid matrix factorization. Future Gener. Comput. Syst. **66**, 30–35 (2017)

Recommender Systems in Healthcare: A Socio-Technical Systems Approach

Mila Kwiatkowska

Abstract The design, development, implementation, and evaluation of recommender systems (RSs) in healthcare requires a multifaceted and multidisciplinary approach. Healthcare systems by their very nature are complex and dynamic, and their structure and functioning are determined by social values, conventional methods, and economical aspects. This chapter describes healthcare as a socio-technical system comprising of interacting human and technical agents. Thus, any change to the system, such as an introduction of RS tools or methods, requires careful consideration of the technical and social aspects. The chapter presents the main issues which should be considered in the deployment of RS-based tools and techniques in healthcare: (1) adherence to the medical regulations for medical software (e.g., Software as Medical Device), (2) compliance with the medical data privacy, (3) provisioning for transparency and trustworthiness of recommendations, (4) analysis of short-term and long-term ethical issues, such as belief formation and behavior modification, and (5) consideration for the patient empowerment (patient-centered care), doctor-patient relationship (relationship-centered care), and human aspects (human-centered care).

1 Introduction

Since the first implementation of computers in the 1960s, humans have been designing, developing, and using software systems to support various aspects of the healthcare system. The first implementations were driven by the needs of storing medical data and processing health records (Electronic Health Records and Personal Health Records), of supporting assessments and diagnoses (medical expert systems and decision support systems), and of aiding in healthy living (virtual health assistant). The developments of internet, web-based applications, mobile applications, and the extensive use of social media brought computer software to all aspects of daily life.

M. Kwiatkowska (✉)
The Department of Computing Science, Thompson Rivers University, 805 TRU Way, Kamloops, British ColumbiaV2C 0C8, Canada
e-mail: mkwiatkowska@tru.ca

Z. W. Ras et al. (eds.), *Recommender Systems for Medicine and Music*, Studies in Computational Intelligence 946,
https://doi.org/10.1007/978-3-030-66450-3_2

At the same time, in the last fifty years, research in Artificial Intelligence in Medicine (AIM) and Machine Learning (ML) have significantly progressed, and AI and ML methods have been used and accepted in many subfields of healthcare [30], for example, medical image interpretation, skin lesion classification, and microbiology. Moreover, the availability of small, inexpensive sensors and wearable devices blurred the lines between in- and out-of-clinic medical testing and data collection. In addition, healthcare can be now provided remotely via telemedicine and eHealth at patients' homes, which in turn changes the context of the healthcare delivery. With the ubiquity of smartphones and other computer devices, patients gained online access to their own health records (personal health records). Patients have established patient-lead support groups and organized patient-lead research. These initiatives are changing the very concept of the role of a patient: from being a passive patient (an object of medical procedures) to being an informed participating patient—an empowered-patient or e-patient. These drastic changes, happening in the last thirty years, triggered a significant top-down redesign of the entire healthcare system. There are many international and national projects aiming towards healthcare system design and redesign. For example, one of the main approaches focuses on patient-centered design [13].

The dramatic changes in healthcare delivery require a top-down perspective on the design of complex, dynamic, multiscale open systems. Moreover, the design of contemporary healthcare systems necessitates modeling of the human (social) and technical (technological) aspects. Since both aspects are intertwined in a complex interactive system of both human and technological agents, the design must take a systemic approach. This means that the design of technological aspects must incorporate the design of human agents and vice versa the design of human agents must take into consideration technical aspects. The design methodology must recognize the fact that the healthcare systems are socio-technical systems. For these reasons, this chapter describes recommender systems and their potential utilization in healthcare using a socio-technical systems approach. This approach views the healthcare system as a highly complex system that requires interaction with human and technical agents. The main premise of the chapter is that the potential healthcare-related applications of the new technological developments from computing science must be carefully assessed from the socio-technical perspective originated from healthcare research and practice. This chapter assumes a top-down analysis of systems while focusing on human agents (patient-centered approach) and presenting some general aspects of technological agents. The socio-technical approach presented in this chapter has its roots in multiple disciplines: sociology, behavioral psychology, and interdisciplinary studies of systems theory. The interdisciplinarity of the presented concepts leads, on the one hand, to some ambiguity of terminology, but, on the other hand, it provides grounds for inter—and transdisciplinary ways of designing and developing software systems.

The remainder of this chapter is organized as follows. Section 2 gives an overview of recommender systems (RS) and examples of RS implementations in health-related domains. Section 3 provides a short introduction to socio-technical systems and their design considerations. Section 4 details the main aspects of the socio-technical design of RS system applications in health-related domains. It discusses the technical regulatory aspects of the use of software as medical devices (SaMD) and an overview of the key issues concerning the social aspects of a healthcare system. The final section, Sect. 5, includes a general discussion on the system-based approach in RS development and lists the key requirements for the design and development of RS applications in healthcare.

2 Recommender Systems

The information overflow and problems with finding relevant or interesting items speared the efforts to create filtering systems to search for the best matching items. Recommender systems help users to find items and help item providers to deliver items to users. In a handbook on recommender systems, Ricci, Rokach, and Shapira define recommender systems (RSs) as "software tools and techniques providing suggestions for items to be of use to a user" [29]. The history of recommender systems or recommendation systems goes back to the 1990s. The first RSs centered around the recommendation of books to buy and read, music to listen, movies and news to watch, and documents to study. Their development was based on the idea of real-life individuals buying, reading, and watching based on the recommendations of their friends or domain experts, for example, movie reviews done by film critics. RSs quickly became a vast research area and were used in practical industrial applications. The first commercial recommender system, Tapestry, designed in 1992 [16], used "collaborative filtering" to recommend documents taken from newsgroups to a group of users. The next well-known commercial applications of RSs were GroupLens and MovieLens in 1997 [19]. The development of RSs was accelerated by the fast-growing e-commerce sites offering an immense number of items and by the needs of the users who were faced with an overwhelming selection and difficulties with decision-making. This situation was alleviated by the websites offering various filtering mechanisms. Initially, two algorithmic approaches were used: collaborative filtering (CF) which analyzes the usage data across users and finds well-matched user-item pairs [6] and content-based (CB) recommendation which matches the historical user's data with the item specification to find the best matches. The user's data and user's profile can be elicited explicitly from the users (e.g., using questionnaires) or can be obtained implicitly (e.g., from the user's browsing behavior). The CF and CB approaches have also been combined to form a hybrid approach using, for example, merging techniques to produce a final ranked list or an adaptive weighted average where the weight of an item increases with the number of users accessing that item. Several extensions were proposed to refine the recommendations. Adomavicius et al. proposed incorporation of additional contextual information (e.g., for movie watching, the additional dimensions would be time of viewing, place, and companion) into a multidimensional model (MD model) [1]. Various contextual information can be utilized in the context-aware recommenders based on multiple dimensions, profiles, aggregations [3], temporal, and spatial information. These CF, CB, and MD filtering mechanisms were further expanded by several machine learning techniques such as

Bayesian classifiers, clustering, decision trees, and artificial neural networks [26], by deep neural networks and by addition of the domain knowledge and knowledge-based techniques, such as case-based reasoning (CBR) and multiple AI techniques [29].

The development and the fast spread of RS implementations have been driven by companies such as Amazon, Google, and Facebook to provide personalization of content displayed to their users. It is important to emphasize that one of the strong driving forces of the RS development is financial gain. As stated by Milano et al., "it is evident that applications of RS have been driven by online commerce and services, where the emphasis has tended to be on commercial objectives" [22].

With the proliferation of RSs in all aspects of our daily life, the importance of the research on the social impact of RSs is becoming paramount. The popularity of RSs in social media and online social networks raises several questions about online opinion formation and social interactions. For example, studies in social psychology show that homophily, i.e., greater interaction between like-minded individuals, results in increasing polarization of opinions. Although several RS algorithms have been presented to manage polarization and disagreement in social media [23], there are still many unaddressed ethical concerns.

In a recent paper, Milano et al. present a framework describing the ethical challenges of RSs. The authors define the task of recommendation as "finding good items" [22]. Three parameters are used for the operationalization of the concept "task of recommendation": the space of options (types of items), the definition of the term "good" in the context of the recommendation (good from the user's perspective or/and good from the service prover's perspective), and the RS's performance evaluation (expected outcome). Using this framework, they specify six areas of ethical concerns in RS: content, privacy, autonomy and personal identity, opacity, fairness, and social effects.

2.1 Technological and Social Issues in Recommender Systems

This subsection presents a brief overview of the main technological and social challenges in RSs. This presentation has three noticeable limitations: (1) interdependence between technological and social issues, which results in repetition of the discussion on the intertwined issues, for example, privacy; (2) diversity of interpretations of ethical and social terms having its roots in multidisciplinary nature of the discussion; and (3) absence of a definite classification of the ethical issues in RSs, which could be ascribed to overall recency of RS ethical research [22, 25].

The research on recommender systems (RSs) covers several well-known technical limitations and a number of wide-ranging social concerns. Adomavicius and Tuzhilin describe five basic technical limitations of RSs: new user problem (common to all RS types), new item problem and sparsity (specific to CF) and limited content analysis and over-specification (specific to CB) [2]. The other important technical issue (which can be seen as a limitation) is the scalability of RSs. With the exponential growth of data in terms of items, users, and user profiles, the response time of the RSs has to be kept at an acceptable level. These technical issues are finding their solutions in new algorithms [34], however, many social issues remain unsolved. Some RS concerns involve both the technological and human aspects, for example, explainability (transparency), trustworthiness, and privacy. Some concerns are purely ethical, for example, biases (e.g., RS designed towards selling more expensive items based on the profile of the user) and behavior manipulation (e.g., RS designed towards long-term addiction forming). These issues are important concerns for all RSs, but they become the primary concerns when RSs (or RS methods) are applied in healthcare.

2.1.1 RS Privacy

One of the key issues in developing RSs for healthcare is data privacy. Several examples of violation of privacy are described in the subject literature. Milano et al. present three types of issues: unauthorized data collection and storage, data leaks, and unauthorized inferences (user profiling) [22]. The issue of data privacy is especially challenging since RSs are based on the explicit and implicit usage of the users' data and users' profiles. Xin argues that "there is an inherent trade-off between the accuracy of recommendations and the extent to which users are willing to release information about their preferences" [34]. Improvements in the accuracy and utilization are achieved via personalization, however, personalization of filtering contradicts the privacy of data. Ramakrishnan, Keller, and Mirza pointed out that "recommender system users who rate items across disjoint domains face a privacy risk analogous to the one that occurs with statistical database queries" [27]. In recommender systems, a person who rates products across several different types of domains (a unique and unusual rating) is called "a straddle." Information about the straddlers [27] could be used in conjunction with other data to identify individuals and compromise the privacy of their data. Data privacy is a major concern in all RSs, but medical data privacy is of paramount concern in healthcare systems, and in many countries requires adherence to country-specific legal regulations. For example, HIPAA regulation is used in the US to govern the privacy and security of personal health information, and PIPEDA is used in Canada to govern all private data including health information.

2.1.2 RS Social Impacts

The RS engines, depending on their designs, could utilize diverse forms of social influence, for example, peer-to-peer pressure, coercion, deception, and persuasion. These mechanisms could be used in ethical or unethical ways. Moreover, some of the long-term social impacts of RSs, such as belief formation and behavior manipulation could be intentional or unintentional. These concerns are currently studied and should be a part of the design methods for RSs. Unfortunately, the social and ethical aspects of socio-technical systems are often overlooked. Due to the complexity of RSs and the multifaceted nature of the ethical issues, there is no standardized terminology or formalized ways to evaluate whether an RS engine is performing in an ethically or unethically acceptable way.

The subject literature describes several examples of ethical concerns, and it provides some initial classifications to organize the diverse social and ethical concepts. For example, Ramos et al. describe cases of the possibility of bribery, buying positive reviews from influential leaders in social networks, and extreme limitation of choices in tightly linked small social groups [28]. Burr et al. describe the social consequences of interactions between technological agents (intelligent software agents) and human agents [8]. The analysis presented by Burr et al. classifies the ethical concerns of intelligent software agents (e.g., recommender systems) into the first-order effects: coercion (e.g., no opting out), deception (e.g., clickbait), and persuasion (e.g., trading and nudging) and second-order effects. The second-order effects of RSs are defined as unintended long-term changes of the human user's beliefs (e.g., increased polarization of opinions) and changes of the human user's behaviors (e.g., possible behavioral addictions, for example, to social media) as a result of a long-term interaction [8]. These ethical issues are related to trustworthiness in RSs, but they have even more important implications for the implementation of RSs in healthcare. The users in healthcare (patients) are in an especially vulnerable position and can be easily influenced and coerced into wrong decisions.

2.2 Applications of Recommender Systems in Healthcare

Current literature on recommender systems (RSs) presents multiple understandings of the role of RSs in healthcare. The definition of a RS, "software tools and techniques providing suggestions for items to be of use to a user," allows for at least three interpretations: (1) application of the recommender software tools in healthcare, (2) application of the recommendation techniques in healthcare, and (3) application of specialized recommender systems designed for health-related areas. This subsection focuses on two issues: (1) the necessity of system-based analysis for the problems in healthcare and (2) the necessity of risk-benefit analysis in the design of RS intended to be used in health-related domains. The first issue is illustrated by an example of RS implementation in healthcare to support patients' understanding of their medical records.

Wiesner and Pfeifer define a health recommender system (HRS) as a specification of an RS system [33]. The HRS distinction is based on the recommended item, which is defined by them as "a piece of non-confidential, scientifically proven or at least generally accepted medical information, which in itself is not linked to an individual's medical history." Furthermore, the authors limit the use of an individual's health data such as a personal health record (PHR) to the internal use of the recommender's software. Wiesner and Pfeifer describe a specific application of HRS, which provides a layperson (patient) with relevant information for the interpretation of PHRs [33]. However, there is a possible contradiction between the proposed HRS definition of the HRS and this particular implementation. Since the described RS implementation in healthcare is presenting the layperson with a specific "translation" of their medical records, it could still be seen as medical data. The use of PHRs by the patients (lay people) should be seen as a larger issue in the design of the healthcare system. Thus, some RS techniques could be used in the solution, but the design of the entire PHR system should consider several critical issues: data ownership, privacy, security, interoperability, and the required level of health literacy.

The discussion on the implementation of RSs in healthcare must include the analysis of risk factors. The risks associated with erroneous recommendation in the traditional areas of RS implementations, such as movie recommender, music recommender or book recommender, are very low. However, the inaccurate or erroneous recommendations in healthcare may have morbid or even mortal consequences. The user of a traditional RS faced with an uninteresting book to read could be bored or frustrated, but the user of an RS used for health recommendation of physiotherapy exercise could further damage an injured spine. The same might happen to a naïve user of a food recommender, who could have a serious allergic reaction to a newly recommended food item. In summary, the design of any component of the healthcare systems must perform a risk-benefit analysis from the patient perspective. The healthcare systems are by their very nature quality-critical, security-critical, and safety-critical.

3 Socio-Technical Systems and Their Design

The term "socio-technical systems" was introduced in 1960, by Eric Trist, Ken Bamforth, and Fred Emery to describe the interaction between people and technology in the workplace [12]. The term has its roots in organizational and clinical psychology. In this context, "technical" is used in a broader sense of techniques, procedures, and related knowledge, in a sense of the ancient Greek word "techne". The term socio-technical system (also spelled as sociotechnical) has been adopted by diverse fields with various interpretations, and therefore, its multiple definitions will be not discussed here. However, in the context of this chapter the term "socio-technical system" describes a system that is composed of people and technology. The design, development, and evaluation systems of such a complex social and technological nature requires its own design methods. Baxter and Sommerville proposed a pragmatic framework for socio-technical systems called socio-technical systems engineering (STSE) which is intrinsically multidisciplinary in its nature [5]. The design methods for socio-technical systems consider human, social, organizational, and technical factors.

Thus, for example, the design of an assistive living support system should consider the users (human aspects), the organizational aspects (home environment), and the technical factors. Several approaches to the socio-technical systems have been discussed in the literature. Baxter and Sommerville list seven approaches: soft system methodology, cognitive work analysis, the socio-technical methods for designing work systems, ethnographic workplace analysis, contextual design, cognitive systems engineering, and human-centered design [5]. Out of this list, two methods seem to be the most suitable for the design of systems in the healthcare domain: (1) socio-technical methods for designing work systems, which focus on function allocation and identification of tasks that are allocated to humans and tasks allocated to machines and (2) human-centered design, which bases the design on an explicit understanding of users (including social and cultural factors), their tasks, and their environment (including working practices and organizational standards).

3.1 Healthcare System as a Socio-Technical System

Healthcare systems are characterized by their high complexity, dynamic nature, and highly technical nature. Effken defines a healthcare system as "a system in which groups of people cooperate for patient care and are faced with numerous contingencies that cannot be fully anticipated" [11]. Moreover, the groups of people involved in the healthcare system have different perspectives and the healthcare organizations may have conflicting values (e.g., financial objectives vs humanitarian objectives). Further complexity is added by numerous illnesses and a variety of high-risk healthcare processes. This great complexity requires a systemic approach to the healthcare design. Therefore, the socio-technical design encompasses the human tasks, medical devices, decision support systems, and other technical agents, and it is guided by several safety standards and regulations.

3.2 Autonomous Agents in a Socio-Technical System

In history, humans used numerous technological agents to solve their daily life problems [10]. Examples of technological agents vary from simple mechanical devices, such as a typewriter, through communication devices, such as telephones, sophisticated word processors and, finally, smartphones. Development of technological agents involves three aspects: problem constraints, human limitations, and available technology. In parallel with the development of more sophisticated and more complex technology, technological agents are becoming progressively more autonomous. As noted by Eccles and Groth, the utilization of autonomous technological agents has paradoxical effects: "There is an important shift in system characteristics when autonomous technological agents are introduced to problem-solving systems. Problem-solving systems become characterized by collaboration between multiple autonomous agents, human and technological, each performing their own operations" [10]. Thus, the main problem in design lies in the coordination among the constituent human and technological agents.

3.3 Workload Analysis in a Socio-Technical System

One of the main objectives of computerization and digitalization is the improvement of system efficiency. Therefore, the workload, its changes, and distribution among the technical and human agents are the key research topics in organizational science. For example, Eccles and Groth analyzed an additional workload risk in designing socio-technological systems comprising of multiple human and technological agents [10]. Their findings suggest that the workload analysis (analysis of the risk of additional workload) is crucial for the efficiency. Moreover, they stated that in poorly designed or inappropriately implemented systems the workload cost could be greater than the workload saving.

4 Design Considerations for RS in Healthcare: A Socio-Technical Approach

The design of software systems for healthcare applications has multifaceted aspects. Some of the design issues stem from the healthcare practitioners' perception on the role of the technology in healthcare. The healthcare publications discuss various technical breakthroughs and improvements in care, as well as the problems with increased workloads, ineffective workflows, safety, and privacy. They also convey ethical perspectives on the use, misuse, and overuse of technology. Technological advances bring some solutions to the problems in the healthcare system, but are not the solutions to all problems. Often, unsuitable design, deficiency in interoperability, or cognitive overload in overcomplex systems introduce new problems to the healthcare workflow. Hofmann in his paper "The myth of technology in health care" presents the perspective in which the technology should be demystified and not used as "a paradigm to be applied to all healthcare challenges" [18]. The design of healthcare systems faces multiple socio-technical problems. The technological components (technical agents) are created, used, and integrated in daily workflows by people, who often have different views on the role of such systems in healthcare practice. Baxter and Sommerville state that "the problems of developing technology for healthcare lie not with the complexity or novelty of the technology itself, but in the complex ways healthcare is practiced and organized" [5].

Sittig and Singh proposed a framework for the development and evaluation of healthcare systems using eight dimensions: (1) hardware and software, (2) clinical content (framework including data, information, and knowledge required for the clinical application), (3) human–computer interface, (4) clinical workflows and communication, (5) internal organizational policies, procedures, and culture, (6) external rules, (7) regulations and pressures, (8) system measurement and monitoring [31]. This socio-technical framework has been used to evaluate many eHealth initiatives. For example, Hagglund and Scandurra describe a project providing online access to Electronic Health Records (HER) in Sweden, a Patient Accessible EHR (PAEHR) [17].

This section presents three main aspects of the socio-technical systems approach to healthcare: (1) organizational: adherence to the medical regulations for medical software (Software as a Medical Device), (2) human relationship and communication: consideration for the doctor–patient relationship (relationship-centered approach) and patient empowerment (patient-centered approach), and (3) human aspects: provisioning for human dignity and empathy.

4.1 Technical Agents: Regulations in Healthcare

Software systems used in healthcare are components (technical agents) in a larger socio-technical system. The following requirements highlight some of the key considerations in the design and maintenance of software used in healthcare: integration with clinical workflows, information security standards for medical data, functional safety, and the life cycle requirements for medical software. These standards are similar to other safety-critical software development standards.

The International Medical Device Regulatory Forum, IMDRF, [15] divides software into three groups: (1) software to run medical hardware devices (e.g., software to activate an MRI equipment), (2) commercial off-the-shelf software (e.g., standard document processing, MS Word), and (3) a specialized software used for medical purposes. The last group is classified as "Software as Medical Device", SaMD, and therefore, must be approved by the regulatory authorities. Recently, in response to the increased applications of AI and Machine Learning techniques, IMDRF created a special category of AI/ML-based SaMD [14]. Software systems excluded from the SaMD and AI/ML-based SaMD regulations include software used for administrative support (e.g., patient scheduling), maintaining a healthy lifestyle, formatting and displaying data, and providing some limited clinical decision support.

Software as a Medical Device, SaMD, is defined as "software intended to be used for one or more medical purposes that perform these purposes without being part of a hardware medical device." The medical purpose is defined by IMDRF as diagnosis, prevention, monitoring, treatment or alleviation of disease. FDA documents provide the following definition of SaMD as [14, 15]:

> A SaMD can best be described as software that utilizes an algorithm (logic, set of rules, or model) that operates on data input (digitized content) to produce an output that is intended for medical purposes.

SaMDs are categorized by two aspects: (1) significance of the provided results to the healthcare decision and (2) health status of the patient. The medical purposes of SaMD are specified as (1) treat or diagnose, (2) drive clinical management, and (3) inform clinical management. IMDRF proposed a framework defining categories of risks: critical (disease or condition is life-threatening, users are specialists, patients are fragile), serious (disease or condition is moderate in progression, intervention is not time critical, patients are not fragile, users are specialists or laypersons), and nonserious (slow progression or minor chronic illness, users are laypersons). The risks and considerations are categorized into four levels, in which Category IV has the highest impact and Category I has the lowest impact. The following are the SaMD examples of Category I: collecting the data from wearable sensors ECG rate, walking speed, heart rate, walking distance to monitor an exercise-based cardiac rehabilitation; analysis of data from healthy individuals to assess risk for developing migraine; storing historical blood pressure information to be later reviewed by the healthcare provider. In addition, these SaMD regulations are applicable to traditional software with specified and unchanging behavior. However, these regulations were not designed for adaptive artificial intelligence and machine learning techniques utilizing the incoming data for continuous learning. Therefore, IMDRF came with regulatory specifications [14] for the AI/ML-based SaMD.

This paper argues that any application of RSs in healthcare should be regulated, for example, using the safety regulations such as the IMDRS's SaMD and AI/ML-based SaMD.

4.2 *Human Agents: Empowerment, Patient- and Relationship-Centered Care*

The fast spread of digital communication through the healthcare system, the dynamic growth of the online patients' communities, the unrestricted online access to a health-related realm of data-information-knowledge, and the availability of portable health monitoring devices have changed the traditional approach towards patient empowerment, the role of the patient in the patient-centered care, and decision-making process in the relationship-centered care.

The doctor–patient (word doctor in the term doctor–patient represents all healthcare practitioners) relationship and communication are significantly changing in the digital age. Although many of the changes are the results of the introduction of the new technologies (technical agents), the changes must be analyzed in the context of medical and social sciences models of doctor–patient relationship. Current literature describes three models of doctor–patient relationship depending on the locus of control: paternalistic, guidance-cooperation, and mutual participation. In the mutual participation model, as discussed by Mesko et al., both doctor and patient "are involved and are participating in the treatment and the decision-making process, and they share information and express their preferences" [21].

The model of the doctor–patient relationship and communication are the fundamental concepts for the design of the technological agents such as RS-based agents supporting the decision-making process.

4.2.1 Patient Empowerment

The patient empowerment has been a research topic of numerous studies and clinical trials [20]. For example, Lamas et al. describe two notions emerging in the digital era: (1) patients lead research which represents a bottom-up approach to data generation and research studies and (2) laypersons initiating the discovery of crowd-sourced knowledge [20]. As stated by Lamas et al. in the new era of the internet and social media, the patients participate in interactions with the patients' communities and have free access to real-time updated scientific information [20]. The traditional approach of healthcare professionals towards patient empowerment has already changed or must change to recognize the new role of a patient. Lamas et al. state "We believe that the development of digital networks has meant a revolution in the possibilities for empowering patients and communities in the care of their health and bodies" [20].

4.2.2 Patient-Centered Care

The patient-centered care becomes an intrinsic part of quality care, and it considers strategies for informing, educating, and involving patients in their own care. There are several studies describing these strategies. Berwick presents a partnership system which includes all stakeholders: healthcare providers, patients, and their families [7]. He defines "patient-centered care" as a patient's experience in which the patient is informed, treated with recognition, respect, and dignity, and in which the patient has choices "related to one's person, circumstances, and relationships in health care." Accordingly, Berwick postulates that the design of a health care system should incorporate the following aspects: patient-centered care as a quality dimension, locus of control, transparency (transparency including science, costs, outcomes, processes, and errors), individualization and customization of care [7].

4.2.3 Relationship-Centered Care

The patient-physician relationship is in the center of the healthcare system, the relationship-centered care (RCC) involves all relationships with caregivers and between caregivers caring for the same patient. Weiner and Biondich state that "the development and maintenance of relationship in healthcare depend on effective flows of information, both objective or subjective, whether verbal, visual, emotional, or tactile" [32]. Information technology can facilitate relationships in healthcare by giving free access to health-related information. This shared access for the patients and practitioners may facilitate the sharing of concepts, terminology, and helps in the management of disease. Advancements in computer-based asynchronous communication (e-mails, voice messages) and synchronous communication (videoconferencing, chatting,) can facilitate self-management of disease including education and counseling. However, technology can create a barrier to a good patient–physician relationship. The increasing complexity of health systems requires a careful design of the tasks which could be automated such as assessing contraindications to drugs, providing education to patients, and generating standardized treatment for preventive care. However, some tasks are people-oriented and their automation will negatively influence RCC. Thus, Weiner and Biondich posit that studies of new IT implementations should include measures of impact on relationships [32]. On the one hand, the use of technological solutions allows for several improvements in diagnostics, patients' safety, and efficiency of care by aiding human cognition. However, technology should not be used "as a crutch for humanistic deficiencies such as lack of compassion, commitment, empathy, or togetherness." Therefore, the design of IT solutions in healthcare must carefully analyze the impact on the interpersonal relationships.

4.3 Human Agents: Human-Driven Care

Human-driven care incorporates intrinsically human factors such as patient's dignity, healthcare provider's empathy, friendliness and reassurance towards patients, psychological vulnerability of people, and their cultural and linguistic differences. Although, technological agents are able to demonstrate behavior based on rational bases; however, they lack the very human capacity of having and expressing human feelings—human feelings can only be felt by human beings. Empathy is one of the core elements of doctor–patient communication and it is viewed as a major indicator of successful therapeutic outcome. The interface for the digital tools can be designed with consideration for empathy [24], but fundamentally, empathy is a human capacity (human agent capacity) and the technical agent has no capacity for those feelings. Thus, empathy, respect, kindness, dignity, compassion, understanding, and courtesy are all important concepts in the design of the human agents' roles in the socio-technical system.

Furthermore, the doctor–patient relationship in itself can be viewed as a healing factor. Thus, an introduction of intermediary technical agents should be carefully evaluated in terms of their possible negative effect on human-to-human contacts. In his book published in 1957, "The Doctor, his patient, and the Illness," Michael Balint introduced the concept "doctor as a drug" which defines the role of the doctor as an important "enhancer" to the prescribed medication [4]. As stated by Curran, Balint's fundamental ideas of the doctor–patient relationship are still valid [9].

5 Discussion

This chapter provided an overview of the important aspects of the application of new technologies in the healthcare domain. It argued that healthcare systems must be designed or re-designed using a socio-technical systems approach and the technical components of such a complex system are intertwined with the social (human) components and cannot be designed in separation. Therefore, the implementation of recommender systems (RSs) in healthcare requires careful analysis of the interactions of human and technical agents within their specific environment. The discussion in this section presents three main design considerations: (1) RS-based tools should be governed by appropriate regulations and data standards, (2) RS-based tools should have mechanisms for their evaluation in the context of the socio-technical system, and (3) RS-based tools should provide mechanisms for transparency and should be designed with clear ethical guidelines.

The RS-based software implementation should be governed by specific regulations that overlook the design, development, implementation, maintenance, and evaluation of the RSs as tools and as specific methods used with other AI methods. The presented earlier IMDRF's regulations for Software as Medical Devices, SaMD and AI/ML-based SaMD provide several strict guidelines for the deployment of software intended for healthcare use. Furthermore, RS implementations, due to their data-driven nature, should be governed by the appropriate data privacy restrictions. Thus, there should be a comprehensive security plan to protect the medical data, and at the same time, to provide dynamic and efficient access to data. For example, the design must make provisions for emergency procedures for data access: "break the glass", which grants one-time access to health information or emergency access, which grants access to a predefined group of caregivers.

In terms of social aspects, RSs should be transparent to the professional users and provide a clear explanation of recommendations to the laypersons (patients). Furthermore, the explanation should be linguistically, culturally, and emotionally appropriate for the specific user in the context of their specific health situation. This socially-sensitive design requires more research on the communication in healthcare, analysis of the role of the technical (intelligent and autonomous) agents in socio-technical systems, and their long-term impact on humans.

Moreover, this chapter invites a further discussion on the concerns related to the design and deployment of RSs in healthcare. First, it suggests a systemic top-down approach to the analysis of a healthcare system, which should be viewed as an open, dynamic, and highly complex system of interacting human and technical agents. Second, it argues for a multifaceted and multidisciplinary socio-technical systems approach to the design, development, implementation, and maintenance and inclusion of an explicitly designed evaluation mechanism. Third, it posits that there is not much of a parallel between the users and items in the RSs and the patients and the doctor–patient relationship and communication in healthcare. Therefore, it suggests a cautionary and highly disciplined approach to the deployment of the RS tools or techniques in such a complex high-risk system as healthcare.

References

1. Adomavicius, G., Sankaranarayanan, R., Sen, S., Tuzhilin, A.: Incorporating contextual information in recommender systems using a multidimensional approach. ACM Trans. Inform. Syst. (TOIS) **23**(1), 103–145 (2005)
2. Adomavicius, G., Tuzhilin, A.: Toward the next generation of recommender systems: a survey of the state-of-the-art and possible extensions. IEEE Trans. Knowl. Data Eng. **17**(6), 734–749 (2005)
3. Adomavicius, G., Tuzhilin, A.: Context-aware recommender systems. In: Recommender systems handbook, pp. 217–253. Springer (2011)

4. Balint, M.: The doctor, his patient and the illness (1957)
5. Baxter, G., Sommerville, I.: Socio-technical systems: from design methods to systems engineering. Interact. Comput. **23**(1), 4–17 (2011)
6. Ben-Shimon, D., Tsikinovsky, A., Rokach, L., Meisles, A., Shani, G., Naamani, L.: Recommender system from personal social networks. In: Advances in Intelligent Web Mastering, pp. 47–55. Springer (2007)
7. Berwick, D.M.: What 'patient-centered'should mean: confessions of an extremist: a seasoned clinician and expert fears the loss of his humanity if he should become a patient. Health Aff. **28**(Suppl1), w555–w565 (2009)
8. Burr, C., Cristianini, N., Ladyman, J.: An analysis of the interaction between intelligent software agents and human users. Minds Mach. **28**(4), 735–774 (2018)
9. Curran, J.: The doctor, his patient and the illness. Bmj **335**(7626), 941–941 (2007)
10. Eccles, D.W., Groth, P.T.: Problem solving systems theory: implications for the design of socio-technological systems. Technol. Instruct. Cognit. Learn. **3**(3/4), 323 (2006)
11. Effken, J.A.: Different lenses, improved outcomes: a new approach to the analysis and design of healthcare information systems. Int. J. Med. Inform. **65**(1), 59–74 (2002)
12. Emery, F.E., Trist, E.L.: Socio-technical systems. management sciences, models and techniques. Churchman C.W. et al (1960)
13. Epstein, R.M., Street, R.L.: The values and value of patient-centered care (2011)
14. FDA: U.s. food and drug administration: proposed regulatory framework for modifications to artificial intelligence/machine learning (ai/ml)-based software as medical device (samd)
15. FDA: U.s. food and drug administration: What are examples of software as a medical device?
16. Goldberg, D., Nichols, D., Oki, B.M., Terry, D.: Using collaborative filtering to weave an information tapestry. Commun. ACM **35**(12), 61–70 (1992)
17. Hägglund, M., Scandurra, I.: A socio-technical analysis of patient accessible electronic health records. Stud. Health Technol. Inform **244**, 3–7 (2017)
18. Hofmann, B.: The myth of technology in health care. Sci. Eng. Eth. **8**(1), 17–29 (2002)
19. Konstan, J.A., Miller, B.N., Maltz, D., Herlocker, J.L., Gordon, L.R., Riedl, J.: Grouplens: applying collaborative filtering to usenet news. Commun. ACM **40**(3), 77–87 (1997)
20. Lamas, E., Salinas, R., Coquedano, C., Simon, M.P., Bousquet, C., Ferrer, M., Zorrilla, S.: The meaning of patient empowerment in the digital age: the role of online patient-communities. Stud. Health Technol. Inform. **244**, 43–7 (2017)
21. Meskó, B., Radó, N., Győrffy, Z.: Opinion leader empowered patients about the era of digital health: a qualitative study. BMJ open **9**(3), e025267 (2019)
22. Milano, S., Taddeo, M., Floridi, L.: Recommender systems and their ethical challenges. AI & SOCIETY pp. 1–11 (2020)
23. Musco, C., Musco, C., Tsourakakis, C.E.: Minimizing polarization and disagreement in social networks. In: Proceedings of the 2018 World Wide Web Conference, pp. 369–378 (2018)
24. NM, G.: Framework for designing digital health tools with empathy, journal of participatory medicine
25. Paraschakis, D.: Recommender systems from an industrial and ethical perspective. In: Proceedings of the 10th ACM conference on recommender systems, pp. 463–466 (2016)
26. Pazzani, M., Billsus, D.: Learning and revising user profiles: the identification of interesting web sites. Mach. Learn. **27**(3), 313–331 (1997)
27. Ramakrishnan, N., Keller, B.J., Mirza, B.J., Grama, A.Y., Karypis, G.: When being weak is brave: Privacy in recommender systems. arXiv preprint cs/0105028 (2001)
28. Ramos, G., Boratto, L., Caleiro, C.: On the negative impact of social influence in recommender systems: a study of bribery in collaborative hybrid algorithms. Inform. Proces. Manag. **57**(2), 102058 (2020)
29. Ricci, F., Rokach, L., Shapira, B.: Introduction to recommender systems handbook. In: Recommender systems handbook, pp. 1–35. Springer (2011)
30. Shortliffe, E.H.: Artificial intelligence in medicine: weighing the accomplishments, hype, and promise. Yearb. Med. Inform. **28**(1), 257 (2019)

31. Sittig, D.F., Singh, H.: A new socio-technical model for studying health information technology in complex adaptive healthcare systems. In: Cognitive informatics for biomedicine, pp. 59–80. Springer (2015)
32. Weiner, M., Biondich, P.: The influence of information technology on patient-physician relationships. J. General Intern. Med. **21**(1), 35–39 (2006)
33. Wiesner, M., Pfeifer, D.: Health recommender systems: concepts, requirements, technical basics and challenges. Int. J. Environ. Res. Public health **11**(3), 2580–2607 (2014)
34. Xin, Y., et al.: Challenges in recommender systems: scalability, privacy, and structured recommendations. Ph.D. thesis, Massachusetts Institute of Technology (2015)

Computer Methods for Localization of the Subthalamic Nucleus During Deep Brain Stimulation Surgeries for Treatment of Parkinson Disease

Konrad A. Ciecierski

Abstract In the neurobiological mechanism of Parkinson's Disease (PD), a certain part of the brain called the Subthalamic Nucleus (STN) becomes overactive. This pathologically increased activity inhibits other regions of the brain, causing many symptoms observed in PD patients. The hyperactivity of the STN can be lowered using a special electrical stimulating electrode. In the neurosurgical treatment of Parkinson's Disease (PD), the goal is the precise placement of such electrode within the Subthalamic Nucleus. As STN does not significantly differ from adjacent structures on images provided by the CT or MRI, these standard techniques of medical imaging can provide only the approximate localization of the STN. The final localization of the STN has to be pinpointed during surgery. For this, typically, three to five very thin electrodes are inserted into the patient's brain and advanced towards the expected STN location given by CT and MRI. Electrodes in measured steps approach, traverse, and exit out of the STN. At each step, the neurobiological activity of brain tissue surrounding the leads of the electrodes is recorded. By careful analysis of recordings provided by these electrodes, it is possible to discriminate which recordings were recorded within the STN. This, in turn, gives the extent of the STN in the 3D space on trajectories of the recording electrodes.

1 Description of the Problem

As the hyperactivity of the STN plays a significant role in the etiology of major PD symptoms [1], it is widely used as the target in the surgical treatment of major PD symptoms [2–7]. The challenge of this surgical procedure is that the STN is a small (nine by four by seven mm) structure [2, 8] that frequently is not easily distinguished at Computer Tomography (CT) or Magnetic Resonance Imaging (MRI) [2, 8–12]. Misdetection of the STN may also cause very severe adverse effects as a result of the inhibition of the surrounding structures (sensory, motor, and autonomic) [13].

K. A. Ciecierski (✉)
Research and Academic Computer Network, ul. Kolska 12, 01-045 Warszawa, Poland
e-mail: konrad.ciecierski@gmail.com

Z. W. Ras et al. (eds.), *Recommender Systems for Medicine and Music*,
Studies in Computational Intelligence 946,
https://doi.org/10.1007/978-3-030-66450-3_3

For example, while a dorsolateral portion of the STN is the motor part being the target for the surgery for PD [6], the ventromedial part of the STN plays an important role in the cognition process [14]. Inhibition of ventromedial portion can result in deterioration of the cognition functions [14]. Inhibition of the anteroventral part of the STN, the limbic portion [15], can result in mood alterations like depression or mania [15–17].

Very precise identification of the STN borders is thus both difficult and obviously extremely important [18]. To facilitate the localization of the STN, a two-step procedure is applied. Firstly using fused CT with MRI scan, the expected localization of the STN is given. In the second phase, the precise STN localization is obtained during surgery by analyzing the neurosurgical microrecording. During microrecording, an array of 3 to 5 parallel microelectrodes is inserted into the patient's brain using the stereotactic guidance system [19]. The electrodes are then advanced towards the expected localization of the STN. From the depth that is roughly about 10 mm dorsal to the STN, electrodes are advanced in measured steps. At each step, a multiunit simultaneous recording is obtained from all of the electrodes. Typically, the time span of the recording is 10 s. After the recording is done, the set of electrodes is advanced ventrally by 1 mm. Such steps are repeated for around 16 mm, i.e., until the electrodes safely traverse the ventral border of the STN. The electrodes are not advanced further if the recording typical for Substantia Nigra Pars reticulata (SNr) [2, 8, 19, 20] is observed. Due to the distinct STN activity [1, 3, 9, 21–25], an experienced neurosurgeon can distinguish whether given recording has been recorded within the STN or not. Such discrimination is, however, by definition, subjective and difficult in cases when the STN hyperactivity is not clearly pronounced. The main goal of computer-based methods that can be used during DBS surgery for the PD is to provide a fast and objective assessment if any given recording has been recorded within STN or not. Having such information for all recordings from all microelectrodes helps the neurosurgeon to visualize the 3D extent of the STN on tracks of these microelectrodes. Such information increases the safety of the neurosurgical procedure [18] and allows it to be performed in a shorter time. This is especially important due to the necessity of obtaining awake brain recordings and the interaction with the patient [26, 27], as the general anesthesia cannot be used and the patient is conscious throughout the neurosurgical part of the procedure.

The required minimal values for the computer classification as measured by sensitivity and specificity depends on the subject for which it is applied. In some non-medical applications, the sensitivity and specificity of values above 0.75 are deemed to be satisfactory [28]. In medical sciences, depending on the specialty, the good and applicable sensitivity and specificity values should be around 0.85 [28]. Such values, while sufficient for many medical applications, might still be not high enough for neurosurgery. Classifications given in this work, in tenfold cross-validation [29] against surgical protocols, have achieved the sensitivity of 0.95, specificity 0.95, and the ROC area 0.99.

2 Characteristics of Microelectrode Recorded Signal

Microelectrode records the brain activity with a sampling rate of 24 kHz, and each recording is at least 10 s long. The recorded signal is noisy; it contains both the noise that is of neurological nature and noise that is unwanted, i.e., various artifacts caused by external sources. Disregarding the unwanted noise, the signal is characterized by spikes of voltage produced by neuron cells located near the recording electrode and background noise being the summary of the activity of neurons that are farther away from the electrode.

2.1 Action Potentials

Neural tissue is electrically active. This is due to the difference in concentration of ions between the inner and outer side of the neuron's cell membrane. This difference in concentrations of ions is actively maintained by the neuron cells. In the wall of the neuron cells are located special ion channels responsible for ion transportation. Some of these channels in a single cycle pull into the cell two K^+ ions while pushing outside three Na^+ ions. At the same time, negatively charged ions cannot leave the cell because they are too large to pass through the mentioned ion channels. This, in time, leads to a situation where there are more positive ions outside than inside of the cell. Outside of the cell becomes positively charged while the inside becomes negatively charged. The ion pumps maintain the negative charge within the cell at a level of about −70 mV. This difference in electrical charge allows the neuron to be electrically active [30].

As an effect of certain external stimulation, this electrical equilibrium for a brief time can change. In such a situation, some of the dedicated and normally closed channels that allow a flow of Na^+ into the cell start to open. The negative charge maintained within the cell starts to weaken, and upon reaching a threshold of about −55 mV, the inbound channels for Na^+ massively open. At this moment, within the cell are K^+ ions that were originally pulled here by ion pumps and newly come Na^+ ions. The cell membrane re-polarizes, the internal potential reaches around +100 mV, and a voltage spike occurs. At this moment, inbound $Na+$ channels close, outbound K^+ channels open, and K^+ ions massively flow out. After K^+ flown out, the internal potential of the cell becomes negative, even more than the original −70 mV. At this stage, channels allowing outflow of K^+ ions also close, and ion pumps start over to pull two K^+ ions while pushing three Na^+ ions outside. Cell returns to equilibrium at −70 mV.

In simplified form, this process could be described as follows:

- The cell is at equilibrium, internal charge around −70 mV.
- The cell is externally stimulated, some of the inbound Na^+ channels start to open.
- The cell internal negative charge lessens.
- The negative charge within the cell reaches potential around −55 mV.

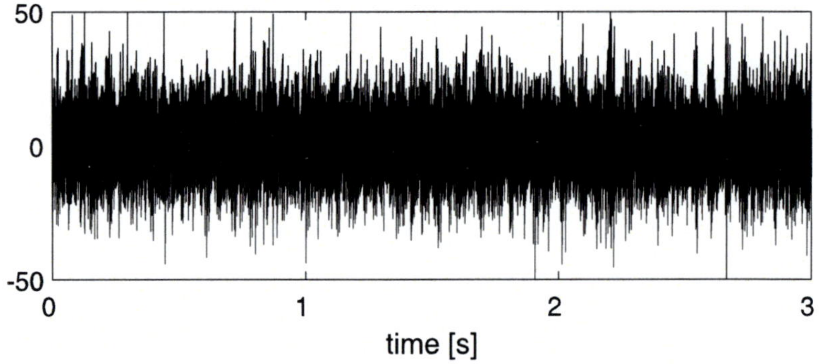

Fig. 1 Fragment of the microelectrode recording

- The inbound Na^+ channels open massively.
- The internal charge of a cell reaches around +100 mV.
- The inbound Na^+ channels close.
- The outbound K^+ channels open, the K^+ ions massively flows out.
- The outbound K^+ channels close, the outflow of K^+ changed the internal charge to below −70 mV.
- The ion pumps in each cycle pulls two K^+ ions inside while pushing three Na^+ ions outside to maintain the internal charge of the cell at a level of around −70 mV.

In different neuron cells, the amount and distribution of ion channels vary [2, 30]. This means that the speed of progression through described stages differs from cell to cell. As a consequence, the shape of the voltage spike produced by the neuron cell is its fingerprint as it originates from the cell morphology.

From this, when in a single recording, one observes spikes with different shapes, it is safe to assume that these spikes originated in different neuron cells. Meanwhile, the spiking activity of more distant neurons summarily forms the background activity present in every recording acquired by the in-brain-placed electrode.

The recording electrode can record the activity of neurons within a radius of about 50 μm [31]. Depending on the brain region, within this radius of 50 μm, one might find well over 100 neurons [2]. Knowing that the STN is a structure that characterizes by large amounts of densely packed neurons [2, 8] It should be then expected, that the signal acquired within the STN would reflect this in its properties.

In Fig. 1 one can see the three-second long recording taken from a microelectrode. There can be clearly seen the spiking and background activity. Many spikes can already be observed as their amplitude is much larger than the background. Both the amplitude of the background noise and the amplitude of the spikes are in some measure dependent on the location at which the signal was acquired.

To see the individual spikes, the signal must be observed in great magnification. The single spike is an electrical impulse that lasts for about one millisecond.

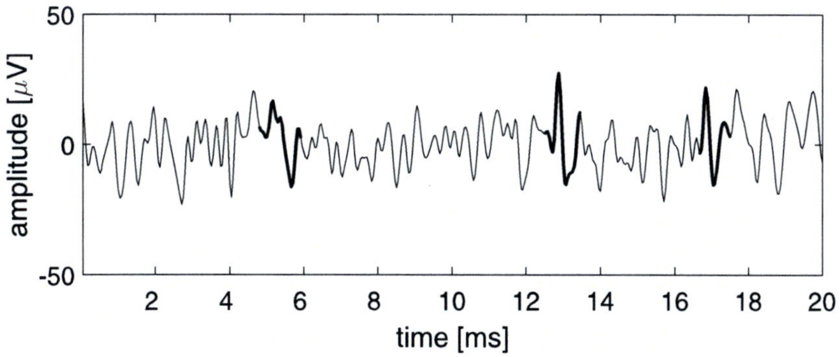

Fig. 2 Fragment of the microelectrode recording with highlighted spikes

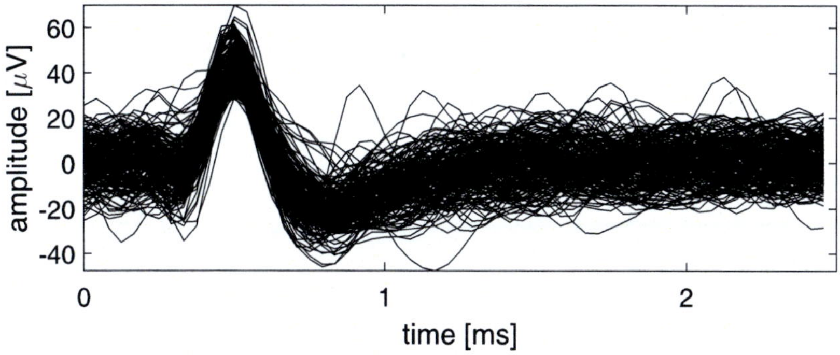

Fig. 3 Spikes registered from a single neuron, shape class 2

Part of the signal shown in Fig. 1 is shown in Fig. 2. Here the whole time span of the figure is only 20 ms. Few selected spikes have been highlighted using a bold line. What is immediately noticeable is the ever-present noise from which spikes arise with their high amplitudes.

As the shape of the spike carries important information, spikes are often grouped according to their shape [32, 33], this procedure is called the spike sorting. Below, in Fig. 3 and Fig. 4, one can see the example of two spike shape classes taken from single recordings, spikes in classes are aligned according to their maximal amplitude.

In the recording from which spike shape classes shown in Figs. 3 and 4 were taken, there were active six distinct neurons. In Fig. 5, one can see times at which these neurons were spiking.

Neuron two, with spikes shown in Fig. 3 is active throughout most of the time, while neuron three, with spikes shown in Fig. 4 is active only at certain times.

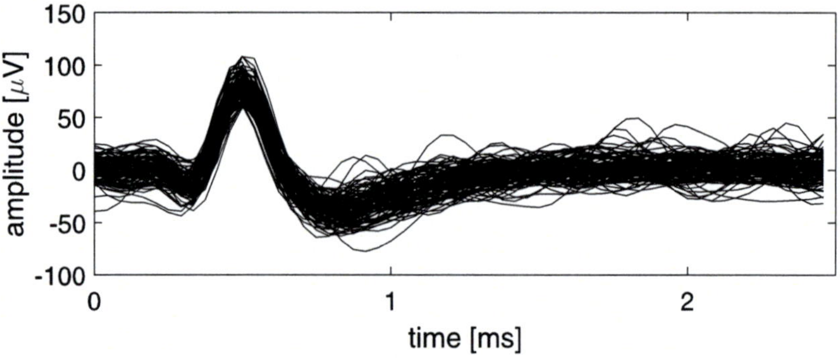

Fig. 4 Spikes registered from a single neuron, shape class 3

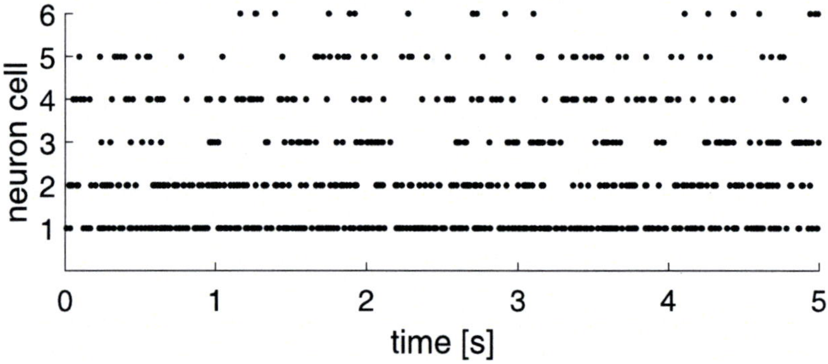

Fig. 5 Times of occurrence of spikes from different shape classes

2.2 *Background Activity*

The activity of the neuron cell being near the electrode's recording lead is registered as a spike of voltage reaching 100 mV or more. The more distant is the spiking neuron, the lower is the voltage of the registered spike. Finally, all distant neurons in the vicinity of the electrode extending beyond the 50 μm radius, summarily contribute to the background activity. This activity forms a noise that can be observed, for example, in Fig. 1. The problem with analyzing the background activity lies in the fact that not all noise present in the recorded signal is of microbiological origin. As the background noise of the recorded signal fits below 50 mV, the recording hardware uses great amplification, and the recording procedure is very sensitive to external contamination. Such minuscule intrusions as touching the stereotactic frame, patient moving, speaking during the recording process, or even his heartbeat cause the presence of high amplitude artifacts in the recordings [2]. From this, any artifacts, i.e., contamination, must be removed from the original recorded signal before it can be used for inferring any information useful for recording classification.

3 Attributes

Classification of the recordings is based on attributes that are calculated from the recordings. Quality of these attributes is of great importance as even the best classification algorithm will not achieve good results using poorly discriminating attributes. Here attributes can be divided into two categories: spike activity-based attributes and background activity-based attributes. Both sets of attributes require the input signal to be filtered. This process is, however, very different for both these cases.

3.1 Spike Activity-Based Attributes

Attributes basing on spike activity require in the first place the detection of spikes in the analyzed recording.

Spikes can be detected using simple amplitude thresholding. For spikes to be detected, it is required that its maximal voltage value exceeds a certain threshold and that its shape fits the general shape described in Sect. 2.1 and in [22]. The raw, recorded signal cannot be, however, effectively used for such a purpose. This is because it contains low-frequency components, see Fig. 6. One can see, for example, the mean amplitude around time index 80 ms is larger than around time index 70 ms. For such a signal, thresholding by amplitude value would miss spikes in regions where low-frequency components of the signal have small values. The low-frequency component of the signal can be removed using wavelet decomposition, filtering, and synthesis [35].

Preprocessing

As the original signal is sampled with 24 kHz, that means that set of wavelet coefficients; S_5 represents the original signal in frequencies 375 Hz [35]. By decomposing the original signal five times with wavelet forward transform, setting all wavelet coefficients in S_5 to zero, and finally performing five times the wavelet inverse transform, one obtains original signal with frequencies 375 Hz filtered out. The signal shown in Fig. 6, after the filtering process is shown in Fig. 7.

For such a signal, there can be defined a proper threshold value for spike detection. This value is set to $4\sigma_N$ [22] where σ_N is a special formula for the standard deviation used for neurological recordings [34]. The σ_N for recording $X = \{x_1, \ldots, x_n\}$ is given by Eq. 1.

$$\sigma_N = \frac{median(|x_1|, \ldots, |x_n|)}{0.6745} \tag{1}$$

When spikes are all detected, they are sorted into shape classes [32, 33]. For electrode e registering brain activity at depth d one can define

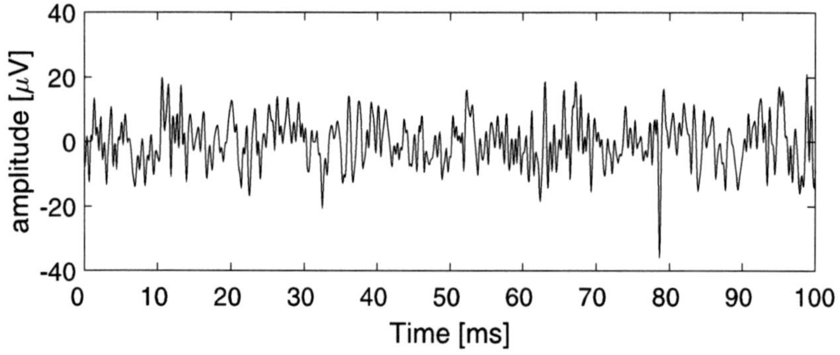

Fig. 6 Example of signal with low-frequency components

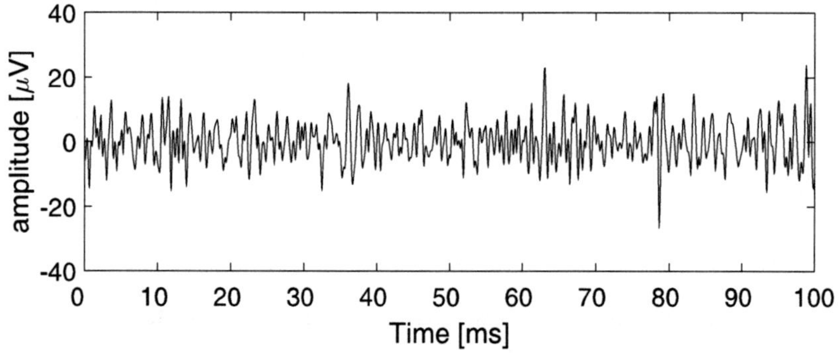

Fig. 7 Example of signal with low-frequency components removed

Definition 1 Let $D = \{-10000, -9000, \ldots, 0, \ldots, ..., d_E\}$ be the set of depths at which electrodes record brain activity.

Definition 2 $mer(e, d)$ as recording of brain activity made by electrode e at depth d with sampling frequency of 24 kHz.

Definition 3 $reclen(mer(e, d))$ as length of recording $mer(e, d)$ in seconds.

Definition 4 $spkcnt(mer(e, d))$ as number of all spikes detected in recording $mer(e, d)$.

Definition 5 $shps(mer(e, d))$ as set of spike shapes detected in recording $mer(e, d)$.

Definition 6 $spkcnt.sc(mer(e, d), s)$ as number of all spikes of shape class s detected in recording $mer(e, d)$.

Definition 7 $intcnt(mer(e, d))$ as number of all interspike intervals detected in recording $mer(e, d)$.

Definition 8 $intcnt.b(mer(e, d))$ as number of shorter than 33 ms interspike intervals detected in recording $mer(e, d)$.

Definition 9 $intcnt.sc(mer(e, d), s)$ as number of interspike intervals between spikes of shape s detected in recording $mer(e, d)$.

Definition 10 $intcnt.sc.b(mer(e, d), s)$ as number of shorter than 33ms interspike intervals between spikes of shape s detected in recording $mer(e, d)$.

Finally, four attributes based on observed spikes can be defined.

spike activity-based attributes

Definition 11 Define spike activity-based attributes as

$$AvgSpkRate(e, d) = \frac{spkcnt(mer(e, d))}{reclen(mer(e, d))}$$

$$AvgSpkRateScMax(e, d) = \max_{s \in shps(mer(e,d))} \frac{spkcnt.sc(mer(e, d), s)}{reclen(mer(e, d))}$$

$$BurstRatio(e, d) = \frac{intcnt.b(mer(e, d))}{intcnt(mer(e, d))}$$

$$BurstRatioScMax(e, d) = \max_{s \in shps(mer(e,d))} \frac{intcnt.sc.b(mer(e, d), s)}{intcnt.sc(mer(e, d), s)}$$

3.2 *Preprocessing for Background Activity-Based Attributes*

The preprocessing and definitions in case of spike-based attributes are simple and straightforward. In case of background activity-based attributes, both preprocessing and definition of attributes are much more complicated.

In case of background-based attributes, the role of preprocessing is the removal of the artifacts contaminating the signal. An example of a typical signal with artifacts is shown in Fig. 8.

The artifacts are visibly located in the signal between time indexes 3 [s] and 6 [s]. The value of RMS calculated for the first three seconds of the recording is 10.465, while the RMS for the full recording is 19.856; increases by a factor of 90%.

As the amplitude fits into interval $[-4\sigma_N, 4\sigma_N]$ for over 99.99% of samples, the most naive approach is just to threshold the amplitude. After all the samples having an absolute value larger than $12\sigma_N$ has been zeroed, the RMS value of the whole recording has decreased to 15.593. This value is still 49 % larger than the reference taken from the first three seconds. Additionally, by zeroing samples one is

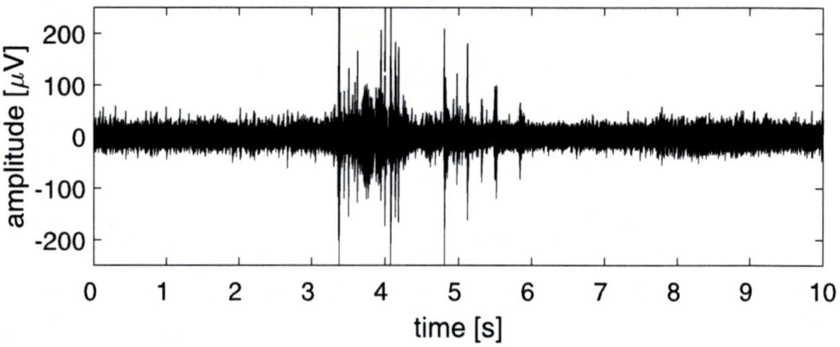

Fig. 8 Microelectrode recorded signal containing artifacts

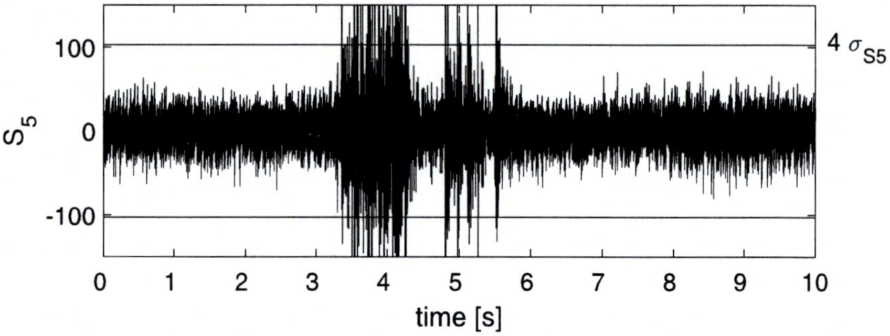

Fig. 9 Coefficient of the S_5 set in the time

effectively introducing new frequencies into the signal [35] and decreases the number of its samples. Using the amplitude approach, this is close to the possible limit of filtering. Lowering the threshold further starts to clip the spikes of voltage produced by neurons, and the usefulness of the resulting recording quickly degrades.

Much better results can be achieved, approaching the problem of artifacts removal in the frequency domain. After decomposition of the original signal sampled with frequency 24 kHz, one obtains a set of wavelet coefficients S_5 and D_5. The S_5 set represents the original signal in frequencies 375 Hz. The D_5 set represents the original signal in frequencies 375 Hz 750 Hz. Figures 9 and 10 are shown amplitudes of S_5 and D_5 in time. Plots also show the value of 5σ calculated for these coefficients.

One can now notice two things. Firstly, the time of occurrence of artifacts in sets S_5 and D_5 matches the time of artifact occurrence in the original signal. This is a very useful feature of wavelet transformation while showing signal in the given frequency band; it retains information about time.

Secondly, the artifacts seen in S_5 and D_5 are much more pronounced and easier to the threshold.

One can easily find all coefficients from S_5 and D_5 that are above the threshold of $5\sigma_N$ and put zero to samples these coefficients map to. It is important to notice

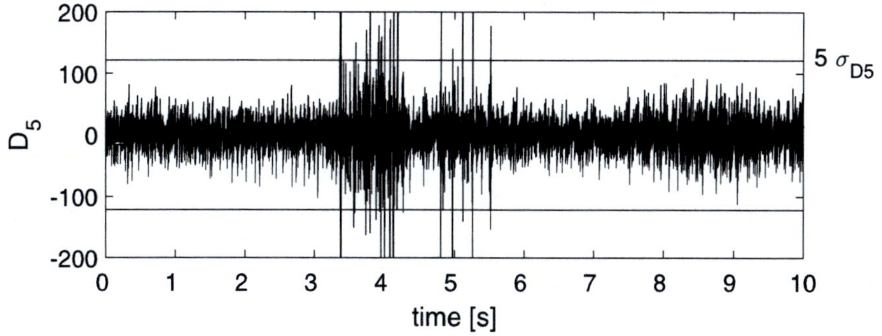

Fig. 10 Coefficient of the D_5 set in the time

that every single coefficient from S_5 or D_5 set maps to consecutive 2^5 samples in the original signal [35]. Signal obtained in this way has RMS value 14.731, much closer to reference 10.465. Still, this method, by setting the value of certain samples to zero, introduces new frequencies into the original signal.

The final approach does not affect the original samples directly, but is more computationally demanding. In this approach, modifications are made in each set of wavelet coefficients obtained after five steps of wavelet forward transform. For each set from $\{S_5, D_5, D_4, D_3, D_2, D_1\}$, the value of σ is calculated, and all coefficients with absolute value exceeding $5\sigma_N$ are set to zero. After all six sets of wavelet coefficients are modified, using the inverse wavelet transform, the filtered signal is obtained. This method does not set values of the original signal, nor is it reducing the number of its effective samples. Additional calculation of inverse wavelet transform is, however, necessary. The final filtered signal has RMS 12.311, which is the closest to the reference value. Final, filtered, and free of artifacts signal is shown in Fig. 11.

Artifact filtering is extremely important as without it value of various attributes described further can be greatly increased by randomly occurring artifacts. Artifacts occur randomly but frequently. In many cases, as many as half of the recordings from given surgery contain them. It is impossible to create even a mediocre classification method when the attributes it is basing on change randomly by such large values. Preprocessing, in the case of background activity-based attributes, is by this an essential part of their definition.

Definition 12 For recording $mer(e, d)$, its artifact free, filtered version is denoted as

$$artrem(mer(e, d))$$

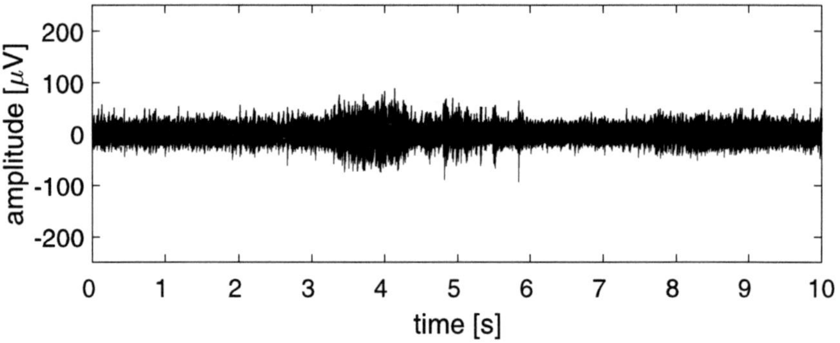

Fig. 11 Microelectrode recorded signal after artifacts removal

3.3 Background Activity-Based Attributes

There are four attributes basing directly on the background activity of the signal. Input for these attributes is always artifact filtered.

Normalization

In case of spike activity-based attributes, they were naturally normalized. In case of background activity-based attributes, the normalization is performed at two levels.

The first level of normalization—if required—acts on the single recording level and assures that value of the attribute does not depend on the length of the recorded signal. Signals in most cases are 10 s long, but there are both shorter and longer ones.

The second level of normalization act on the level of all recordings registered by a given electrode. The electrical properties of the electrode, the amplification, and other conditions may vary. To take these possible variations into account, to make sure that data obtained using different electrodes is comparable, the normalization of the second level is done.

As the recording procedure starts at levels that are ten millimeters above the expected center of the STN, the first five depths at which electrode registers brain activity is the white matter [2], which is characterized by the low background noise. For background-based attribute, average taken from these depths can be thus used as a basing referencing level for normalization.

Definition 13 For input signal $mer(e, d)$, define a function $f(mer(e, d)) \in \mathbb{R}$. Define also set of base depths $D_B = \{d \in D : d < -5000\}$.
Let the base value of function f_B be defined as

$$f_B(e) = \underset{d \in D_B}{avg}\, f(mer(e, d)) \tag{2}$$

then the normalized value of function f for $mer(e, d)$ is

$$f_N(e, d) = \frac{f(mer(e, d))}{f_B(e)} \tag{3}$$

Definition 14 Assume that the original signal S_0 is sampled with frequency f_0 Hz, and has n samples (n being a power of 2). Then, for $k = 1, \ldots, log_2 n$, there are: S_k as a tuple of $\frac{n}{2^k}$ wavelet coefficients representing the signal S_0 in frequencies $(0, \frac{f_0}{2^{k+1}}]$ D_k as a tuple of $\frac{n}{2^k}$ wavelet coefficients representing the signal S_0 in frequencies $(\frac{f_0}{2^{k+1}}, \frac{f_0}{2^k}]$. Full decomposition is therefore represented as the following set:

$$WD(S_0, f_0) = \{S_{log_2 n}, D_{log_2 n}, \ldots, D_1\} \tag{4}$$

Definition 15 For original signal sampled with frequency f_0 Hz, the frequency coverage of a S_k tuple can be defined as $FC_S(f_0, k) = (0, \frac{f_0}{2^{k+1}}]$, while the frequency coverage of a D_k tuple can be defined as $FC_D(f_0, k) = (\frac{f_0}{2^{k+1}}, \frac{f_0}{2^k}]$. Finally, for original the signal S_0 sampled with a frequency f_0 Hz, and for a given continuous, left open, frequency interval $\mathbb{F}$, a defined function returning a set of tuples of wavelet coefficients that fit into its range can be created.

$$\begin{aligned} FC(S_0, f_0, \mathbb{F}) = \\ & \{S_k \in WD(S_0, f_0) : k = log_2 n \wedge FC_S(f_0, k) \subseteq \mathbb{F}\} \\ & \cup \\ & \{D_k \in WD(S_0, f_0) : k \leq log_2 n \wedge FC_D(f_0, k) \subseteq \mathbb{F}\} \end{aligned} \tag{5}$$

$$PWR(mer_{e,d}, f_0, f_b, f_e) = \frac{\sum_{T \in FC(mer_{e,d}, f_0, (f_b, f_e])} \sum_{x \in T} x^2}{\frac{|mer_{e,d}|}{f_0}}$$

background activity-based attributes

Definition 16 Define background attributes as

$$prc80(e, d) = vprc80_N(mer(e, d))$$

$$rms(e, d) = vrms_N(mer(e, d))$$

$$lfb(e, d) = vlfb_N(spkr(mer(e, d)))$$

$$hfb(e, d) = vhfb_N(spkr(mer(e, d)))$$

where

$$vprc80(mer(e, d)) = P_{80\%}(abs(artrem(mer_{e,d})))$$

$$vrms(mer(e,d)) = \sqrt{\frac{1}{|mer(e,d)|} \sum_{x \in artrem(mer(e,d))} x^2}$$

$$vlfb(mer(e,d)) = PWR(artrem(mer_{e,d}), 24000, 0, 500)$$

$$vhfb(mer(e,d)) = PWR(artrem(mer_{e,d}), 24000, 500, 3000)$$

The $spkr(mer(e,d))$ function, removes from recording $mer(e,d)$ all spikes detected using method described in Sect. 3.1 and in [22].

3.4 Moving Average-Based Attributes

For each of the background activity-based attributes: PRC80, RMS, LFB, and HFB, the one-padded moving average is calculated. In this manner, four moving average-based filters are defined: MPRC80, MRMS, MLFB, and MHFB.

Definition 17 Let for input signal $mer(e,d)$, function $f(mer(e,d)) \in \mathbb{R}$, define its one-padded form as

$$f_{PAD1}(e,d) = \begin{cases} f(e,d), & \text{if } d \in D \\ 1, & \text{otherwise} \end{cases} \tag{6}$$

moving average-based attributes

Definition 18 Define moving average attributes as

$$prc80_M(e,d) = prc80_{PAD1}(mer(e,d))$$

$$rms_M(e,d) = rms_{PAD1}(mer(e,d))$$

$$lfb_M(e,d) = lfb_{PAD1}(mer(e,d))$$

$$hfb_M(e,d) = hfb_{PAD1}(mer(e,d))$$

The role of these attributes is to provide smoothed information about changes of primary background activity-based attributes.

3.5 Temporal Attributes

For each of the background activity-based attributes: PRC80, RMS, LFB, and HFB, four temporal attributes are defined.

The temporal filters reflect maximal observed positive or negative changes in the values of a certain attribute. The changes are observed by comparing the value of the attribute at current depth with values of attribute at 1000 and 2000 μm above it.

Definition 19 Let for input signal $mer(e, d)$, function $f(mer(e, d)) \in \mathbb{R}$ representing an attribute, be defined

$$dlt(f, e, d, step) = \begin{cases} 0, & \text{if } d - step < min(D) \\ f(mer(e, d)) - f(mer(e, d - step)), & \text{otherwise} \end{cases} \quad (7)$$

$$dlt_{MAX}(f, e, d, step) = \max_{d_i \le d} dlt(f, e, d_i, step) \quad (8)$$

$$dlt_{MIN}(f, e, d, step) = \min_{d_i \le d} dlt(f, e, d_i, step) \quad (9)$$

temporal attributes

Definition 20 Define temporal attributes for $prc80$ attribute as

$$prc80_{1U}(e, d) = dlt_{MAX}(prc80, e, d, 1000)$$

$$prc80_{2U}(e, d) = dlt_{MAX}(prc80, e, d, 2000)$$

$$prc80_{1D}(e, d) = dlt_{MIN}(prc80, e, d, 1000)$$

$$prc80_{2D}(e, d) = dlt_{MIN}(prc80, e, d, 2000)$$

Following 12 temporal attributes defined for remaining three background activity-based attributes are analogous both in naming and definition.

3.6 Narrow Frequency Band-Based Attributes

These attributes reflect the power of the artifact filtered signal in narrow frequency bands. While there are already defined attributes LFB and HFB, which reflect the signal's power, these two attributes span rather broad frequency ranges. Calculation of signals power for an arbitrary frequency range is also technically difficult when using the DWT approach (see Definition 15 in Sect. 3.3).

It would be useful to have additional attributes describing the signal's frequency-based properties in a more detailed way. For this, the frequency range below 300 kHz has been equally split into 30 frequency intervals, each having width 100 Hz.

Definition 21 Let for input signal $mer(e, d)$, function $bpf(mer(e, d), f_b, f_e) \in \mathbb{R}$, denotes recording $mer(e, d)$ filtered with band-pass filter passing only frequencies between f_b Hz and f_e Hz. The normalized power of the recording $mer(e, d)$ in frequency band between f_b Hz and f_e Hz is then given by:

$$bpfn(mer(e, d), f_b.f_e) = \frac{\sum_{x \in bpf(artrem(mer(e,d)), f_b.f_e)} x^2}{reclen(mer(e, d))}$$

where the band-pass filtering is done using a Matlab R2020a implementation of minimum-order filter having a stopband attenuation of 60 dB.

The Definition 21 already assures that narrow frequency band-based attributes are normalized according to the length of the recording. The normalization on the electrode level is done in a way that is similar to this described in Definition 13 in Sect. 3.3.

Definition 22 For input signal $mer(e, d)$, a function $f(mer(e, d)) \in \mathbb{R}$ and set of base depths $D_B = \{d \in D : d < -5000\}$ be defined

$$BVS(e) = \{f(mer(e, d) : d \in D_B\} \tag{10}$$

Let now

$$BVS_m(e) = BVS(e) \setminus (min(BVS(e)) \cup max(BVS(e))) \tag{11}$$

then the normalized value of function $f(mer(e, d)$ for $mer(e, d)$ is

$$f_\chi(e, d) = \frac{f(mer(e, d))}{mean(BVS_m(e))} \tag{12}$$

The exclusion of the smallest and the largest values from the $BVS(e)$ set reduces the influence of variance in the value of an attribute in the first millimeters of the recording procedure.

narrow frequency band-based attributes

Definition 23 Define narrow frequency band-based attributes as follows:

For $j = 0 \ldots 29$

$$pwr_j(e, d) = bpfn_\chi(mer(e, d), 100 * j, 100 * (j + 1))$$

For example: $pwr_{13}(e, d)$ represents power of the signal $mer(e, d)$ in range 1300 Hz 1400 Hz.

4 Evaluation and Interpretation

notation

For simplicity in the following classification results, instead of referring to the attribute pwr_j that gives normalized power for the band $100 * j \sim 100 * (j + 1)$ Hz, the description of this band itself is used. That is, for example, by results basing on band 1600–1700 Hz it is meant that these results base on attribute pwr_{16}.

All classification results presented in this paper were obtained using Matlab R2020a. Data used for classification consist of 18349 recordings registered during 175 DBS surgeries for Parkinson's Disease. Each recording was registered using sampling frequency 24 kHz and lasts for at least 10 s. Out of 18349 recordings, the 3693 (20.13%) were labeled as recorded within the STN.

Classifications have all been made using classifier AdaBoostM1 with 500 trees, minimal leaf size 5 and learning rate 0.1. AdaBoost has been chosen as it is particularly well suited for imbalanced data [36, 37]. All presented results have been obtained using a tenfold cross-validation schema [29].

4.1 Spike Activity-Based Attributes

STN is characterized by high spiking activity, and this is the reason why spike activity-based attributes have good sensitivity in finding recordings registered within this nucleus. The problem with spiking activity is that STN is not the only region on track of the electrode that can and does produce many spikes. There are other very active regions located both above and beneath the STN. Above leads to classifier basing solely upon spiking activity to be poor in specificity.

Spike activity-based attributes were sorted according to their influence on Area under ROC (AuROC) value. The changes in sensitivity, specificity, and AuROC values that occur as a following attributes are added to the classification pool, are shown in Table 1.

While these attributes themselves are clearly not sufficient, they do carry some additional information and can be used together with other attributes as additional confirmation of the STN detection. The detection of spikes is also used in construction of some of the background-based attributes as shown in Sect. 3.3.

Table 1 Classification measures change with the addition of subsequent spike activity-based attributes

Attributes	Attribute added	Sensitivity	Specificity	AuROC
1	AvgSpkRate	0.873	0.591	0.780
2	BurstRatio	0.880	0.580	0.797
3	AvgSpkRateScMax	0.848	0.667	0.819
4	BurstRatioScMax	0.833	0.701	0.829

4.2 Narrow Frequency Band-Based Attributes

Analysis of classification results obtained using narrow band-based attributes is very important. The ROC based ordering of these attributes gives information about the frequency fingerprint of the STN. The changes in sensitivity, specificity, and AuROC values that occur as following narrow band-based attributes are added to the classification pool, are shown in Table 2 and in Fig. 12.

Very interesting finding present in Table 2 is that frequencies typical for the STN start with the band 1600 Hz 1700 Hz, to later grow as a continuous frequency range up to full interval below 3 kHz.

It is also worth noticing that, already using only the frequency band 1600 Hz 1700 Hz one can discriminate the STN recordings with sensitivity and specificity above 0.9. The frequency band 1600 Hz 1700 Hz, can thus be described as the core STN frequency.

The main advantage of these attributes is that while providing sensitivity and specificity above 0.9, their construction does not require deep knowledge in the area of neurophysiology.

In Fig. 12, it is shown how measures of classification quality change as subsequent attributes (in the order shown in Table 2) are added. One can notice that AuROC value after initial increase has a plateau at 0.974 till more than 25 attributes are used for classification.

It is also evident that frequencies below 1 kHz are not well suited for the STN discrimination in view of the AuROC value. Compare the ROC curves shown in Fig. 13 for the difference between 100–200 Hz band and one between 1600–1700 Hz. The ROC curve for 100–200 Hz band shows that the sensitivity and specificity are never both above 0.8. The classifier with such ROC curve might be deemed satisfactory in some research areas. In case of neurosurgical application, it is, however, not acceptable. In Fig. 14, it is shown how measures of classification quality change as subsequent attributes (in the order shown in Table 3) are added. Classifier with ROC curve shown in Fig. 15b is good, the sensitivity and specificity exceed 0.9, and such a classifier could be used for a decision support system.

Still, as it is shown in the following section, even better results might be achieved.

Table 2 Classification measures change with the addition of subsequent narrow band-based attributes

Attributes	Band added	Band covered	Sensitivity	Specificity	AuROC
1	1600–1700	1600–1700	0.926	0.912	0.956
2	1700–1800	1600–1800	0.931	0.901	0.966
3	1500–1600	1500–1800	0.937	0.901	0.968
4	1800–1900	1500–1900	0.924	0.915	0.970
5	1900–2000	1500–2000	0.929	0.916	0.970
6	1400–1500	1400–2000	0.929	0.919	0.971
7	2000–2100	1400–2100	0.924	0.925	0.972
8	2100–2200	1400–2200	0.926	0.924	0.972
9	1300–1400	1300–2200	0.927	0.924	0.973
10	2200–2300	1300–2300	0.929	0.925	0.973
11	1200–1300	1200–2300	0.923	0.931	0.973
12	2300–2400	1200–2400	0.934	0.920	0.973
13	2400–2500	1200–2500	0.925	0.931	0.973
14	1100–1200	1100–2500	0.933	0.923	0.974
15	2500–2600	1100–2600	0.936	0.918	0.974
16	1000–1100	1000–2600	0.931	0.925	0.974
17	2600–2700	1000–2700	0.925	0.927	0.974
18	2700–2800	1000–2800	0.924	0.931	0.974
19	2800–2900	1000–2900	0.923	0.933	0.974
20	900–1000	900–2900	0.930	0.926	0.974
21	2900–3000	900–3000	0.933	0.926	0.974
22	800–900	800–3000	0.932	0.928	0.974
23	700–800	700–3000	0.928	0.932	0.974
24	600–700	600–3000	0.930	0.930	0.974
25	500–600	500–3000	0.934	0.927	0.974
26	400–500	400–3000	0.937	0.926	0.976
27	300–400	300–3000	0.934	0.932	0.977
28	200–300	200–3000	0.935	0.932	0.978
29	100–200	100–3000	0.940	0.929	0.978
30	<100	<3000	0.935	0.931	0.978

4.3 Attributes Based-On and Derived-From Background Activity

In this section, the focus is on attributes described in Sects. 3.3, 3.4, and 3.5, i.e., on attributes basing directly or indirectly on the background activity of the recording. These attributes, in contrast to narrow band-based ones, are derived from neurophysi-

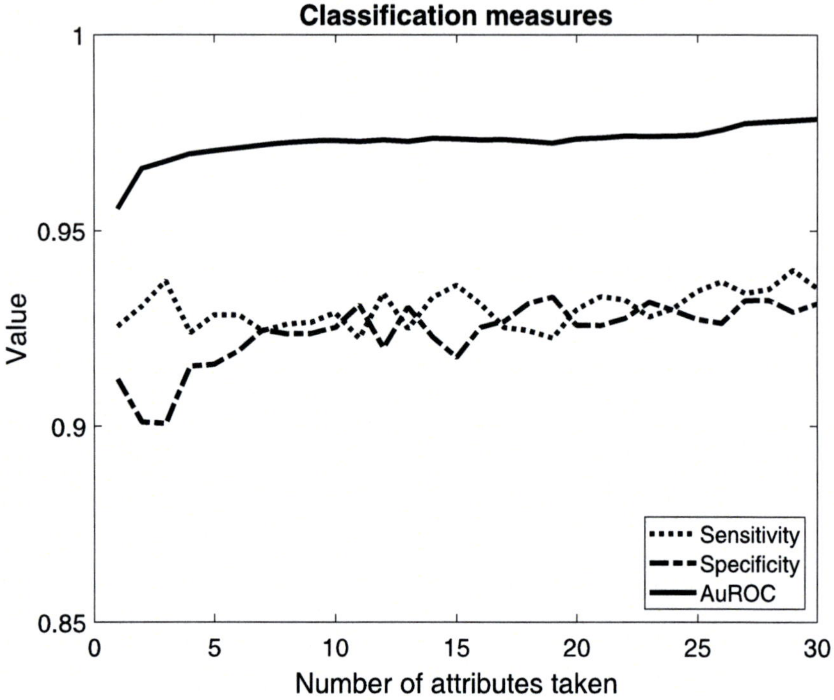

Fig. 12 Classification measures according to the number of attributes taken

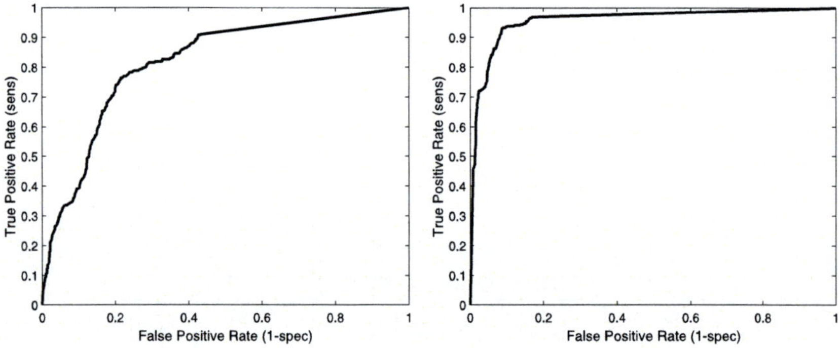

(a) 100 ~ 200 Hz (b) 1600 ~ 1700 Hz

Fig. 13 ROC plots for classification based on different bands

ological features of brain tissue in the STN [2, 8]. As it is shown below, these attributes achieve results where both sensitivity and specificity are above 0.95. Table 3 shows how the addition of subsequent attributes affects the classification results. All results shown in Tables 1, 2, and 3 were obtained using tenfold cross-validation procedure.

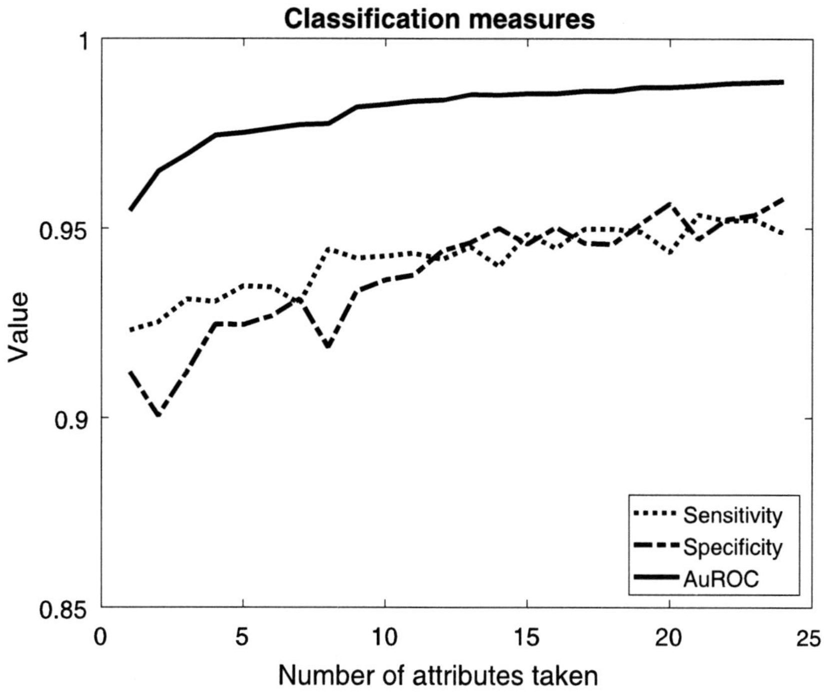

Fig. 14 Classification measures according to the number of attributes taken

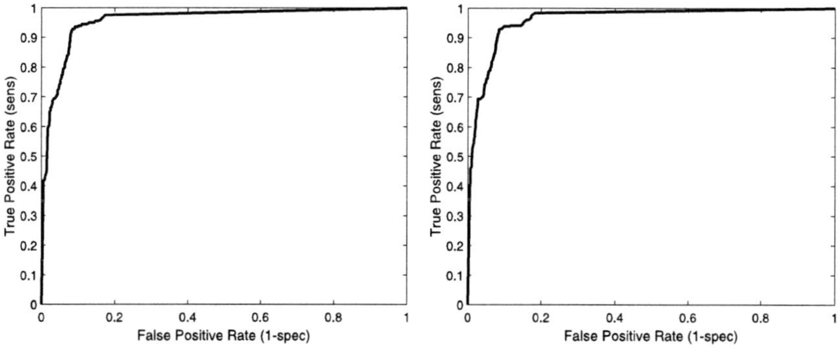

(a) 100 ~ 200 Hz (b) 1600 ~ 1700 Hz

Fig. 15 ROC plots for classification based on different bands

Table 3 Classification measures change with the addition of subsequent background-derived attributes. Sensitivity and specificity of at least 0.95 are highlighted using a gray background

Attributes	Attribute added	Sensitivity	Specificity	AuROC
1	$prc80$	0.923	0.912	0.955
2	rms	0.925	0.900	0.965
3	hfb	0.931	0.912	0.969
4	$prc80_M$	0.931	0.925	0.974
5	rms_M	0.935	0.925	0.975
6	hfb_M	0.934	0.927	0.976
7	lfb	0.930	0.931	0.977
8	lfb_M	0.944	0.919	0.978
9	hfb_{2U}	0.942	0.933	0.982
10	$prc80_{2U}$	0.943	0.936	0.983
11	hfb_{1U}	0.943	0.938	0.983
12	rms_{2U}	0.942	0.944	0.984
13	$prc80_{1U}$	0.945	0.946	0.985
14	rms_{1U}	0.940	0.950	0.985
15	lfb_{2U}	0.949	0.946	0.986
16	lfb_{1U}	0.945	0.950	0.986
17	lfb_{1D}	0.950	0.946	0.986
18	hfb_{1D}	0.950	0.946	0.986
19	lfb_{2D}	0.949	0.951	0.987
20	rms_{1D}	0.944	0.957	0.987
21	$prc80_{1D}$	0.954	0.947	0.988
22	hfb_{2D}	0.952	0.952	0.988
23	rms_{2D}	0.952	0.954	0.989
24	$prc80_{2D}$	0.949	0.958	0.989

It is also interesting that when ranking is made using all background-derived attributes together with narrow frequency band-base attributes, the sensitivity and specificity do not reach the value 0.95.

5 Conclusions

In this chapter, it has been shown that there are at least two valid approaches to discrimination of recordings made within the STN. Using just a simple band-pass filtering-based approach, one can obtain good classification results.

Regardless of the chosen method, the recorded signal must be first filtered from artifacts. Artifacts—very common in neurosurgical microrecordings—if not removed, cause the value of the narrow frequency band-based and background activity-based attributes to be distorted to the point of being unusable.

The first approach, based upon the analysis of signal's power in narrow frequency bands, is computationally repetitively straightforward, and the signal is cleaned out of artifacts, band-pass filters are applied, and normalized power of such filtered signal is calculated to obtain attributes. These attributes can later be used for the construction of the AdaBoost classifier. Such a classifier achieves sensitivity and specificity above 0.9. It has been shown that STN distinct activity is most evident in frequencies around 1600 Hz 1700 Hz band.

The second approach is based upon handpicked and defined neurobiologically-based features. The calculation of these features requires complex calculations. For example, it requires the detection and removal of neuronal spikes before the calculation of some of the attributes. The more complex calculation of the attributes proves, however, to be worth the effort. The sensitivity and specificity are, in this case, both above 0.95.

This is a very good performing classification, especially knowing that surgical protocols are filled basing upon subjective decisions of a neurosurgeon. Additionally, in case of recordings made on the verge of the STN, the decision is difficult and the great majority of misclassifications occur in these borderline areas.

Acknowledgements I would like to express my gratitude to T. Mandat, MD, PhD of Maria Sklodowska–Curie Memorial Oncology Center in Warsaw, for providing invaluable medical expertise.

References

1. Parent A, Hazrati L-N.: Functional anatomy of the basal ganglia. II. The place of subthalamic nucleus and external pallidium in basal ganglia circuitry. Brain Res Rev. **20**, 128–154 (1995). Elsevier
2. Israel, Z., Burchiel, K.J.: Microelectrode recording in movement disorder surgery. Thieme (2011)
3. Shamir, R.R., Zaidel, A., Joskowicz, L., Bergman, H., Israel, Z.: Microelectrode recording duration and spatial density constraints for automatic targeting of the subthalamic nucleus. Stereotact. Funct. Neurosurg. **90**, 325–334 (2012). Karger Publishers
4. Moran, A., Bar-Gad, I., Bergman, H., Israel, Z.: Real-time refinement of subthalamic nucleus targeting using Bayesian decision-making on the root mean square measure. Mov. Disord. (2006). https://doi.org/10.1002/mds.20995
5. Winestone, J.S., Zaidel, A., Bergman, H., Israel, Z.: The use of macroelectrodes in recording cellular spiking activity. J. Neurosci. Methods. **206**, 34–39 (2012). Elsevier
6. Zaidel, A., Spivak, A., Shpigelman, L., Bergman, H., Israel, Z.: Delimiting subterritories of the human subthalamic nucleus by means of microelectrode recordings and a Hidden Markov Model. Mov Disord. **24**, 1785–1793 (2009). Wiley Online Library
7. Pizzolato, G., Mandat, T.: Deep brain stimulation for movement disorders. Front. Integr. Neurosci. 6, 2 (2012). Frontiers

8. Nieuwenhuys, R., Voogd, J., Van Huijzen, C.: The Human Central Nervous System: A Synopsis and Atlas. Springer Science & Business Media (2007)
9. Hutchison, W.D., Allan, R.J., Opitz, H., Levy, R., Dostrovsky, J.O., Lang, A.E., et al.: Neurophysiological identification of the subthalamic nucleus in surgery for Parkinson's disease. Ann Neurol. **44**, 622–628 (1998). Wiley Online Library
10. Massey, L.A., Miranda, M.A., Zrinzo, L., Al-Helli, O., Parkes, H.G., Thornton, J.S., et al.: High resolution MR anatomy of the subthalamic nucleus: imaging at 9.4 T with histological validation. Neuroimage. 59, 2035–2044 (2012). Elsevier
11. Starr, P.A.: Placement of deep brain stimulators into the subthalamic nucleus or globus pallidus internus: technical approach. Stereotact. Funct. Neurosurg. **79**, 118–145 (2002). Karger Publishers
12. Benazzouz, A., Breit, S., Koudsie, A., Pollak, P., Krack, P., Benabid, A.-L.:Intraoperative microrecordings of the subthalamic nucleus in Parkinson's disease. Mov. Disord. 17 (2002). Wiley Online Library
13. Schmahmann, J., Pandya, D.: Fiber pathways of the brain. OUP USA (2009)
14. Temel, Y., Blokland, A., Steinbusch, H.W.M., Visser-Vandewalle, V.: The functional role of the subthalamic nucleus in cognitive and limbic circuits. Prog. Neurobiol. **76**, 393–413 (2005). Elsevier
15. Mallet, L., Schüpbach, M., N'Diaye, K., Remy, P., Bardinet, E., Czernecki, V. et al.: Stimulation of subterritories of the subthalamic nucleus reveals its role in the integration of the emotional and motor aspects of behavior. Proc Natl Acad Sci. Nat. Acad. Sci. 104, 10661–10666 (2007)
16. Mandat, T.S., Hurwitz, T., Honey, C.R.: Hypomania as an adverse effect of subthalamic nucleus stimulation: report of two cases. Acta Neurochir (Wien). 148, 895–898 (2006). Springer
17. Anderson, P.B., Rogers, M.H.: Deep Brain Stimulation: Applications, Complications and Side Effects. Nova Biomedical Books (2009)
18. Priori, A., Egidi, M., Pesenti, A., Rohr, M.: Do intraoperative microrecordings improve subthalamic nucleus targeting in stereotactic neurosurgery for Parkinson's disease? J. Neurosurg. Sci. 47, 56 (2003). Edizioni Minerva Medica
19. Schaltenbrand, G.: Atlas for stereotaxy of the human brain. Georg Thieme (1977). Stuttgart
20. Hendelman, W.: Atlas of Functional Neuroanatomy. CRC Press (2015)
21. Levy, R., Hutchison, W.D., Lozano, A.M., Dostrovsky, J.O.: High-frequency synchronization of neuronal activity in the subthalamic nucleus of parkinsonian patients with limb tremor. J Neurosci. Soc Neurosci. **20**, 7766–7775 (2000)
22. Ciecierski, K., Mandat, T., Rafał, R., Raś, Z.W., Przybyszewski, A.W.: Konrad Ciecierski, Tomasz Mandat, Rafał Rola, Zbigniew W. Raś AWP. Computer aided subthalamic nucleus (STN) localization during deep brain stimulation (DBS) surgery in Parkinson's patients. Annales Academiae Medicae Silesiensis, pp. 275–283 (2014)
23. Mandat. T., Tykocki, T., Koziara, H., Koziorowski, D., Brodacki, B., Rafał, R., Bonicki, W., et al.: Subthalamic deep brain stimulation for the treatment of Parkinson disease. Neurol. Neurochir. Pol. 45, 32–36 (2011). Elsevier
24. Novak, P., Daniluk, S., Ellias, S.A., Nazzaro, J.M.: Detection of the subthalamic nucleus in microelectrographic recordings in Parkinson disease using the high-frequency (> 500 Hz) neuronal background. J Neurosurg. 106, 175–179. American Association of Neurological Surgeons (2007)
25. Kano, T., Katayama, Y., Kobayashi, K., Kasai, M., Oshima, H., Fukaya, C. et al.: Detection of boundaries of subthalamic nucleus by multiple-cell spike density analysis in deep brain stimulation for Parkinson's disease. Adv. Funct. Repar. Neurosurg, 33–35 (2006). Neurosurgery
26. Saleh, S., Swanson, K., Lake, W.: Functional KS-S and, 2015 undefined. Awake neurophysiologically guided versus asleep MRI-guided STN DBS for Parkinson disease: a comparison of outcomes using levodopa equivalents. karger.com. https://www.karger.com/Article/Abstract/442425
27. Ho, A., Ali, R., Connolly, I.: JH-JNN, 2018 U. Awake versus asleep deep brain stimulation for Parkinson's disease: a critical comparison and meta-analysis. jnnp.bmj.com. http://jnnp.bmj.com/content/early/2018/01/31/jnnp-2016-314500.abstract

28. Freeman, E.A., Moisen, G.G.: A comparison of the performance of threshold criteria for binary classification in terms of predicted prevalence and kappa. Ecol. Modell. **217**, 48–58 (2008). Elsevier
29. Ijcai, R.K-.: 1995 undefined. A study of cross-validation and bootstrap for accuracy estimation and model selection. pdfs.semanticscholar.org. https://pdfs.semanticscholar.org/0be0/d781305750b37acb35fa187febd8db67bfcc.pdf
30. Koch, C.: Biophysics of Computation: Information Processing in Single Neurons. Oxford University Press (2004)
31. Pettersen, K.H., Einevoll, G.T.: Amplitude variability and extracellular low-pass filtering of neuronal spikes. Biophys J. **94**, 784–802 (2008). Elsevier. https://doi.org/10.1529/biophysj.107.111179
32. Ciecierski, K., Raś, Z.W.: Przybyszewski AW. Spike sorting based upon PCA over DWT frequency band selection
33. Quiroga, R.Q., Nadasdy, Z., Ben-Shaul, Y.: Unsupervised spike detection and sorting with wavelets and superparamagnetic clustering. Neural Comput. **16**, 1661–1687 (2004). MIT Press. https://doi.org/10.1162/089976604774201631
34. Donoho, D.L.: De-noising by soft-thresholding. IEEE Trans. Inf. Theor. IEEE **41**, 613–627 (1995). https://doi.org/10.1109/18.382009
35. Jensen, A., la Cour-Harbo, A.: Ripples in Mathematics: the Discrete Wavelet Transform. Springer Science & Business Media (2001)
36. Lior, R.: Data Mining with Decision Trees: Theory and Applications. World scientific (2014)
37. Sun, Y., Kamel, M.S., Wong, A.K.C., Wang, Y.: Cost-sensitive boosting for classification of imbalanced data. Pattern Recognit. **40**, 3358–3378 (2007). https://doi.org/10.1016/J.PATCOG.2007.04.009. Pergamon

Stutter Detection and Remediation in Speech

Ayman Hajja and Pierre Arbajian

1 Introduction and Background

The quality of life is negatively impacted when individuals are chronically unable to express themselves due to a lack of speech fluency. Stuttering, also referred to as stammering, is a condition that is exhibited in bad fluency of speech. The onset of stuttering generally occurs during childhood years, and in one-fourth of cases, this speech impediment persists throughout life [1, 2].

Automatic speech disfluency detection offers many advantages, ranging from time-saving, constant speech monitoring to reducing the subjectivity of manual disfluency identification [3, 4]. Manually identifying "episodes" of stutter is a tedious and time-consuming task; introducing a machine-learning approach that automatically detects, ranks, and isolates episodes of stutter provides great and immediate benefits to both the research and speech therapy communities [3–5]. The reliable identification of segments that contain stutters, such as pauses, blocks, interjections, and hesitations, is a natural first step to further address the speech disfluency problem; this will allow speech cleanup by removing blocks and interjections, smoothing the hesitation segments, and shortening the prolongations [6–8].

The state of the art is rich with papers which describe various prosodic- and semantic-based machine learning approaches and algorithms for the detection of disfluent speech [2, 9–12]. Building a system capable of detecting stutter in speech, however, exhibits some characteristics that make the task rather challenging. One of these properties is with regards to the auditory nature of the data we are concerned

A. Hajja (✉)
College of Charleston, 66 George Street, Charleston, SC 29424, USA
e-mail: hajjaa@cofc.edu

P. Arbajian
UNC Charlotte, 9201 University City Blvd, Charlotte, NC 28223, USA
e-mail: pierrenclt@yahoo.com

Z. W. Ras et al. (eds.), *Recommender Systems for Medicine and Music*,
Studies in Computational Intelligence 946,
https://doi.org/10.1007/978-3-030-66450-3_4

with, which makes it difficult to collect and construct labeled datasets efficiently; this problem will be addressed in Sect. 4, where we present an open-source system developed by the authors of this chapter that will aid in the process of generating such (labeled) dataset. The second problem is concerning the subjectivity in what is defined or perceived as "stutter"; stutter exists in many forms and in varying degrees. Even for the human ear, an audio segment of a soft-spoken person can be confused with stutter, which makes the task even more challenging for a machine learning classier. Our approach has taken these challenges into consideration, and we placed a substantial amount of emphasis and effort on making sure that we incorporate this key-point into our methodology, which involved providing our classifier segments of non-stutter low-volume utterances to prevent our system from resulting in excessive False Positives by over-classifying audio segments as stutter.

The material presented in this chapter is primarily the result of the doctoral dissertation of the second author, Pierre Arbajian [13, 14]. In this chapter, we will be exclusively addressing the problem of classifying audio segments that contain stutter. This is a binary classification problem involving the two following classes: "stutter" and "no stutter"; therefore, "stutter" will be considered as the "positive" class, and "no stutter" will be considered as the negative class. In other words,

- "True Positive (TP)" occurs when the classifier classifies a "stutter" (positive) audio segment **correctly** as "stutter" (positive),
- "False Positive (FP)" occurs when the classifier classifies a "non-stutter" (negative) **incorrectly** as "stutter" (positive),
- "True Negative (TN)" occurs when the classifier classifies a "non-stutter" (negative) **correctly** as "non-stutter" (negative), and
- "False Negative (FN)" occurs when the classifier classifies a "stutter" (positive) **incorrectly** as "non-stutter" (negative).

Going back to the abovementioned nature of the stutter data, it is safe to assume that the False Positive numbers will tend to be high when classifying such data; since again, many low-volume non-stutter data-points will be classified as "stutter".

> One can always adjust the sensitivity of the model to reduce the number of False Positives, but that will have a negative effect on the True Positives (i.e. reduction in the True Positives, and therefore lower accuracy); such false classification will introduce an undesired trade-off situation. If the sensitivity or recall of the model is high (i.e. leaning toward classifying low-volume segments as "stutter"), then our model will result in high numbers of both True Positives and False Positives; a model with low-sensitivity to stutter, on the other hand, will result in low numbers of both True Positives and False Negatives. In both cases, the accuracy is compromised.

It is worth noting here that this problem is not confined to stutter detection; however, the problem is usually amplified when most of the positives (or "stutter") data-points can easily be confused with a specific type of negative (or "non-stutter") data-points, as it is the case with stutter detection. Also, one should keep in mind that this attribute is not always true the other way around, and certainly not in our case; most non-stutter data-points are not easily confused with stutter. Again, this attribute can be observed in many datasets and it is not unique to stutter. Think of wolves and dogs, for example; most wolves can be confused with a dog breed, since some dog breeds (such as the Husky) resemble wolves, but most dogs are not confused with wolves, since most dogs do not look like wolves.

The dataset of speeches that we used was obtained from the UCLASS series of recordings [1]. UCLASS, which stands for the University College London Archive of Stuttered Speech, is a database of stuttered speech recordings with individual speech and speaker metadata. UCLASS contains a collection of over one hundred speeches from which we chose fifteen for our research study.

The approach that we adopted was to begin by scanning each speech for potentially stuttered segments according to varying intensity thresholds and lengths of audio segments; by doing so, we are identifying segments that we will refer to in this chapter as "potentially undesired". These "potentially undesired" segments that are extracted using primitive features (which will be discussed later) are considered candidates for removal because of the selection criteria used; however, and as the word "candidate" implies, in numerous cases, these candidate segments contain semantic speech and therefore should not be omitted from the original speech. Determining which candidate segments are truly undesired candidates and which segments are not is done through a second-phase classification system that will be discussed later; this machine learning system is able to distinguish "true undesired" (or "stutter") from "false undesired" (or "non-stutter").

The features that are used for training this second-phase classifier include data extracted from both the frequency domain (voice formants and pitch), and from the time domain (intensity). In addition to that, a combination of speaker and speech metadata is also used to improve the trained classifier; a more elaborate description of the feature list used will be presented in the next section.

The difference between the quality of the best possible remediation (or "gold standard") of a given speech compared to the quality of the machine learning classifier enhanced speech after having every "potentially undesired" segment being classified is used to evaluate the quality of our system. The results with respect to the classifier performance are tabulated in the findings section according to the extraction parameters. We will also provide a brief discussion on the process efficiency improvements utilized to minimize manual labeling effort as well as segment deletion redundancy.

2 Stutter Detection System

The method presented in this chapter, which was adopted from Dr. Arbajian's dissertation work, consisted of selecting a set of speeches to be examined from a group of disfluent speeches available from UCLASS. UCLASS speeches exhibit a wide variety of speakers and stuttering conditions, yet the vast majority of the speeches are distinctly stuttered and quite disfluent. Fifteen speeches (roughly one hour of stuttered speech) were selected as the foundation for this research.

Our goal in this chapter is to present a system capable of automatically identifying stuttered speeches for the purpose of detecting undesired segments, then later enhance the overall speech quality through the elimination of the segments that are classified as "disfluent". In this work, we developed a script for initially identifying the potential candidate segment to be removed from the stuttered speech; the initial goal of the work presented here was to build a system capable of distinguishing the "true undesired" from the "false undesired" for all candidate segments. In the following section, we provide an elaborate description of the workings of this initial step design.

2.1 Identifying Potentially-Undesired Audio Segments

Fifteen speeches from the UCLASS repository were selected as the stuttered speeches of interest, where each speech is scanned with a total of 8 extraction parameters. The extraction parameters determine what the sound intensity threshold and the minimum duration theshold of those segments should be. The minimum durations that we used to iterate through our speeches are 0.6, 0.8, 1.0, and 1.2 s, and the speech intensity thresholds are at 95 and 90% of the entire speech intensity in decibels; for example, if the average intensity of a given speech is 50 decibels, then the intensity thresholds that correspond to 95% and 90% are 47.5 db and 45 db, respectively.

For each possible pair combination of segment duration and intensity threshold (total of 8 unique combinations), the entire speech is scanned and the "potentially undesired" candidates are detected according to the corresponding threshold pair combination. The minimum segment duration ensures that no excessively-short segments are extracted as potential candidates for deletion, which would disrupt the flow of normal speech and unfavorably affect the speech cadence. Note that the extracted segments from each unique pair will not overlap, and that only such overlapping is possible (and rather likely to happen) when examining segments extracted from different pairs. In other words, a particular intensity-duration combination (say the intensity of 90% and minimum duration of 1.2 s) will only extract non-overlapping segments.

We provide a demonstration of how the segments may look like in Fig. 1. For example, according to Fig. 1, extracting potentially undesired segments from the fourth row (0.6 s minimum duration with 95% intensity threshold) will result in three different segments (B, G, and K); since segment B's length is 0.8 s, which satisfies the minimum duration threshold for the third row, then the same segment will also be identified as a "potentially undesired" segment on the third row; however, since the length of the segment is not 1.0 s (or more), that segment will not be identified in the second (or first) row in Fig. 1.

Each extracted candidate segment results in a waveform audio file accompanied by five additional vectors that serve as the segment inherent features, three out of which

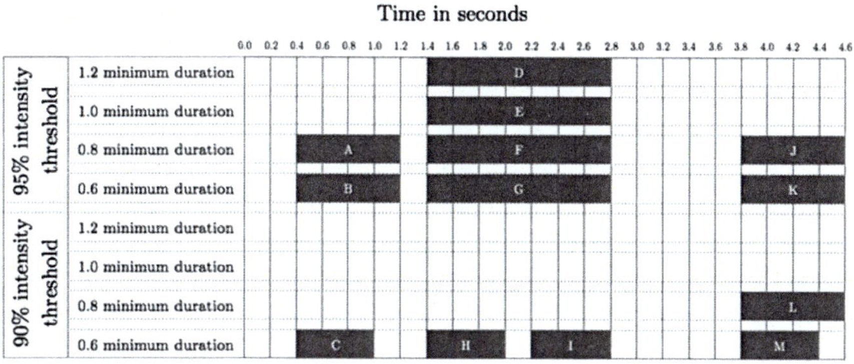

Fig. 1 Extracting potentially undesired candidate segments

contain the values of formant 1, formant 2, and formant 3, and the remaining two vectors contain the pitch and the intensity values. All formants were computed with a 50 ms Gaussian analysis window with a 12.5 ms offset. The pitch values were taken at 10 ms interval and computed (using "Praat" [15]), which performs an acoustic periodicity detection on the basis of an accurate autocorrelation method as described in [16]. The intensity values were computed by squaring and then convolving the sound values within a Gaussian analysis window of 50 ms length. The waveform audio files will be later used for manually labeling the candidate segment, and the set of inherent features (in addition to a set of derived features, which will be presented in Subsection 2.3) will be used to build our classifier.

2.2 Labeling Potentially Undesired Segments

In the previous subsection, we illustrated how, by using the intensity and minimum duration, we were able to identify potentially-undesired segments. These segments represent the majority of undesired segments; however, a substantial portion of these segments was "desired" (i.e. "non-stutter"). For all of the segments that were identified as potentially-undesired, a manual labeling phase takes place in which we assign each audio segment one of the following audio labels:

1. delete and analyze (denoted by the letter "G", for Good),
2. leave in the speech and analyze (denoted by the letter "B", for Bad), and
3. no analysis, but delete from the speech; these segments of speech represent external sounds such as when the interviewer was attempting to speak softly.

In an attempt to avoid redundant labeling efforts and minimize the number of segments which must be manually reviewed, we have sorted the list of segments to be reviewed such that if a segment "s" is marked for deletion, then all other segments that are contained within "s" (start with, or after, "s"; and end when "s" ends, or anytime before that) will also be deleted. The reasoning behind our approach is that if some segment "s" is void of semantic meaning, then any other segment contained in "s" must also be void of semantic meaning. Note here that it is not the case that the opposite is true; given that some segment "s" contains some semantic meaning, we cannot conclude that all other segments contained in "s" must also contain semantic meaning. This approach has allowed us to reduce review time by a factor of five.

We will use Fig. 1 to demonstrate the process explained above. The first step is to sort all "potentially undesired" segments according to their start time, from top to bottom. This means that based on Fig. 1, the list of candidate segments will be sorted as follows: A, B, C, D, E, F, G, H, I, J, K, L, and M. The first candidate segment that will be listened to is "A"; if the segment "A" is marked as "true undesired" (no semantic value), then all other subsets that are contained in "A" are also marked "true undesired", which are "B" and "C". Similarly, if segment "D" is labeled as "true undesired", then segments "E", "F", "G", "H", and "I" are also labeled "true undesired". If however, segment "D" was marked as "false undesired" (contains semantic value), then this only implies that segments "E", "F", and "G" are also "false undesired" (since they are essentially the same as segment "D"), but we cannot conclude that segment "H" nor "I" is also "false undesired"; therefore, we would need to listen to the two segments "H" and "I" to determine what the label of each of them should be.

The dataset used in our classification exhibited two possible class values: "G" (or "no stutter"), which meant that the candidate sound must be deleted; and "B" ("stutter"), which meant that the sound segment should not be deleted.

2.3 Constructing the Classifiers

In addition to the label feature, the dataset used to train our classifiers will contain two additional types of features: 1) a set of derived attributes extrapolated from the set inherent features, and 2) speaker and speech metadata [17]. The inherent features that are associated with each candidate segment are formant 1, formant 2, and formant 3 (sampled at 50 ms intervals with the time step being 12.5 ms), pitch (sampled at 10 ms), and intensity (sampled at 8 ms). The derived features that are used in our classifier training are all extrapolated from the inherent features and will serve as a set of data-points that provide information about the entire segment as opposed to an exact point in time (due to sampling).

We start by calculating the derivatives of each one of the five inherent features; the reason for calculating the derivatives is to assess the variance of our inherent features, which is vital for detecting stutter. Then, for each one of the inherent features and their derivatives, we calculate the average, median, standard deviation, percentiles (25, 50, and 75), minimum value, maximum value, peak-to-peak amplitude measurement, and variance. The speaker and speech metadata we included in our dataset consisted of those data features provided with the UCLASS dataset; Table 1 shows these metadata features, along with their possible values.

Table 1 Metadata features and their possible values

Feature	Possible values
Speaker gender	Male or female
Speaker handedness	Left, right, or unknown
Speaker past history of stuttering in the family	Yes or no
Speaker age of stuttering onset	Numeric value
Speaker age at the time of recording	Numeric value
Location of recording	Clinic, UCL, or home
Recording conditions	Quiet room or sound-treated room
Type of therapy received	Family-based or holistic treatment
Time between therapy and recording time	Duration in days
Speaker hearing problems	Yes or no
Speaker history of language problems	Yes or no
Speaker special educational needs	Yes or no
Recording background acoustic noise level	Numeric value
Recording environmental noise level	Numeric value
Recording clarity	Numeric value
Recording interlocutor intrusiveness	Numeric value

The resulting dataset containing signal statistics, metadata, and labels consisted of 126 features and was used to train eight different classifiers, each for a unique pair combination of minimum duration and intensity threshold (see Algorithm 1). Recall that the minimum duration threshold is the minimum length of "potentially undesired" segments, and that the intensity (percentage) threshold is measured by examining the averaged speech intensity. We used the "R-Caret" package in order to streamline the classifier testing process and cover a wide range of classifiers.

Algorithm 1: Summary of our proposed algorithm

for *every segment duration and intensity threshold pair* **do**
  Extract potentially undesired candidate segments from a given speech;
  Manually label each candidate as *true undesired* or *false undesired*;
end
training and testing phase;
for *every segment duration and intensity threshold pair* **do**
  Train a classifier using a portion of the labeled candidate segments;
  Test the remaining segments using the classifier built above;
  Evaluate the resulting labels by comparing them to the "gold standard";
end

There are three different courses of action for segment removal that are examined in this research work, each producing a different level of stutter remediation:

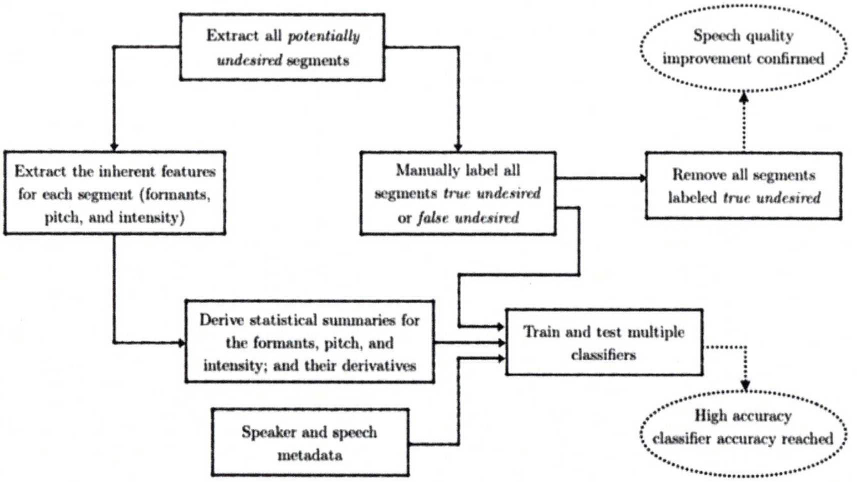

Fig. 2 Depiction of our proposed method

1. Remove all candidate segments without human intervention (this approach does not require manual labeling).
2. Remove only the candidate segments that are manually labeled "true undesired" (resulting speech is referred to by the "gold standard").
3. Classify all candidate segments using our trained classifier, and only remove the candidates that are classified "true undesired".

Each segment removal course of action yields a certain "enhanced" speech file; the enhanced files are then examined and compared. Our goal is to build a classifier that generates an audio file (course of action number 3) that is as close as possible to the golden standard audio file (generated from the course of action number 2).

In the case of speech remediation, it is more important to avoid deleting semantically meaningful segments than to miss deleting semantically meaningless segments. In other terms, when evaluating our classifier performance, false negatives (deleting what should not be deleted) should be considered more undesirable than false positives (missing to delete segments which must be deleted). The "R" classifiers that we trained and tested are C5.0, Neural Networks, Recursive Partitioning, Random Forests, Polynomial SVM, and AdaBoost.

In Fig. 2 below, we show the process flow starting at the top left: "Extraction" of the candidate segments followed by two independent paths (1) Feature extraction, and (2) Labeling. The results of the two flows provide the digital signal processing predictors and manual label results which will be combined with the metadata to create the complete dataset.

3 Experiments and Results

Our approach proved to be effective in eliminating the vast majority of voice blocks when applied to stuttered speech. The results of disfluent speech remediation consisted of the elimination of anomalous speech and a reduction in speech length between 60% for the most severe stuttered speech to about 25% for mildly stuttered speeches.

The effectiveness of our remediation process was highly dependent on the threshold of the speech intensity tolerance during the potentially undesired segment identification. As we have stated earlier, we used two different thresholds for the sound intensity for the initial phase—not to be confused with the voting threshold. On the one hand, the lower threshold (90% of average) resulted in considerably less undesired candidates as shown in Table 2; although most of the undesired candidates extracted using the lower threshold were actually true undesired, there were many instances where stutter segments were not detected (due to the low threshold). On the other hand, the higher threshold (95%) resulted in a much higher number of potentially undesired segments, some of which were false undesired; however, most of the stuttered segments were detected in the first phase. Therefore, the value of the second phase (training and testing phase), which identifies true undesired and false undesired from potentially undesired segments, is most useful when the threshold is high, and when most of the actual stutter segments are detected, even if that means potentially marking some segments as potentially undesired while in reality they are false undesired, during the first phase.

We have subsequently added a component to this system of remediation which helped us to enhance the usability of the system. Because a good remediation process should lose little to no semantic meaning, we implemented a "False Positives" restricting subsystem which relies on a voting cutoff approach. This enhancement would only tag a segment for removal if the vote for removal is nearly unanimous among all qualifiers. Although our accuracy was negatively affected by this component, the results of this experimentation proved to be effective in reducing "False Positives".

The second threshold value that we used during the extraction of the potentially undesired sound segments was the minimum time duration, starting with 0.6 s and ending with 1.2 s. It is worth noting that we tried shorter duration time frames with

Table 2 Segment count of the eight different minimum duration and intensity threshold pairs

	90% of speech avg sound volume threshold	95% of speech avg sound volume threshold
0.6 s	195	211
0.8 s	149	159
1.0 s	114	130
1.2 s	83	93

Table 3 Results obtained from building a single classifier using all of segments

	True positive rate (%)	True negative rate (%)	Accuracy (%)
C5.0	100	94	97.4
Neural networks	75.6	55.9	67.7
Recursive partitioning	92.6	94.2	93.2
Random forests	98.4	91.7	95.8
Polynomial SVM	89.9	75.6	84.4
AdaBoost	98.3	93.8	96.4

little success, but this caused the comprehensibility of the speech to be diminished; we found 0.6 s minimum silence duration to be the lowest value that can be used in our experiments.

We used two different approaches for treating our data with each classifier. The first approach is to build one classifier for our data after balancing the labels regardless of the minimum duration and intensity threshold values; in other words, we combine all the segments extracted from all eight different unique pairs of minimum duration and intensity threshold, and build our classifier accordingly. The balancing approach we chose to apply for the balancing of the data consisted of randomly excluding data tuples of the over-represented class G.

The second approach was to build a single classifier for each unique pair, then average the accuracy and confusion matrix results. Table 3 shows the results obtained using the first approach, while Table 4 shows the results obtained by using the second approach for the two classifiers that performed the best using separate classifiers for every unique pair: Random Forests and C5.0.

Using tenfold cross validation, we trained six different classifiers: C5.0, Neural Networks, Recursive Partitioning, Random Forests, Polynomial SVM, and AdaBoost. During the training of our classifiers, we used the "R-Caret" package because of its built-in tuning functionality. The parameters to build the respective models were chosen based on highest accuracy. We have listed the "R-Caret" package chosen parameters below.

Neural Network (NNet): Tuned model parameters when training on the balanced dataset: size = 5 and decay = 0.1. Tuned model parameters when training on the entire dataset: size = 1 and decay = 0.1. Size represents the number of units in the hidden layer and can be zero if there are skip-layer units. The decay parameter represents weight decay.

Random Forest (RF): Tuned model parameters when training on the balanced dataset: mtry = 2. Tuned model parameters when training on the entire dataset: mtry = 56. The parameter mtry represents the number of variables randomly sampled as candidates at each split.

SVM Polynomial (SVMPoly): Tuned model parameters when training on the balanced dataset: degree = 3, scale = 0.01, and C = 1. Tuned model parameters when training on the entire dataset: degree = 3, scale = 0.01, and C = 1. The degree

Table 4 Results obtained from using a single classifier for each pair of minimum duration and intensity threshold, and averaging the results

	Random forest	C5.0 Classifier
True positive rate (Averaged)	95.3 %	94.8%
True negative rate (Averaged)	82.3 %	76.6%
Classifier with highest true positive rate	1.2 minimum duration, 90% intensity threshold	0.8 minimum duration, 90% intensity threshold
Classifier with highest true negative rate	1.2 minimum duration, 90% intensity threshold	1.2 minimum duration, 90% intensity threshold
Classifier with lowest true positive rate	1.2 minimum duration, 95% intensity threshold	1.0 minimum duration, 95% intensity threshold
Classifier with lowest true negative rate	1.0 minimum duration, 95% intensity threshold	1.0 minimum duration, 95% intensity threshold

parameter represents the polynomial degree of the kernel function. The scale is the scaling parameter of the polynomial and tangent kernel. C is the cost regularization parameter.

Adaptive Boosting (AdaBag): Tuned model parameters when training on the balanced dataset: mfinal = 100 and maxdepth = 3. Tuned model parameters when training on the entire dataset: mfinal = 150 and maxdepth = 3. The mfinal parameters represent the number of iterations for which boosting is run or the number of trees to use. Maxdepth is the maximum depth of any node of the final tree.

Recursive Partitioning (RPart): Tuned model parameters when training on the balanced dataset: cp = 0.03797468. Tuned model parameters when training on the entire dataset: cp = 0.05970149. Cp is the complexity parameter; any split that does not decrease the overall lack of fit by a factor of cp is not attempted. The main role of this parameter is to save computing time by pruning off splits that are evidently not worthwhile.

As can be seen in Table 3, when we balance our data we reduce the number of samples in the dataset; this big reduction in the number of tuples seems to have a detrimental impact on our neural network classifier model, since neural network training is best accomplished with large datasets.

4 Crowdsourcing Stutter Labels Web-Platform

In Sect. 1, we stated that one of the reasons that makes stutter detection rather difficult is the lack of labeled datasets. This is primarily due to the auditory nature of our data; it is difficult to listen to a speech that contains stutter segments and accurately mark (and isolate) these segments that contain stutter. In this section, we will present a web-based platform developed by the authors of this chapter, which will allow individuals and research teams to crowdsource large sums of labeled audio segments efficiently and effectively [18]. We believe that this web-platform will be filling a growing need for an easy-to-use, open-source and freely-available tool that can be used by the machine learning research community; the source code for this project is hosted on GitHub (https://github.com/grifffin/Web-Platform-for-Labeling-Audio).

Voice-based analysis solutions can be grouped into two categories: lexical- and semantic-based analysis, and prosodic-based analysis. In the lexical analysis category, the speaker's voice is first transcribed into words and sentences, then text analysis is performed [19, 20] whereas in the prosodic variant, researchers are interested in exploiting the tonality of voice such as pitch, pauses, rhythms, relative emphases, and certain forms of stutter [21, 22]; for instance, when analyzing prosodic aspects of a voice recording, one could detect fear or anger, even if the semantic meaning is void of any indications for such emotional state.

The prosodic analysis of voice is a broad and rich field with interesting implementation possibilities [23, 24]; it encompasses important audio traits such as voice quality, which is fundamental to human communication not only for conveying meaning, but also for expressing feeling and disposition. One can easily argue that humans (and many animals for that matter) are particularly superior to machines at detecting emotional states of other beings; that said, with the help of large sums of labeled data, we believe that a well-trained machine learning model would be able to make some of these vocal-based distinctions, somewhat successfully.

We envision that the rich set of possibilities for the detection of soft speech content (fear, conviction, anger, etc.) would be of particular interest to our targeted audience; as a result, we expect that potential users of our system will consist of researchers and research teams who are particularly interested in the development of automatic intelligent speech emotion detection systems, many of whom we believe will be attracted from the social science fields such as psychology.

4.1 System Overview

In this section, we will describe the functionalities that this platform provides, along with screenshots for the most important user interfaces. Through the use of this developed system, study administrators are able to create customized crowdsourcing studies that enable them to collect data quickly and efficiently according to a set of user-defined rules, which will be further used by the algorithm to optimize the data-collection process. The developed web-platform will allow users to upload audio files from which the segments will be extracted, specify the duration of segments and the potential labels for each segment, and define other study-related features that will be covered in the following subsections. Once a study is created through the GUI of the system, other users can be invited (by study administrators) to partake in the data collecting process by labeling the audio segments; we will refer to users that label audio segments by the term "workers".

One of the main novelties of this platform stems from the fact that audio segments are dynamically (and in real time) assigned to workers based on the previous labels (for the same segment) provided by other workers. As will be demonstrated below, by dynamically assigning workers audio segments, the system optimizes the data-collection process in such a way that it minimizes human effort and maximizes the amount of usable labeled data-points; we say "usable" because some data-points will be discarded with accordance to the study rules set by the administrators. Finally, once a study is completed, administrators are able to download comma-separated values (CSV) files to be used for further analysis and model building. In addition to being able to download CSV files, administrators can also download folders containing the labeled audio segments (grouped by labels).

4.2 *Creating a Crowdsourcing Study*

In this subsection, we will provide a summary of all the pieces of information that a study administrator needs to provide to create a crowdsourcing study; we will also discuss the impact that each value has on the resulting study. Here is the list of information with their description:

Segment size: As mentioned in Sect. 1, one of the motives that led us to develop this system is to facilitate the process of labeling short segments of audio files. The segment duration (in seconds) needs to be provided by the study administrators when the study is created, and our system will automatically present workers with audio segments accordingly. The choice of this value will highly depend on the domain of the study. For example, if an administrator wants to label audio segments for stutter detection, then a reasonable segment size would be between 0.5 and 2 s [25]; if on the other hand, the goal of the study is to label audio segments for the purpose of emotions-in-speech detection, then a much bigger segment size would be needed [26].

Stride size: The stride size can be defined as the distance between (the beginning of) any two consecutive segments, and will consequently determine whether there will be an overlap in the segments or not, and what the exact ratio of the overlap is. In addition to having a direct impact on the overlap ratio, the stride size (in conjunction with the audio file(s) duration) will also determine the number of candidate segments generated for labeling. Next, we will provide an example of a hypothetical study to demonstrate the effects of the stride size.

Let us assume that we have a single 18-second audio file; let us also assume that the user-defined stride size in our study is 2 s, which means that the beginning of each segment that will be presented to workers will be a multiple of 2 (0, 2, 4, ..., 16). Now, if the duration of each segment that needs to be labeled happens to be also 2 s (equal to the stride size), then the generated segments will exhibit no overlap between them. Figure 3 shows the segments that the workers will be prompted to label.

If, for example, the segment duration is greater than the stride size (say segment size is equal to 3, and stride size is equal to 2), then the resulting segments will contain an overlap in the segments that the workers will be prompted to label. Figure 4 shows the segments that the workers will be prompted to label.

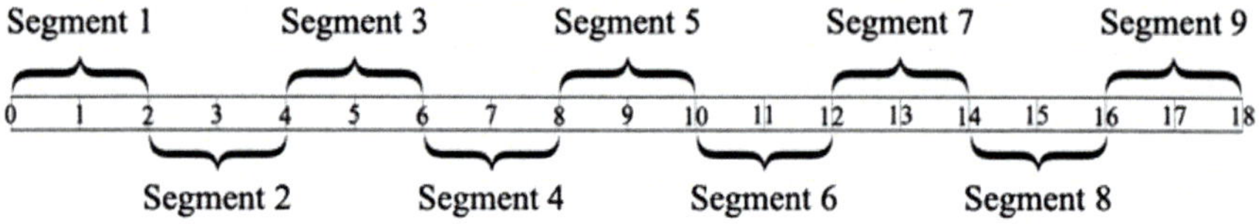

Fig. 3 Resulting segments when segment size and stride size are both 2 s

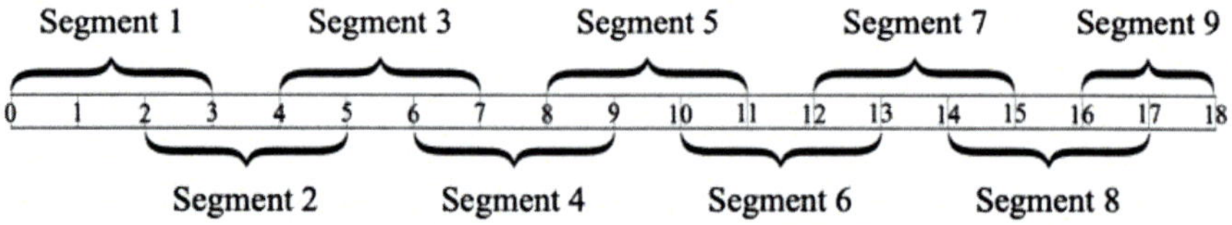

Fig. 4 Resulting segments when segment size is 3 s and stride size is 2 s

As can be shown in Fig. 4, we notice here that there is a 1/3 overlap between each of two consecutive segments. This can be useful, and rather necessary, when the start and end times of a label need to be precise, such as in the case of stutter detection. The ratio of overlap p can be defined as

$$max\left(0, 1 - \frac{\text{stride size}}{\text{segment size}}\right)$$

.

An upper bound (0) needed to be introduced to prevent our ratio of overlap from resulting in a negative value when the stride size is greater than the segment size.

The number of unique segments n can be defined as

$$\sum_{i=1}^{m} \left\lfloor \frac{\text{duration of file i}}{\text{stride size}} \right\rfloor$$

where m is the number of files associated with the given study.

Labels: There is no limit on the number of different labels that workers can be prompted with for a given study; our system allows study administrators to define as many labels as their study requires. In one of the stutter-related studies that we conducted, we prompted users to classify the type of stutter; in that study, we had four different labels: "Blocking", "Prolongation", "Repetition", and "Interjection".

Maximum number of overall responses: Study administrators can set a limit on the total number of responses gathered from workers; this value can be useful to define when a study would end, or to limit expenses in the event where workers are compensated. When this value is not specified, there will be no limit on the number of responses, and the study will remain open indefinitely.

Maximum (and minimum) number of responses for a segment: These two values are crucial to the success of any study, and they play a major role (jointly with the stop threshold value, which will be explained next) in the optimization and adaptable data-collection process executed by the platform. Our system will determine the exact number of responses (within the minimum and maximum range) that will satisfy the stop threshold value for every unique segment, as will be explained next.

Stop threshold for a single segment: The stop threshold can be defined as the minimum percentage of agreeability that study administrators require for any segment to be marked useful (or credible) for further analysis. As soon as a particular segment becomes *credible*, and as long as the number of responses for that segment is within the minimum and maximum range, then our system will not present this segment for additional labeling.

Let us demonstrate how the stop threshold, the minimum and maximum responses, and the number of labels affect the labeling process when they are used altogether in a single study. Let us assume that the number of unique labels for a given study is 4, the minimum and maximum number of responses for a single segment is 3 and 10, respectively, and that the stop threshold value is 70%.

Since any segment needs to be labeled by at least 3 (minimum responses) unique workers to become *credible*, our system will start by prompting 3 unique workers to label some random segment s, which will result in three different potential responses:

1. The three workers will agree on one label (label with the highest percentage is 100%)
2. Only two workers will agree on one label (label with the highest percentage is 66.67%)
3. Each worker will choose a different label (label with the highest percentage is 33.33%)

Notice here that the third scenario is only possible because the number of labels in this study is greater than two.

If the first case scenario occurs, then our system would mark the segment s as *credible*, and no additional labeling will be needed for that segment. If, on the other hand, either scenario 2 or 3 occur, then our system will need to ask a fourth worker to label segment s, which would result in the three following potential responses:

1. Three (out of four) workers agree on one label (the highest percentage is 75%)
2. Two (out of four) workers agree on one label (the highest percentage is 50%)
3. The four workers choose a different label each (the highest percentage is 25%)

Again, notice here that the third scenario is only possible because the number of labels in our study is greater than three (4). Also, we notice here that we cannot have all four workers agree on a single label, since for this to occur, the three original workers would have agreed on the same label initially, which would have caused our system to mark segment s as credible, and stop presenting for further labeling.

Based on the three possible scenarios listed above, only if the first one occurs, our system would mark segment s as credible. If either the second or third scenario occurs, then our system will prompt two more workers to label segment s.

Table 5 The number of responses that can yield credible segments per our example

# of total responses for a given segment	3	4	5	6	7	8	9	10
Min. # of responses needed to satisfy stop threshold (70%)	3	3	4	5	5	6	7	7
Can segment potentially be marked *credible*?	✓	✓	✗	✗	✓	✗	✗	✓

The reason why our system will ask for two additional responses instead of one is because, in this case, it would be impossible for segment s to become *credible* by obtaining only one other response, due to the value of the stop threshold specified (70%). Here are the two scenarios that we would end up with if we ask for only one additional response:

1. Three (out of five) agree on one label (the highest percentage is 60%)
2. Only two (out of five) agree on one label (the highest percentage is 40%)

Neither of the two cases listed above satisfies the stop threshold.

Table 5 shows the number of responses that we can obtain "credible" segments in. Notice here that the minimum number of responses that satisfies the stop threshold also depends on the number of labels in our study. Our website will dynamically (and on-the-fly) show whether a segment can be "credible" or not for all the number of responses between the minimum and maximum values provided. Figure 5 shows a screenshot of a filled study.

Workers who join a study can request audio segments (simply by visiting the study page), which would be provided by the platform according to the study rules and specifications, and in accordance with the algorithm described above. After a worker listens to the audio segment, he or she can select one of the pre-defined labels by clicking on the corresponding button; a worker also has the option of re-playing the segment if desired, as shown in Fig. 6.

The results of the study are made available in a CSV file format, containing the filename, start and end segment times, distribution of workers' responses, and percentage of most-agreed-upon labels; administrators can also play the audio segment from the results page. Figure 7 shows a screenshot of the results page.

In addition to being able to download a CSV file with the study results, study administrators can download the set of all labeled audio segments as WAV files for further analysis. Our system will group audio segments in folders based on the *final label* value of the files, and will compress all the folders in a single downloadable zip file. For convenience, audio segments are named based on the identification numbers of the segments provided in the table (or CSV file).

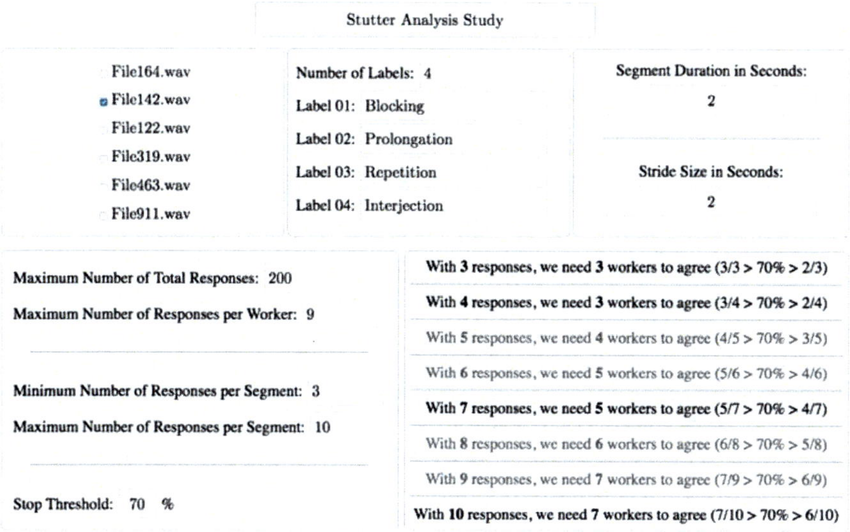

Fig. 5 Interface for creating a new crowdsourcing study

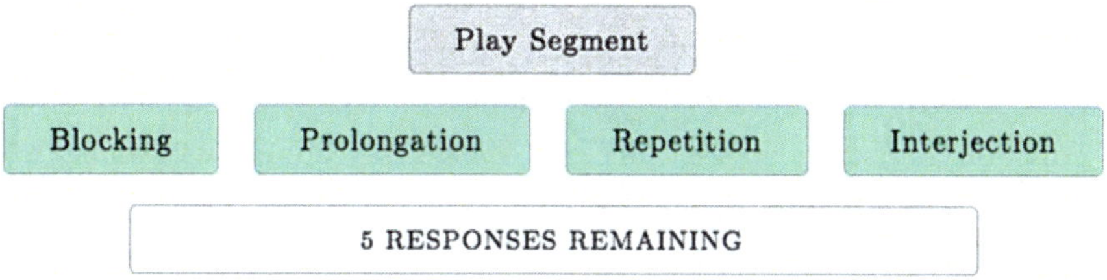

Fig. 6 Worker interface that shows available functions for a stutter analysis study

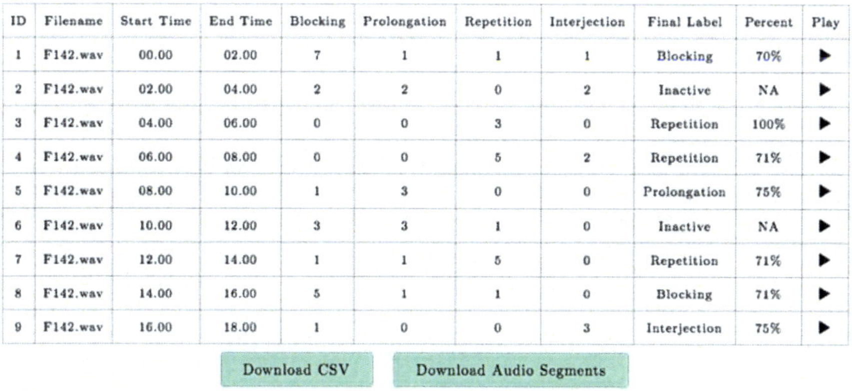

ID	Filename	Start Time	End Time	Blocking	Prolongation	Repetition	Interjection	Final Label	Percent	Play
1	F142.wav	00.00	02.00	7	1	1	1	Blocking	70%	▶
2	F142.wav	02.00	04.00	2	2	0	2	Inactive	NA	▶
3	F142.wav	04.00	06.00	0	0	3	0	Repetition	100%	▶
4	F142.wav	06.00	08.00	0	0	5	2	Repetition	71%	▶
5	F142.wav	08.00	10.00	1	3	0	0	Prolongation	75%	▶
6	F142.wav	10.00	12.00	3	3	1	0	Inactive	NA	▶
7	F142.wav	12.00	14.00	1	1	5	0	Repetition	71%	▶
8	F142.wav	14.00	16.00	5	1	1	0	Blocking	71%	▶
9	F142.wav	16.00	18.00	1	0	0	3	Interjection	75%	▶

Download CSV   Download Audio Segments

Fig. 7 Screenshot of sample results from a stutter detection analysis study

4.3 Logic Behind Segment-Worker Label Assignment

In this section, we will provide an explanation of the logic employed to optimize the data-collection process; before we present the algorithm however, we need to define a few terms. Each audio segment has a start time, end time, and a file associated with it; in addition, every segment exhibits one of these four states:

1. **Credible**: a credible segment is a segment that (a) has been labeled x number of times, where x is between the minimum and maximum number of responses provided by the study administrator(s), and (b) the percentage of the most-agreed-upon label by the workers satisfies the stop threshold provided.
2. **Inactive**: as soon as our system determines that a particular segment cannot reach the stop threshold defined, even if that segment has not reached its maximum number of responses, that segment would be marked as "Inactive", and our system will no longer present that segment to workers for further labeling.
3. **High Priority**: high priority segments refer to segments that have been labeled at least once, and they still have the potential of becoming "credible".
4. **Low Priority**: a low priority segment is a segment that has not been labeled by anyone yet. A random "low priority" segment will be assigned to a worker only if there are no "high priority" segments available for labeling for that particular worker.

The reason for our introduction of the "low priority" and "high priority" labels is to introduce a way to minimize the partially labeled segments. In Algorithm 2, we provide a summary of the segment-worker assignment algorithm deployed by this platform.

Algorithm 2: Summary of our implemented algorithm

start by creating the audio segments based on the stride size and the files associated with the study, and mark all of them as *low priority*;
for *every worker w requesting an audio segment for labeling* **do**
  populate the set H_w with all the *high priority* segments, excluding the ones that have been already labeled by worker w;
  if *$|H_w|$ is greater than or equal to 1* **then**
    randomly choose segment $h : h \in H_w$ and return to worker w;
    after worker w labels segment h, update the status of segment s to either *Credible* or *Inactive* if necessary, according to the label provided by worker w;
  else
    randomly choose and return to worker w segment $h : h \in L$, where L is the set of segments that exhibit status *low priority*;
    after worker w labels segment h, update the status of segment h to either *High prioriy* or *Credible* (in the case where the min. responses is equal to 1)
  end
end

5 Conclusion

In this chapter, we started by providing a review of the most relevant literature on stutter detection; we then presented a two-phase machine learning system capable of identifying stutter segments in a speech. As has been shown above, the system presented here was successfully able to reduce stutter speech disfluency by removing certain potentially undesired speech segments. The work presented in this chapter was primarily adopted from the dissertation work of Dr. Pierre Arbajian.

We then expanded our discussion of the topic to include an elaborate description of a web-platform developed by the authors of the chapter. The motivation for developing such a system is to provide researchers with the ability to efficiently and effectively collect pre-labeled audio information for further analysis. The system allows streamlined data management with easy scope extension. We have developed this system in support of an ongoing research in the area of stuttered speech detection.

References

1. Howell, P., Davis, S., Bartrip, J.: The university college london archive of stuttered speech (uclass). J. Speech Lang. Hear. Res. (2009)
2. Liu, Y., Shriberg, E., Stolcke, A., Harper, M.: Comparing hmm, maximum entropy, and conditional random fields for disfluency detection. In: Ninth European Conference on Speech Communication and Technology (2005)
3. Fook, C.Y., Muthusamy, H., Chee, L.S., Yaacob, S.B., Adom, A.H.B.: Comparison of speech parameterization techniques for the classification of speech disfluencies. Turk. J. Electr. Eng. Comput. Sci. **21**(1), 1983–1994 (2013)
4. Hariharan, M., Chee, L.S., Ai, O.C., Yaacob, S.: Classification of speech dysfluencies using LPC based parameterization techniques. J. Med. Syst. **36**(3), 1821–1830 (2012)
5. Chee, L.C., Ai, O.C., Yaacob, S.: Overview of automatic stuttering recognition system. In: Proc. International Conference on Man-Machine Systems, no. October, Batu Ferringhi, Penang Malaysia, pp. 1–6 (2009)
6. Honal, M., Schultz, T.: Correction of disfluencies in spontaneous speech using a noisy-channel approach. In: Eighth European Conference on Speech Communication and Technology (2003)
7. Honal, M., Schultz, T.: Automatic disfluency removal on recognized spontaneous speech-rapid adaptation to speaker-dependent disfluencies. In: Proceedings (ICASSP'05). IEEE International Conference on Acoustics, Speech, and Signal Processing (2005)
8. Lease, M., Johnson, M., Charniak, E.: Recognizing disfluencies in conversational speech. IEEE Trans. Audio Speech Lang. Process. **14**(5), 1566–1573 (2006)
9. Ai, O.C., Hariharan, M., Yaacob, S., Chee, L.S.: Classification of speech dysfluencies with MFCC and LPCC features. Expert Syst. Appl. **39**(2), 2157–2165 (2012)
10. Km, R.K., Ganesan, S.: Comparison of multidimensional MFCC feature vectors for objective assessment of stuttered disfluencies. Int. J. Adv. Netw. Appl. **2**(05), 854–860 (2011)
11. Ravikumar, K., Rajagopal, R., Nagaraj, H.: An approach for objective assessment of stuttered speech using MFCC. In: The international congress for global science and technology, p. 19 (2009)
12. Świetlicka, I., Kuniszyk-Jóźkowiak, W., Smołka, E.: Hierarchical ANN system for stuttering identification. Comput. Speech Lang. **27**(1), 228–242 (2013)
13. Arbajian, P., Hajja, A., Raś, Z.W., Wieczorkowska, A.A.: Segment-removal based stuttered speech remediation. In: International workshop on new frontiers in mining complex patterns, pp. 16–34. Springer (2017)

14. Arbajian, P., Hajja, A., Raś, Z.W., Wieczorkowska, A.A.: Effect of speech segment samples selection in stutter block detection and remediation. J. Intell. Inform. Syst. **53**(2), 241–264 (2019)
15. Boersma, P.: Praat, a system for doing phonetics by computer. Glot. Int. **5**(9), 341–345 (2001)
16. Boersma, P.: Accurate short-term analysis of the fundamental frequency and the harmonics-to-noise ratio of a sampled sound. In: Proceedings of the institute of phonetic sciences, vol. 17, no. 1193, pp. 97–110. Amsterdam (1993)
17. Czyzewski, A., Kaczmarek, A., Kostek, B.: Intelligent processing of stuttered speech. J. Intell. Inform. Syst. **21**(2), 143–171 (2003)
18. Hajja, A., Hiers, G.P., Arbajian, P., Raś, Z.M., Wieczorkowska, A.A.: Multipurpose web-platform for labeling audio segments efficiently and effectively. In: International Symposium on Methodologies for Intelligent Systems, pp. 179–188. Springer (2018)
19. Snover, M., Dorr, B., Schwartz, R.: A lexically-driven algorithm for disfluency detection. In: Proceedings of HLT-NAACL 2004: Short Papers
20. Taboada, M., Brooke, J., Tofiloski, M., Voll, K., Stede, M.: Lexicon-based methods for sentiment analysis. Comput. Linguist. **37**(2), 267–307 (2011)
21. Ferguson, J., Durrett, G., Klein, D.: Disfluency detection with a semi-markov model and prosodic features. In: Proceedings of the 2015 Conference of the North American Chapter of the Association for Computational Linguistics: Human Language Technologies, pp. 257–262 (2015)
22. Huang, Z., Chen, L., Harper, M.: An open source prosodic feature extraction tool. In: Proceedings of the language resources and evaluation conference (LREC) (2006)
23. El Ayadi, M., Kamel, M.S., Karray, F.: Survey on speech emotion recognition: features, classification schemes, and databases. Pattern Recognit. **44**(3), 572–587 (2011)
24. Scherer, S., Siegert, I., Bigalke, L., Meudt, S.: Developing an expressive speech labeling tool incorporating the temporal characteristics of emotion. In: LREC (2010)
25. Tumanova, V., Zebrowski, P.M., Throneburg, R.N., Kayikci, M.E.K.: Articulation rate and its relationship to disfluency type, duration, and temperament in preschool children who stutter. J. Commun. Disord. **44**(1), 116–129 (2011)
26. Kim, S., Georgiou, P.G., Lee, S., Narayanan, S.: Real-time emotion detection system using speech: Multi-modal fusion of different timescale features. In: Multimedia Signal Processing: MMSP 2007, pp. 48–51. IEEE (2007)

Personalizing Patients to Enable Shared Decision Making

Mamoun T. Mardini, Amal Hashky, and Zbigniew W. Raś

Abstract Shared decision making (SDM) is a process in which clinicians and patients collaboratively work together to reach a shared medical decision, where the best medical evidence is presented, and the preferences and priorities of the patient are respected. In this paper, we developed an evidence-based platform that aims to facilitate communication between patients and clinicians. We mined the Healthcare Cost and Utilization Project dataset (H-CUP) and extracted medical knowledge personalized to the patient's medical characteristics. Our platform is tailored toward the hospital readmission problem. First, we employed machine learning techniques to build models that can predict the readmission and mortality for newly admitted patients at the hospital. Second, we built a graph named *Procedure Graph* to visualize the primary procedures during the course of treatment and show the number of potential readmissions. Third, we personalized the procedure graph to the patient's medical characteristics by applying our developed *Rough Clustering* technique. The developed platform is highly significant and novel within the context of hospital readmission. It can enhance the patient-clinician communication by providing a visualized evidence-based knowledge extracted from the electronic health records and personalized to the patient's level.

M. T. Mardini (✉)
College of Medicine, Dept. of Aging and Geriatric Research, University of Florida, Gainesville, FL 32610, USA
e-mail: malmardini@ufl.edu

A. Hashky
Georgia Institute of Technology, School of Computer Science, Atlanta, GA 30332, USA
e-mail: ahashky@gatech.edu

Z. W. Raś
University of North Carolina at Charlotte, Charlotte, NC 28223, USA
e-mail: ras@uncc.edu

Polish-Japanese Academy of Information Technology, 02-008 Warsaw, Poland

Z. W. Ras et al. (eds.), *Recommender Systems for Medicine and Music*,
Studies in Computational Intelligence 946,
https://doi.org/10.1007/978-3-030-66450-3_5

1 Introduction

Shared decision making (SDM) is a collaborative process in which the clinician and the patient reach a shared medical decision, where the best medical evidence is presented and the preferences of the patient are respected [1]. In SDM, clinicians support and respect patients' informed preferences that are based on high-quality clinical evidence. In 2007, Washington State in the USA passed legislation to galvanize shared decision making as an alternative to the traditional treatment process [2]. In 2016, National Quality Forum issued national certification standards for patient decision aids according to those adopted in Washington State [3]. After these legislations, other entities adopted and announced shared decision making models such as Centers for Medicare & Medicaid Services (CMS), and the Medicare Access and CHIP Reauthorization Act of 2015 (MACRA) [4]. This emphasizes the importance of SDM in clinical practice. Despite the expansion of SDM, clinicians have limited experience and use of decision aids. This limitation undermines the potential of SDM to engage patients in the clinical decision making process in an open and transparent manner.

SDM is based on providing an evidence-based knowledge to the patient. This evidence is based on historical data found in electronic health records. The purpose of this evidence is to provide the patient and the clinician with a reference to all possibilities and consequences along the course of treatment. This would facilitate and enhance the patient-clinician communication. Figure 1 shows the components of the SDM equation. Developing platforms that are easy to use allows clinicians to apply SDM in their medical practice.

SDM is neither about ignoring the basic biomedical science, which is the groundwork in medicine, nor solely following the recommendations from the clinical trials. SDM is a balance between medical practice and patient's preferences [5]. Clinical guidelines are designed for the general population, which is likely to be different from the patient, who has unique conditions, preferences, and priorities. It would be infeasible to provide personalized guidelines. However, acknowledging the need for personalized recommendations in the clinical practice is necessary [5]. This personal-

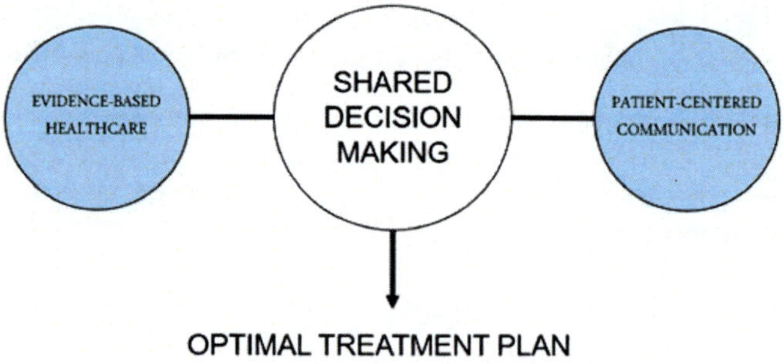

Fig. 1 Shared decision making concept

ization is possible with the advent of machine learning techniques and the availability of electronic health records. Recently, there have been several attempts to develop SDM platforms. For example, Hill and his colleagues [6] designed an interface for SDM to inform risk ratios and visualize quantified treatment outcomes. Shaoibi et al. [7] proposed a Bayesian collaborative filtering (CF) algorithm that amalgamates preferences and patient reported outcomes (PROs) to provide treatment recommendations. Although there is an increase in the number of SDM platforms [8–10], there is a lack of platforms focused on hospital readmission.

According to H-CUP Statistical Brief published in 2014, all-cause hospital readmissions in the United States were associated with $41.3 billion in hospital costs [11]. A hospital readmission is defined as a hospitalization of the patient after being discharged from the hospital. The period in average is 30 days [12]. One of the reasons for hospital readmissions is the wrong diagnosis of patients. It is very important to provide patients with the proper diagnosis in order to avoid future readmissions or minimize their number as well as reduce healthcare spending. SDM is relevant in the context of hospital readmission. Presenting medical evidence can help clinicians to avoid any mistake and enhance the overall patient-clinician communication and shared decision making.

In this paper, we show how to develop an evidence-based healthcare platform that can be used to facilitate communication between clinicians and patients. We mined the Healthcare Cost and Utilization Project (H-CUP) and extracted medical knowledge personalized to the patient's medical characteristics. In our approach, we focused on hospital readmission and mortality problems. First, we built a machine learning model to predict the possibility of readmission and mortality for newly admitted patients at the hospital. Second, we built a graph named *Procedure Graph* to visualize the primary procedures during the course of treatment and showed the number of potential readmissions. Third, we personalized the procedure graph to the patient's medical characteristics by applying our developed *Rough Clustering* technique. The developed system is valuable in clinical practice. It can enhance the patient-clinician communication by providing a visualized evidence-based knowledge extracted from the electronic health records and personalized to the patient's level.

2 Healthcare Cost and Utilization Project (H-CUP)

We mined Florida State Inpatient Databases (SID) that are part of H-CUP. The SID dataset is primarily a state-level discharge data that is collected from non-federal community hospitals, which constitute the majority of hospitals in the USA. SID include patients' demographic data, such as age, gender, and race. In addition to the demographic information, SID include patients' medical data, such as diagnoses and procedures. The main table in SID is the Core table, which is considered as the nucleus of the H-CUP databases. The Core table contains over 280 features (attributes). However, many of those features are repeated with different values according to the

Table 1 Description of the used features

Features	Concepts	Feature margin	Value type
VisitLink	Patient identifier	8(n)	Integer (8)
DaysToEvent	Temporal visit ordering	nnnn	Integer (4)
LOS	Length of stay	0–365	Integer (3)
DXCCSn	*n*th Diagnosis, flexible feature	1–259	Integer (3)
PRCCSn	*n*th Procedure, meta-action	1–231	Integer (3)
DXPOAn	Present on admission indicator	Y/N	Boolean
FEMALE	Indication of sex	1/0	Boolean
RACE	Indication of race	1–6	Integer (1)
AGE	Age in years at admission	0–124	Integer (3)
DIED	Died during hospitalization	1/0	Boolean

patient's status. There are two types of coding schemes used in the Core table for labeling and formatting, which are International Classification of Diseases, Ninth Revision, Clinical Modification (ICD-9-CM), and Clinical Classifications Software (CCS). The ICD-9-CM coding is detailed and uses more codes to label the procedures and diagnoses. On the other hand, CCS is more generalized and a collapsed form of ICD-9-CM. For example, there are 15,072 diagnosis categories and 3,948 procedure categories in ICD-9-CM. CCS collapses these categories into a smaller number of more generalized categories, so there are 285 diagnosis categories and 231 procedure categories. In this work, we used both the ICD-9-CM and the CCS coding schemes, with more focus on the ICD-9-CM coding.

In our experiments, we only used the features listed in Table 1 that are relevant to the examined problem. The Visit Linkage ($VisitLink$) feature is an encrypted identifier for patients. Each patient has a unique identifier among the hospitals within the same state. The Days to Event ($DaysToEvent$) feature provides information about the number of days between two consecutive visits for the same patient identified by the $VisitLink$ feature. The value of this feature is set randomly for the first visit to preserve the privacy of patients. The de-identification of such information can prevent any attempt to track patients. Therefore, some of the values in the dataset are assigned random values initially. The value of the following visit would be the initial random value assigned for the first visit plus the number of days between the admission dates of the two consecutive visits. For example, the patient can be assigned $DaysToEvent$=12 in the first visit, which is an entirely arbitrary number and does not provide us with any information about the actual admission date. The value of $DaysToEvent$ in the second visit will be the first value (12) plus the number of

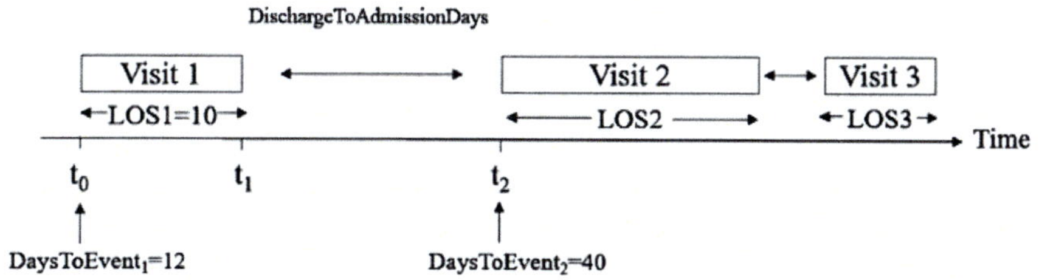

Fig. 2 Depiction showing the timeline of a patient's visits

days between the two visits. If $DaysToEvent$=12 for the first visit and the number of days between the two admission dates is 28 days, then $DaysToEvent$ for the second visit will be 12+28=40 days. It is worth mentioning here that $DaysToEvent$ represents the number of days between the admission dates, and not between the discharge date and the next admission date. $VisitLink$ and $DaysToEvent$ features are encrypted identifiers of the patients. They are used together to track patients across multiple visits within the same hospital or multiple hospitals within the same state without revealing the patient's identity. The *Length of Stay* (LOS) feature represents the number of days a patient stays at the hospital, which is the number of days from the admission date to the discharge date. $VisitLink$ and LOS can be used together to calculate the number of days between the discharge date and the next admission date. Referring back to our example above, depicted in Fig. 2, if $DaysToEvent_1$=12 and LOS=10 for the first visit, and $DaysToEvent_2$=40 for the second visit, then the number of days between these two visits (between the discharge of the first visit to the admission of the second visit) is 40-12-10=18 days. The following is the equation used to calculate the number of days between the discharge date and the next admission date:

$$DischargeToAdmissionDays = DaysToEvent_2 - DaysToEvent_1 - LOS_1 \tag{1}$$

where $DischargeToAdmissionDays$ refers to the number of days between the discharge date and the next admission date, $DaysToEvent$ refers to the number of days between any two consecutive admission dates, and LOS refers to the length of stay at the hospital. The subscript in the variable names indicates the visit number, 1 being the first visit and 2 being the second visit.

Calculating the number of days between the discharge date and the next admission date is of substantial importance, especially when the research concerns hospital readmissions. In order to consider that a patient had a readmission, the result of Eq. 1 should be less than or equal to 30 days for any two consecutive visits, as shown in Eq. 2.

$$ReadmissionIndicator = \begin{cases} Yes, & \text{DischargeToAdmissionDays} \leq 30 \\ No, & \text{DischargeToAdmissionDays} > 30 \end{cases} \tag{2}$$

Table 2 Procedures' categories as listed in H-CUP

Procedure category	Description
Minor diagnostic	Non-operating room procedures (diagnostic)
Minor therapeutic	Non-operating room procedures (therapeutic)
Major diagnostic	Operating room procedures performed for diagnostics
Major therapeutic	Operating room procedures performed for therapeutic

The *Core* table reports up to 31 diagnoses ($DXCCSn$) and up to 31 procedures ($PRCCSn$) per discharge as it has 31 diagnosis columns and 31 procedure columns. It is worth mentioning that it is often the case that patients' examination returns less than 31 diagnoses, and that the number of procedures they undergo is less than 31. Furthermore, even though a patient might have gone through several procedures during a given visit, the primary procedure that occurred at the visit discharge is assumed to be the first procedure ($PRCCS1$). Table 2 shows the different categories of procedures. The Present on Admission ($DXPOAn$) indicator identifies the diagnoses that were present when the patient was admitted. Since the dataset represents discharge data, this feature is useful for identifying the diagnoses that were present at the time of admission rather than the time of discharge. In addition to the features explained above, there are several demographic data that are reported in the *Core* table as well, such as race, age range, sex, and living area.

3 Predicting Medical Outcomes

The prediction of medical outcomes such as mortality, readmission, length of stay, and hospital disposition allows clinicians to identify patients who are at higher risk. Knowing that requires clinicians to provide extra care and take all possible precautions to maintain the patient's health, and avoid any adverse events. Additionally, this will facilitate the patient-clinician communication, especially if critical medical decisions are to be made. This can enhance the satisfaction of patients and their relatives regardless of the medical outcome. In this section, we provide our prediction results on the readmission and mortality outcomes [13]. We applied several supervised machine learning algorithms including Naïve Bayes, Decision Tree, Logistic Regression, Neural Network, and Support Vector Machine. We selected these algorithms due to their relevance to the problem at hand, and their prevalence in the field of machine learning. Overall, the performance of the models was reasonably high in predicting the likelihood of mortality and hospital readmission. Tables 3 and 4 list the accuracy of predicting mortality and readmission, respectively. Each table lists the training and testing accuracy values for each algorithm. As can be noticed, the prediction of mortality is found to be higher than the prediction of readmission.

Table 3 Predicting mortality accuracies

Algorithm	Training accuracy (%)	Testing accuracy (%)
Naïve bayes	87.43	80.47
Decision tree	96.29	80.34
Logistic regression	84.65	65.21
Neural network	84.64	82.78
SVM	95.21	82.68

Table 4 Predicting readmission accuracies

Algorithm	Training accuracy (%)	Testing accuracy (%)
Naïve bayes	62.76	61.98
Decision tree	91.38	56.92
Logistic regression	64.57	63.59
Neural network	64.38	63.1
SVM	76.75	62.71

Additionally, the models built on some algorithms such as the neural networks and support vector machine resulted in slightly better accuracy than others in both the mortality and readmission predictions. Moreover, the model built using decision tree outperformed the other models over the training dataset, which is foreseeable as decision trees tend to over-fit the training data.

The high dimensionality of the dataset usually affects the performance of the prediction model. Our dataset consists of 520 features. Not all of these features contribute the same in predicting the outcome. Instead of using all the available features, a subset was selected. We used three feature selection techniques to assign weights to the most significant features with respect to each prediction problem. These techniques are Entropy-based, Chi-Squared, and Correlation filtering. We could reduce the number of features by [50–70]%. We selected the reduction percentage that gave us the best accuracy. The results did not significantly improve the testing accuracy. However, there was a noticeable improvement in the processing performance. Additionally, we were able to identify the features that are significant in predicting the risk of mortality and readmissions, as shown in Table 5.

Predicting the possibility of medical outcomes such as readmission and mortality can provide a better risk assessment to the patient. Additionally, the identification of the medical features that are significant to each outcome can enhance the evaluation of the patient's medical condition. This will improve the overall patient-clinician discussion, by presenting the possible treatment options and selecting the best option that aligns well with the patient's preferences and priorities.

Table 5 The most significant features in the mortality and readmission predictions. The prefix in the CCS code columns indicates whether the code refers to a procedure (PR) or a diagnosis (DX)

Readmission		Mortality	
CCS Code	Description	CCS Code	Description
DX196	Normal pregnancy and/or delivery	DX131	Respiratory failure; insufficiency; arrest (adult)
DX158	Chronic kidney disease	PR216	Respiratory intubation and mechanical ventilation
DX59	Deficiency and other anemia	DX249	Shock
DX99	Hypertension with complications and secondary hypertension	DX244	Other injuries and conditions due to external causes
PR137	Other procedures to assist delivery	DX2	Septicemia (except in labor)
PR58	Hemodialysis	DX107	Cardiac arrest and ventricular fibrillation
DX55	Fluid and electrolyte disorders	DX157	Acute and unspecified renal failure
PR134	134: Cesarean section	DX55	Fluid and electrolyte disorders
DX181	Other complications of pregnancy	DX122	Pneumonia (except that caused by tuberculosis or sexually transmitted disease)
DX195	Other complications of birth; puerperium affecting management of mother	DX106	Cardiac dysrhythmias

4 Treatment Plan Visualization

Visualizing all possible treatment options is fundamental in selecting the best plan that fits the patient's preference with a balance of medical advantages and disadvantages. We used the H-CUP data to extract all the possible treatment options. We selected one procedure at a time and tracked all the next procedures in the EHR. We called the resulting graph the *Procedure Graph* and each path within the procedure graph is called the *Procedure Path*. A *procedure path* [14, 15], for procedure P, is defined as a sequence of the primary procedures that a newly admitted patient may undertake during the course of treatment. A *procedure graph*, for procedure P, is defined as a tree of all the possible procedure paths that a patient may undertake during the

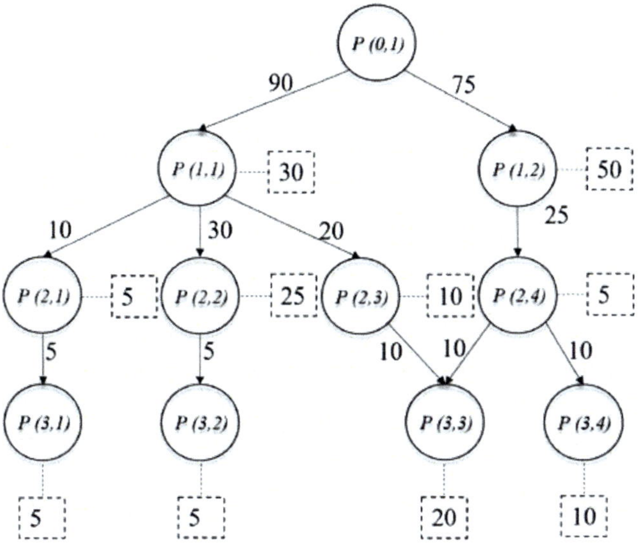

Fig. 3 Depiction of the procedure graph. This is a hypothetical graph showing all the possible procedure paths following procedure $P_{(0,1)}$. Each arrow is labeled with the number of patients who followed that path. The numbers in the dashed squares represent the number of patients who were discharged after performing the procedure and did not have to return. Each node in the tree is given an identifier $P_{(x,y)}$. x represents the level in the tree, and also represents the number of hospital readmissions till that node (or procedure). y is an identifier to distinguish the different paths in the procedure graph

course of treatment. Figure 3 shows a hypothetical example of the procedure graph. As can be noticed, it follows a tree structure, where the root of the tree represents the initial and the primary procedures of interest. The nodes in the tree represent other procedures that were needed in the following hospital readmissions. Procedures vary in their significance from X-ray (minor) to kidney transplant (major), for example. The length of any path in the procedure graph represents the number of hospital readmissions. Each arrow is labeled with the number of patients who followed that path in EHR. The numbers in the dashed squares represent the number of patients who were discharged after performing the procedure and did not have to return. Each node in the tree is given an identifier $P_{(x,y)}$, where x represents the level in the tree and also represents the number of hospital readmissions till that node (or procedure). y is an identifier to distinguish the different paths in the procedure graph. For example, $P_{(2,1)}$ refers to the procedure (node) at level 2 (number of readmissions is 2) and belongs to the first path in the procedure graph. The procedure graph is an invaluable addition to the treatment process, where it allows clinicians to visualize all the possible outcomes after performing a specific procedure (P). This would enhance the patient-clinician communication by exploring the treatment options, and selecting the procedure path that fits the patient's preference, while following the physician recommendations.

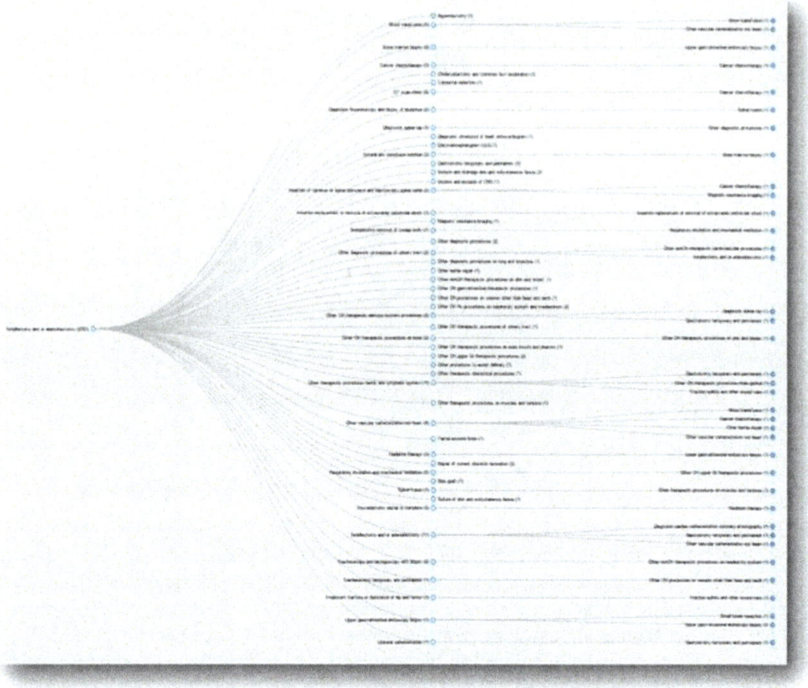

Fig. 4 A depiction showing how complex the procedure graph could be

Visualizing the procedure graph allowed us to realize that there is a high number of unique procedure paths. In other words, it is unlikely to find a common path that the majority of patients follow. For example, the number of patients who underwent *blood transfusion* as their first procedure (the root in the procedure graph) was 72,521. Tracking those patients showed 1,230 unique procedure paths. In contrary, 72,928 patients underwent the *spinal fusion* procedure. Tracking those patients showed 443 unique procedure paths. These differences could be explained due to the significance of the procedure. Minor and common procedures such as *blood transfusion* may result in a high number of unique procedure paths, compared to more complex and specific procedures such as *spinal fusion*. Although there is a difference in the number of unique procedure paths between the two procedures, the number is still considerably high, and this emphasizes the fact that patients do not follow the same path during their course of treatment. This fact can entangle the patient-clinician communication and complicate the selection of the most optimal path. Figure 4 shows a full procedure graph extracted from our dataset. Although it is blurry, the purpose was to show how complex it could be for the generic population.

Table 6 Procedure paths with the highest probabilities for *kidney transplant* (procedure code: 105). 54: Other vascular catheterization, not heart; 70: Upper gastrointestinal endoscopy biopsy; 88: Abdominal paracentesis; 99: Other OR gastrointestinal therapeutic procedures; 110: Other diagnostic procedures of urinary tract; 111: Other nonOR therapeutic procedures of urinary tract; 193: Malignant neoplasm of thyroid gland; 231: Other therapeutic procedures. ICD-10 Clinical Classification Software (CCS) category names were used

Procedure path	Probability (%)
{105, 231}	0.404
{105, 193}	0.231
{105, 70, 54}	0.173
{105, 110, 111}	0.115
{105, 88, 99}	0.058

The selection process of any procedure path follows a probabilistic function that can be calculated by dividing the number of patients at the end of the path by the number of patients at the beginning of the path, as shown in the following equation:

$$prob(path_k) = freq(P_{(l,i)})/freq(P_{(0,1)}) \quad (3)$$

where $prob(path_k)$ refers to the probability of following the k_{th} path, $freq(P_{(l,i)})$ refers to the number of patients at the last node (leaf), and $freq(P_{(0,1)})$ refers to the number of patients at the initial node (root). l refers to the number (or rather level) of readmissions, which is in this case the last level, and the second argument i refers to the procedure identifier at that level.

Table 6 shows the most probable paths for *Kidney Transplant* (procedure code: 105), and the following is an overview of the procedure graph features:

- 1732 patients started with this procedure,
- the shortest path was of length 1,
- the longest path was of length 10, and
- the average path length was 3.11 (average number of readmission was 3.11).

As can be noticed from Table 6, increasing the number of procedures in the procedure path decreases the probability of the path. This was anticipated as there is a large number of unique procedure paths, and the number of patients in any path decreases as we move toward the leaves of the tree. Extracting the procedure graph directly from Electronic Health Records (EHR) is not useful to guide the patient-clinician communication. The procedure graph should be personalized to the patient's medical and demographic characteristics to increase the predictability of a certain procedure path or the predictability of the next procedure [16]. This is viable through clustering patients who share certain features into groups, and then building a personalized procedure graph.

5 Personalizing Treatment Plan

As explained in the previous section, extracting the procedure graph from EHR for the general population is not useful. The resulting graph will be complex, as shown in Fig. 4. Personalizing the procedure graph to the patient's medical characteristics can enhance the patient-clinician communication, and help them in choosing the path that results in the optimum outcome and aligns with the patient's preferences.

In this section, we present our clustering algorithm called *Rough Clustering* [15]. It stems from the *Rough Set Theory* [17]. The rough clustering defines two sets of diagnoses that are used as criteria for whether a new patient belongs to a certain cluster or not, which mimic the upper and lower approximation concept in the rough set theory. Unlike other clustering algorithms, rough clustering groups patients according to the diagnoses they have and the diagnoses they do not have. The first set is called the *Included Set*, which includes the diagnoses that a new patient must exhibit to belong to the specified cluster. The other set is called the *Excluded Set*, which includes the set of diagnoses that a new patient must not exhibit in order to belong to the specified cluster. Diagnoses in this set are labeled with a hyphen (-). The rationale of defining these two sets and using them as affiliation criteria is to emphasize the importance of ensuring the exclusion of certain medical conditions in the treatment process. Not having certain medical conditions can change the course of treatment.

The following cluster extracted from our dataset can elucidate the concept of the *included* and *excluded* sets. The following cluster was extracted for patients who underwent the *spinal fusion* (procedure code: 158) as their first procedure. The extracted cluster is described as follows: $\{98, -49, -138, -211\}$. Accordingly, the included and excluded sets are expressed as follows:

- *Included*: $\{98\}$ and
- *Excluded*: $\{-49, -138, -211\}$.

A newly admitted patient can belong to this cluster, only if he/she exhibits all the diagnoses in the *Included* set: *essential hypertension* (diagnostic code: 98); and if the patient does not exhibit any of the diagnoses in the *Excluded* set: *diabetes mellitus without complication* (diagnostic code: 49), *esophageal disorders* (diagnostic code: 138), and *other connective tissue disease* (diagnostic code: 211).

The construction of the clusters in the rough clustering algorithm follows a hierarchical structure. It starts with all the possible diagnoses in the dataset by creating two one-element sets for each diagnosis: included set {diag} and excluded set {-diag}. In each level in the construction process of clusters, we combined the sets (of size n) in the previous level and generated new clusters (of size n+1). Clearly, a diagnostic code cannot be combined with its negation, for example, *essential hypertension* (diagnostic code: 98) cannot be combined with -98, as this means that the patient has hypertension and does not have it at the same time.

Figure 5 shows some of the clusters extracted from our dataset for patients with kidney disease and gout. Patients with *chronic kidney disease* (diagnosis code: 40391)

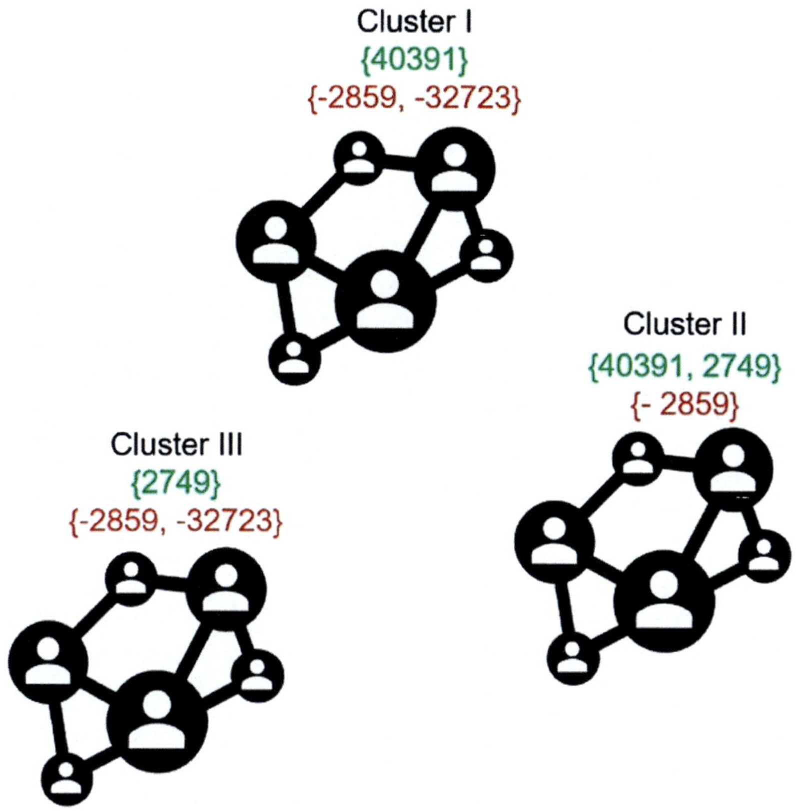

Fig. 5 Extracted clusters by using our *Rough* clustering algorithm. Green represents the *Included set*, and red represents the *Excluded set*. 2749: Gout; 40391: Hypertensive chronic kidney disease; 2859: Anemia; 32723: Obstructive sleep apnea

and *gout* (diagnosis code: 2749) are with higher risk of readmission—two risk factors. However, patients with only *chronic kidney disease* only have a lower risk of readmission. The procedure graph in the case of *Cluster I* would show a smaller average number of edges—less readmissions. On the contrary, the procedure graph in the case of *Cluster II* would show a larger average number of edges—more readmissions. Knowing that a patient belongs to *Cluster II*, having both *chronic kidney disease* and *gout*, allows the physician and the patient to have an overview of the possible future readmissions and the potential procedures needed in each readmission. This level of details is personalized to the patients who have both *chronic kidney disease* and *gout*. This would eliminate several procedure paths that would have appeared in the case of building the procedure graph based on patients who have *chronic kidney disease*. This emphasizes the importance of personalization in the construction of the procedure graph, which provides a precise visualization of the treatment options that are relevant to the patient's medical conditions.

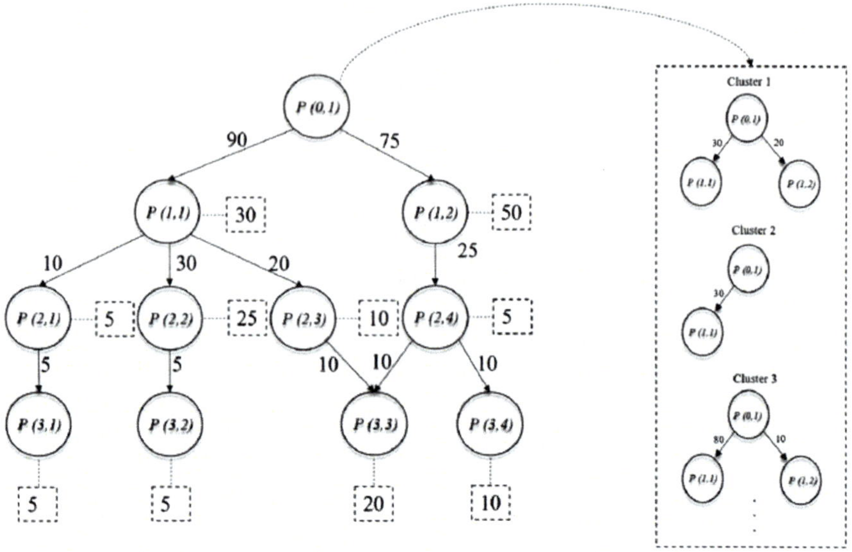

Fig. 6 Illustration of how the clusters from rough clustering are shown in the procedure graph. The clusters are shown in the large dashed box. The nodes after the root represent the next procedures that the patients in that cluster are more likely to follow

Figure 6 shows how the clusters can be embedded in the procedure graph. The clusters are shown in the large dashed box. The nodes after the root represent the next procedures that the patients in that cluster are more likely to follow.

For example, the patients in *Cluster 2* underwent $P_{(1,1)}$, and no one underwent $P_{(1,2)}$. Therefore, if a new patient affiliates with this cluster, then he/she will undergo $P_{(1,1)}$. On the other hand, if a new patient affiliates with *Cluster 3*, then he/she will either undergo $P_{(1,1)}$ or $P_{(1,2)}$, but most probably will undergo $P_{(1,1)}$, since it has higher probability. The distribution of the following procedures implies the most probable procedure that a new patient will undergo after the first primary procedure. As can be noticed, building personalized procedure graphs according to the patient's characteristics eliminates irrelevant procedure paths, and can enhance the probability to follow the most optimal path.

6 Conclusion

In this chapter, we presented a personalized evidence-based platform that aims to facilitate communication between patients and clinicians. We achieved that by mining the Healthcare Cost and Utilization Project (H-CUP) dataset, and extracting medical knowledge personalized to the patient's medical characteristics. Presenting this medical knowledge in a visualized manner, as we have shown by using the *procedure graph*, is highly valuable in clinical practice. Additionally, personalizing these visualizations to the patient's medical characteristics is of more significance. It allows clinicians to present the historical medical knowledge to the patient and discuss the possible treatment options. In the future, we aim to enhance the performance of our rough clustering algorithm and validate our platform in medical practice.

References

1. Grad, R., Légaré, F., Bell, N.R., Dickinson, J.A., Singh, H., Moore, A.E., Kasperavicius, D., Kretschmer, K.L.: Shared decision making in preventive health care: What it is; what it is not. Can. Fam. Phys. **63**(9), 682 (2017)
2. Washington State Legislature, RCW 7.70.060. Consent form-Contents-Prima facie evidence-Shared decision making-Patient decision aid-Failure to use. title 7, chapter 770, section 770060.
3. National Quality Forum: National standards for the certification of patient decision aids (2016)
4. Spatz, E.S., Krumholz, H.M., Moulton, B.W.: Prime time for shared decision making. JAMA **317**(13), 1309–1310 (2017)
5. McCormack, J., Elwyn, G.: Shared decision is the only outcome that matters when it comes to evaluating evidence-based practice. BMJ Evid. Based Med. **23**(4), 137–139 (2018)
6. Hill, B., Proulx, J., Zeng-Treitler, Q.: Exploring the use of large clinical data to inform patients for shared decision making. In: Studies in Health Technology and Informatics, pp. 851–855 (2013)
7. Shaoibi, A., Neelon, B., Lenert, L.A.: Shared decision making: from decision science to data science. Medical Decision Making (2020) 0272989X20903267
8. Puppala, M., He, T., Chen, S., Ogunti, R., Yu, X., Li, F., Jackson, R., Wong, S.T.: Meteor: an enterprise health informatics environment to support evidence-based medicine. IEEE Trans. Biomed. Eng. **62**(12), 2776–2786 (2015)
9. Jin, W., Gromala, D., Neustaedter, C., Tong, X.: A collaborative visualization tool to support doctors' shared decision-making on antibiotic prescription. In: Companion of the 2017 ACM Conference on Computer Supported Cooperative Work and Social Computing, pp. 211–214 (2017)
10. Lee, Y.J., Bryce, C., Jain, S., Kraschnewski, J., McTigue, K.: Patient-centered visualization on supporting patient' decision-making. Eur. J. Pers. Cent. Healthc. **7**(4), 630–639 (2020)
11. Hines, A.L., Barrett, M.L., Jiang, H.J., Steiner, C.A.: Conditions with the largest number of adult hospital readmissions by payer, HCUP Statistical Brief 172 (2011)
12. Silow-Carroll, S., Edwards, J.N., Lashbrook, A.: Reducing Hospital Readmissions: Lessons from Top-Performing Hospitals. CareManagement **17**(5), 14 (2011)
13. Almardini, M., Raś, Z.W.: A supervised model for predicting the risk of mortality and hospital readmissions for newly admitted patients. Foundations of Intelligent Systems, Proceedings of International Symposium on Methodologies for Intelligent Systems in Warsaw, Poland, LNAI, vol. 10352, pp. 29–36 (2017)
14. Almardini, M., Hajja, A., Raś, Z.W., Clover, L., Olaleye, D., Park, Y., Paulson, J., Xiao, Y.: Reduction of readmissions to hospitals based on actionable knowledge discovery and personalization, beyond databases, architectures and structures-BDAS 2016, conference proceedings. Commun. Comput. Inf. Sci. **613**, 39–55 (2016)
15. Mardini, M.T., Raś, Z.W.: Extraction of actionable knowledge to reduce hospital readmissions through patients personalization. Inf. Sci. **485**, 1–17 (2019)

16. Almardini, M., Hajja, A., Raś, Z.W., Clover, L., Olaleye, D.: Predicting the primary medical procedure through clustering of patients' diagnoses, in New Frontiers in Mining Complex Patterns, Post-proceedings of NFMCP, : ECML/PKDD Workshop in Riva del Garda. Italy, LNAI **10312**(2016), 117–131 (2016)
17. Pawlak, Z.: Rough Sets. Int. J. Comput. Inf. Sci 11(5), 341–356 (1982). https://doi.org/10.1007/BF01001956

An LSTM-based Approach for Insulin and Carbohydrate Recommendations in Type 1 Diabetes Self-Management

Jeremy Beauchamp, Razvan Bunescu, and Cindy Marling

Abstract To avoid serious diabetic complications, people with type 1 diabetes must keep their blood glucose levels (BGLs) as close to normal as possible. Insulin dosages and carbohydrate consumption are important considerations in managing BGLs. Since the 1960s, models have been developed to forecast blood glucose levels based on the history of BGLs, insulin dosages, carbohydrate intake, and other physiological and lifestyle factors. Such predictions can be used to alert people to impending unsafe BGLs or to control insulin flow in an artificial pancreas. In past work, we have introduced an LSTM-based approach to blood glucose level prediction aimed at "what if" scenarios, in which people could input the grams of carbohydrates in foods they might eat or units of insulin they might take and then see the effect on future BGLs. Building on these neural models for "what-if" predictions, in this work we derive a novel LSTM-based architecture that can be trained to make either insulin or carbohydrate recommendations to ensure that future BGLs attain the desired level. Experimental evaluations using data from the OhioT1DM dataset show that the neural architecture substantially outperforms the baselines. The promising results suggest that this novel approach could potentially be of practical use to people with type 1 diabetes for self-management of BGLs.

1 Introduction and Motivation

Diabetes self-management is a time-consuming, yet critical, task for people with type 1 diabetes. To avoid serious diabetic complications, these individuals must continually manage their blood glucose levels (BGLs), keeping them as close to

J. Beauchamp (✉) · C. Marling
Ohio University, Athens, OH, USA
e-mail: jb199113@ohio.edu

C. Marling
e-mail: marling@ohio.edu

R. Bunescu
University of North Carolina at Charlotte, Charlotte, NC, USA
e-mail: rbunescu@uncc.edu

Z. W. Ras et al. (eds.), *Recommender Systems for Medicine and Music*,
Studies in Computational Intelligence 946,
https://doi.org/10.1007/978-3-030-66450-3_6

normal as possible. They must avoid both low BGLs, or hypoglycemia, and high BGLs, or hyperglycemia, for their physical safety and well-being. Diabetes self-management entails carefully monitoring BGLs throughout the day, by testing blood obtained from finger sticks and/or by using a continuous glucose monitoring (CGM) system. It also entails making numerous daily decisions about the timing and dosage of insulin and the timing, ingredients, and quantity of food consumed.

Current diabetes self-management may be characterized as *reactive*, rather than *proactive*. When BGLs are too high, individuals may take insulin to lower them, and when BGLs are too low, they may eat a snack or take glucose tablets to raise them. The ability to accurately predict BGLs could enable people with type 1 diabetes to take preemptive actions *before* experiencing the negative effects of hypoglycemia or hyperglycemia. There have been efforts to model BGLs for the purpose of determining insulin dosages dating back to the 1960s [4]. There has been much recent work in BGL prediction for the purpose of providing support for diabetes self-management, including our own [5, 13]. Accounts of some of the most recent BGL prediction efforts can be found in the proceedings of two international BGL prediction challenges [1, 2]. It should be noted that, even with the benefit of accurate BGL predictions, individuals still need to determine how much to eat, how much insulin to take, and what other actions they can take to prevent hypoglycemia or hyperglycemia.

The broad goal of the research presented here is to essentially reverse the BGL prediction problem, and instead predict how many grams of carbohydrate (carbs) an individual should eat or how much insulin they should take in order to achieve the desired BGL target. We have previously introduced an LSTM-based neural architecture that was trained to answer *what-if* questions of the type "What will my BGL be in 60 min if I eat a snack with 30 carbs 10 min from now?" [11]. We show that, by using the BGL target as a feature and the carbohydrates or insulin as labels, a similar architecture can be trained instead to predict the number of carbs that should be consumed or the amount of insulin that should be taken during the prediction window in order to reach that BGL target.

The work by Mougiakakou and Nikita [12] represents one of the first attempts to use neural networks for recommending insulin regimens and dosages. Bolus calculators were introduced as early as 2003 [16], wherein a standard formula is used to calculate the amount of bolus insulin based on parameters such as carbohydrate intake, carbohydrate-to-insulin ratio, insulin on board, and target BGL. Walsh et al. [15] discuss major sources of errors and potential ways to improve bolus advisors, such as utilizing the massive quantities of clinical data collected by the bolus advisors. As observed by Cappon et al. in [6], the standard formula approach ignores potentially useful preprandial conditions, such as the glucose rate of change. They propose a feed-forward fully connected neural network to exploit CGM information and some easily accessible patient parameters. Their experimental evaluations on simulated data show a small, but statistically significant, improvement in the blood glucose risk index. Simulated data is also used by Sun et al. in [14], where a basal-bolus advisor is trained using reinforcement learning in order to provide personalized suggestions to people with type 1 diabetes taking multiple daily injections of insulin.

The data-driven architecture introduced herein is generic in the sense that it can be trained to make recommendations about any variable that can impact BGLs, in particular, carbohydrates and insulin. Carbohydrate recommendations are potentially useful when someone wants to prevent hypoglycemia well in advance or when someone wants to achieve a higher target BGL before physical exercise that is expected to lower it. Bolus recommendations are useful prior to meals and also for lowering BGLs when individuals experience hyperglycemia. In [3], we reported preliminary results only for the task of carbohydrate recommendation, where the aim was to achieve the desired target BGL 30 or 60 min into the future. The timing of the meal was variable within the prediction window and was used as one of the inputs to the model. In this paper, we change the task definition to make the system easier to use and more relevant to the type of situations encountered in the daily life of individuals with type 1 diabetes. As such, the timing of the bolus or meal is now fixed at 10 min into the future, based on the assumption that patients are most interested in using the system right before making a meal or bolus decision. To achieve the desired BGL, the user can specify any time horizon between 30 and 90 min, giving them more flexibility in terms of how fast they want their BGL to change.

The rest of this chapter is organized as follows: Sect. 2 presents three different recommendation scenarios. Section 3 describes the neural architecture as well as the baselines used for comparison. Section 4 describes the dataset and explains how recommendation examples were derived. Section 5 explains the experimental methodology and presents the results of the experiments. Section 6 contains the conclusion and plans for future work.

2 Three Recommendation Scenarios

We assume that blood glucose levels are measured at 5 min intervals through a CGM system. We also assume that discrete deliveries of insulin (boluses) and continuous infusions of insulin (basal rates) are recorded. Subjects provide the timing of meals and estimates of the number of grams of carbohydrates in each meal. Given the available data up to and including the present (time t), the system aims to estimate how much a person should eat or bolus[1] 10 min from now (time $t + 10$) such that their blood glucose will reach a target level τ minutes after that action (time $t + 10 + \tau$). A system that computes these estimates could then be used in the following three recommendation scenarios:

1. **Carbohydrate Recommendations**: Estimate the amount of carbohydrate C_{t+10} to have in a meal in order to achieve a target BG value $G_{t+10+\tau}$.
2. **Bolus Recommendations**: Estimate the amount of insulin B_{t+10} to deliver with a bolus in order to achieve a target BG value $G_{t+10+\tau}$.
3. **Bolus Recommendations given Carbohydrates**: Expecting that a meal with C_{t+20} grams of carbohydrate will be consumed 20 min from now, estimate the

[1] Administer a bolus.

amount of insulin B_{t+10} to deliver with a bolus 10 min before the meal in order to achieve a target BG value $G_{t+10+\tau}$.

These recommendation scenarios were designed to align with decision-making situations commonly encountered by people with type 1 diabetes. In particular, the corresponding recommendation systems would help an individual to estimate how much to eat or bolus for the purpose of raising or lowering their BGL (scenarios 1 and 2, respectively), as well as how much to bolus for a planned meal (scenario 3).

In the following section, we describe a number of baseline models and neural architectures using Long Short-Term Memory (LSTM) networks, all implementing the three types of recommendations. The LSTM-based models will be trained on examples extracted from the OhioT1DM dataset [9], as explained in Sect. 4. Ideally, to match the intended use of these recommendations in practice, training examples should not have any extra meals or boluses in the prediction window $[t, t + 10 + \tau]$. Following the terminology from [11], we call these examples *inertial*. However, to benefit from a larger number of training examples, we also train models on a more general class of *unrestricted* examples, in which other bolus or meal events are allowed to appear in the prediction window. In Sect. 5.1, we show the extent to which models trained on the larger set of unrestricted examples transfer to inertial examples.

3 Baseline Models and Neural Architectures

Given training data containing time series of blood glucose levels, meals with their carbohydrate intake, and boluses with their corresponding insulin dosages, we define the following two baselines:

1. **Global average**: For the carbohydrate recommendation scenario, the average number μ of carbs over all of the meals in the subject's training data is computed and used as the estimate for all future predictions for that subject, irrespective of the context of the example. Analogously, for the bolus and bolus given carbs recommendation scenarios, μ is the average amount of insulin dosage over all boluses in the subject's training data. This is a fairly simple baseline, as it predicts the same average value for every test example for a particular subject.
2. **ToD average**: In this Time-of-Day (ToD) dependent baseline, an average number of carbs or an average amount of bolus insulin is computed for each of the following five time windows during a day:

   - 12am–6am: μ_1 = early breakfast/late snacks.
   - 6am–10am: μ_2 = breakfast.
   - 10am–2pm: μ_3 = lunch.
   - 2pm–6pm: μ_4 = dinner.
   - 6pm–12am: μ_5 = late dinner/post-dinner snacks.

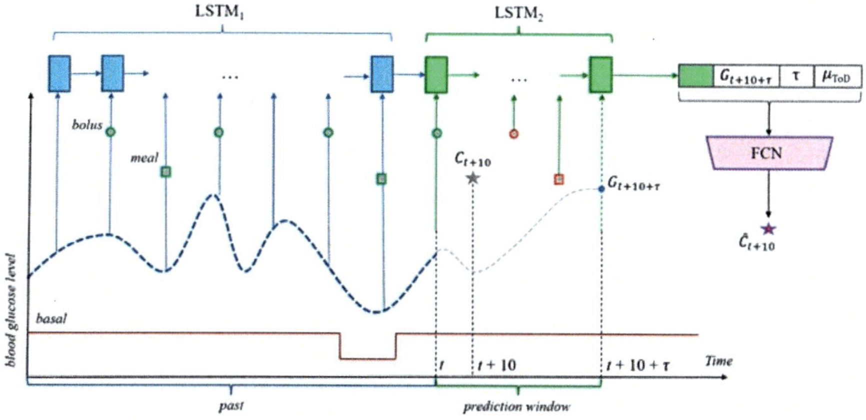

Fig. 1 The general neural network architecture for the carbohydrate recommendation scenario. The dashed blue line in the graph represents a subject's BGL, while the solid brown line represents the basal rate of insulin. The gray star represents the meal at $t + 10$. The other meals are represented by squares, and boluses are represented by circles. Meals and boluses with a red outline cannot appear in *inertial* examples, but are allowed in *unrestricted* examples. The blue units in $LSTM_1$ receive input from different time steps in the past. The green units in $LSTM_2$ receive input from the prediction window. The purple trapezoid represents the 5 fully connected layers, whereas the output node at the end computes the prediction

> The average for each ToD interval is calculated over all of the meals or boluses appearing in the corresponding time frame in the subject's training data. At test time, to make a recommendation for time $t + 10$, we first determine the ToD interval that contains $t + 10$ and output the corresponding ToD average.

Given sufficient historical data, the ToD baseline is expected to perform well for individuals who tend to eat very consistently and have regular diets. However, it is expected to perform poorly for individuals who have a lot of variation in their diets.

For the bolus given carbs recommendation scenario, one may ask why not also implement and evaluate a bolus calculator "baseline", for which insulin dosages would be computed using the actual bolus calculator employed by the subjects in the OhioT1DM dataset every time they had a meal. However, assuming subjects had perfect adherence to using the bolus calculator, this "baseline" would coincide with the ground truth every time, making it inappropriate as a baseline.

While simple to compute and use at test time, the two baselines are likely to give suboptimal performance, as their predictions ignore the history of BGL values, insulin (boluses and basal rates), and meals, all of which could significantly modulate the effect a future meal and/or bolus might have on the BGL. To exploit this information, we use the general LSTM-based network architecture shown in Fig. 1. The first component in the architecture is a recurrent neural network instantiated using Long Short-Term Memory (LSTM) cells [7], which is run over the previous 6 h of data, up to and including the present time t. At each time step (every 5 min), this $LSTM_1$ network takes as input the BGL, the carbs, and the insulin dosages recorded at that

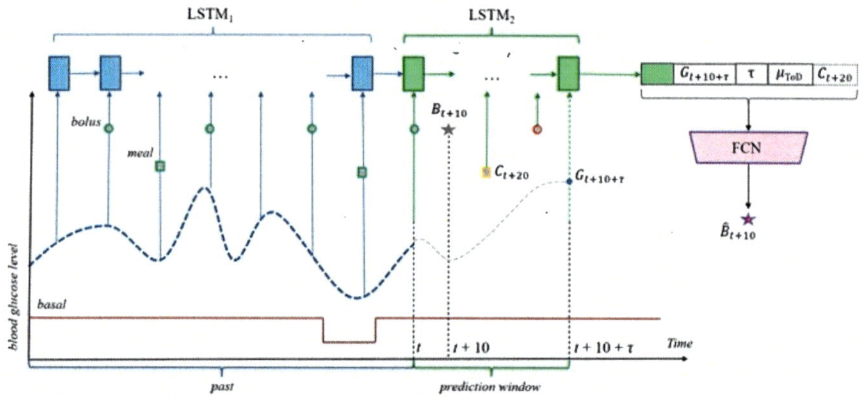

Fig. 2 The general neural network architecture for the bolus and bolus given carbs recommendation scenarios. The architecture itself is similar to that of Fig. 1. The gray star now represents the bolus at $t + 10$. For the bolus recommendation scenario, the events outlined in red or orange are not allowed in *inertial* examples. However, in the bolus given carbs scenario, the meal event C_{t+20} shown with the yellow outline is an important part of each example, be it inertial or unrestricted. As such, in this scenario, the dashed C_{t+20} becomes part of the input to the FCN

time step. While sufficient for processing *inertial* examples, this LSTM cannot be used to process events that may appear in the prediction window $(t, t + 10 + \tau)$ of *unrestricted* examples, because BGL values are not available in the future. Therefore, when training on unrestricted examples, the final state computed by the LSTM_1 model at time t is projected using a linear transformation and used as the initial state for a second LSTM model, LSTM_2, that is run over all the time steps in the prediction window $(t, t + 10 + \tau)$. The final state computed either by LSTM_1 (for inertial examples) or LSTM_2 (for unrestricted examples) is then used as input to a fully connected network (FCN) whose output node computes an estimate of the carbs or bolus insulin at time $t + 10$. In addition to the LSTM final state, the input to the FCN contains the following features:

- The target blood glucose level $\tau + 10$ minutes into the future, i.e., $G_{t+10+\tau}$.
- The prediction horizon τ.
- The ToD average for the time frame that contains $t + 10$.
- For the bolus given carbs scenario only, the planned amount C_{t+20} of carbohydrate becomes part of the input, too.

Each LSTM uses vectors of size 32 for the states and gates, whereas the FCN is built with 5 hidden layers, each consisting of 64 ReLU neurons, and one linear output node.

4 Using the OhioT1DM Dataset for Recommendation Examples

To evaluate the proposed recommendation models, we create training and test examples based on data collected from 6 subjects with type 1 diabetes that is distributed with the OhioT1DM dataset [10]. Time series containing the basal rate of insulin, boluses, meals, and BGL readings were collected over roughly 50 days, although the exact number of days varies from subject to subject. Insulin and BGL data was automatically recorded by each subject's insulin pump. Meal data was collected in two different ways. Subjects self-reported meal times and estimated carbs via a smartphone interface. Subjects also entered estimated carbs into a "Bolus Wizard," or calculator, when bolusing for meals, and this data was recorded by the insulin pump.

While exploring the data, it was observed that self-reported meals and their associated boluses were in unexpected temporal positions relative to each other. For many meals, patients recorded a timestamp in the smartphone interface that preceded the corresponding bolus timestamp recorded in the insulin pump. This was contrary to what was recommended to the subjects by their physicians, which was to bolus shortly before the meal, and no more than 15 min prior to the meal. This discrepancy is likely due to subjects reporting incorrect meal times in the smartphone interface.

Preprocessing of meals: To correct the meal events, we used the data input to the Bolus Wizard in the insulin pump and ran a preprocessing step that changed the timestamp of each meal associated with a bolus to be exactly 10 min after that bolus. For these meals, we also used the number of carbs provided to the Bolus Wizard, which is likely to be more accurate than the estimate provided by the subject through the smartphone interface. To determine the meal event that is associated with a bolus having non-zero carb input, we searched for the meal that was closest in time to the bolus, either before or after. In case there are 2 meals that are equally close to the bolus, we selected the one for which the number of carbs from the smartphone interface is closest to the number of carbs entered into the Bolus Wizard. Experimental results reported in Sect. 5.1 show that this preprocessing of meal events leads to significantly more accurate predictions, which indirectly justifies the preprocessing.

Table 1 shows the number of meals in each subject's preprocessed data, together with statistics such as the minimum, maximum, median, average, and standard deviation for the number of carbs per meal. Table 2 shows the same statistics for boluses and their dosages, expressed in units of insulin. The numbers in Table 1 show that most subjects have a similar average number of carbs in their meals, with the exception of 570 who has a significantly larger number of carbs per meal on average. More importantly, subject 570 also has a much higher standard deviation than the other subjects, which is likely to make the recommendation task more difficult in their case.

The number of boluses varies from subject to subject more so than the number of meals. Most subjects had similar average and standard deviations, with the exception of subject 563, who had a much larger average and standard deviation than the rest of

Table 1 Per subject and total meal and carbohydrate statistics: Minimum, Maximum, Median, Average, and Standard Deviation (StdDev)

	Carbs Per Meal					
Subject	Meals	Minimum	Maximum	Median	Average	StdDev
559	179	8.0	75.0	30.0	34.6	15.1
563	153	5.0	84.0	34.0	35.6	18.4
570	169	5.0	200.0	115.0	106.3	41.6
575	284	2.0	110.0	40.0	40.2	21.9
588	257	2.0	60.0	20.0	22.4	14.6
591	248	3.0	77.0	28.0	31.4	14.1
Total	1290	2.0	200.0	34.0	42.3	33.7

Table 2 Per subject and total boluses and insulin units statistics: Minimum, Maximum, Median, Average, and Standard Deviation (StdDev)

		Insulin Per Bolus				
Subject	Boluses	Minimum	Maximum	Median	Average	StdDev
559	186	0.1	9.3	3.6	3.7	1.9
563	424	0.1	24.7	7.8	8.0	4.2
570	1,345	0.2	12.1	1.3	1.8	2.1
575	271	0.1	12.8	4.4	4.1	3.0
588	221	0.4	10.0	3.5	4.3	2.3
591	331	0.1	9.4	2.9	3.1	1.8
Total	2758	0.1	24.7	1.9	3.5	3.4

the subjects. It is also interesting to note that subject 570 had a lower bolus average than most subjects and far more boluses than any of the others. Subject 570 used many dual boluses, which we did not include as prediction labels, since the scope of the project to date supports only recommendations for regular boluses.

4.1 *From Meals and Bolus Events to Recommendation Examples*

In all recommendation scenarios, the prediction window ranges between the present time t and the prediction horizon $t + 10 + \tau$. For the carbohydrate or bolus recommendation scenarios, the meal or the bolus is assumed to occur at time $t + 10$. For the bolus given carbs scenario, the bolus occurs at time $t + 10$ and is followed by a meal at time $t + 20$, which matches the preprocessing of the meal data. For evaluation purposes, we set τ to values between 30 and 90 min with a step of 5 min, i.e., $\tau \in \{30, 35, 40, ..., 90\}$ for a total of 13 different values. As such, each meal/bolus

Table 3 *Inertial* (*I*) examples by recommendation scenario and prediction horizon

Carbohydrate recommendation				
Horizon	Training	Validation	Testing	Total *I*
$\tau = 30$	700	190	168	1,058
$\tau = 45$	684	188	165	1,037
$\tau = 60$	664	181	163	1,008
$\tau = 75$	632	177	155	964
$\tau = 90$	597	170	150	917
All 13 horizons	8,546	2,356	2,088	12,990
Bolus recommendation				
$\tau = 30$	345	91	107	543
$\tau = 45$	324	88	101	513
$\tau = 60$	293	82	89	464
$\tau = 75$	258	76	81	415
$\tau = 90$	234	67	72	373
All 13 horizons	3,790	1,054	1,176	6,020
Bolus given carbs recommendation				
$\tau = 30$	488	143	142	773
$\tau = 45$	483	142	140	765
$\tau = 60$	474	139	139	752
$\tau = 75$	460	134	136	730
$\tau = 90$	444	133	130	707
All 13 horizons	6,118	1,799	1,789	9,706

event in the data results in 13 recommendation examples, one example for each value of τ. While all 13 examples use the same value for the prediction label, e.g., B_{t+10} for bolus prediction, they will differ in terms of the target BG feature $G_{t+10+\tau}$ and the τ feature, both used directly as input to the FCN module in the architectures shown in Figs. 1 and 2. For the bolus given carbs scenario, the 13 examples are only created when there is a meal that had a bolus delivered 10 min prior. Due to the way the data is preprocessed, it is guaranteed that if a meal had a bolus associated with it, the bolus will be exactly 10 min before the meal.

Table 3 shows the number of *inertial* examples for 5 prediction horizons, as well as the total overall 13 possible prediction horizons. Table 4 shows the number of *unrestricted* examples. Since the same number of *unrestricted* examples are available for every prediction horizon, only the totals are shown. The only exceptions would be if an event was near the end of a subject's data and the prediction horizon $t + 10 + \tau$ goes past the end of the dataset for some value of τ.

For the carbohydrate and bolus given carbs recommendation scenarios, the gap between the number of *inertial* and *unrestricted* examples is not very large, as most examples qualify as inertial examples. However, in the bolus recommendation sce-

Table 4 *Unrestricted* (U) examples by recommendation scenario. Also showing in the last column the total number of non-inertial ($U - I$) examples

Recommendation scenario	Training	Validation	Testing	Total U	Total $U - I$
Carbohydrate	10,899	2,964	2,665	16,528	3,538
Bolus	12,282	3,595	3,810	19,687	13,667
Bolus given carbs	7,407	2,236	2,276	11,919	2,213

nario, there is a very sizable gap between the number of inertial versus unrestricted examples. This is because a significant number of boluses are associated with meals, and since these meals are timestamped to be 10 min after the bolus, the result is that a bolus at time $t + 10$ will be associated with a meal at time $t + 20$. Therefore, for preprandial boluses at $t + 10$, the meal at time $t + 20$ will prohibit the creation of inertial recommendation examples, because by definition inertial examples do not allow the presence of other events in the prediction window $(t, t + 10 + \tau)$.

5 Experimental Methodology and Results

For each of the 6 subjects in the dataset, their time series data is split into three sets, as follows:

- *Testing*: the last 10 days of data.
- *Validation*: the 10 days of data preceding the testing portion.
- *Training*: the remainder of the data, around 30 days.

The blood glucose, carbs, and insulin values are all scaled to be between [0, 1] by using maximum and minimum values computed over training data. When computing the performance metrics at test time, the predicted values are scaled back to the original range. The neural architecture is trained to minimize the mean squared error between the actual event (meal or bolus) value recorded in the training data and the estimated value computed by the output node of the FCN module. The Adam [8] variant of gradient descent is used for training, with the learning rate and mini-batch size tuned on the validation data. To avoid overfitting, early stopping and dropout are used in all experiments. The early stopping has a patience of 10 epochs and the dropout rate is set to 10%.

Before training a personalized model for a specific subject, a generic model is first pretrained on the union of all 6 subjects' training data. The generic model is then fine-tuned separately for each individual subject, by continuing training on that subject's training data only. The pretraining allows the model parameters to be in a better starting position before fine-tuning, allowing faster and better training. The learning rate and batch size are tuned for each subject on their validation data. Once the hyper-parameters are tuned, the final models are then fine-tuned on the union of the training and validation data for each subject for a maximum of 100 epochs. For each subject, the results are aggregated over 5 models that are trained with different seedings of the random number generators.

The metrics used to evaluate the models are Root Mean Squared Error (RMSE) and Mean Absolute Error (MAE). Two scores are reported for each evaluation of the LSTM-based recommendation model:

1. The **Model.mean** score calculates the average RMSE and MAE on the testing data across the 5 models trained for each subject, and then averages these scores across all 6 subjects.
2. The **Model.best** score instead selects for each subject the model that performed best in terms of MAE on the validation data, out of the 5 models trained for that subject. The RMSE and MAE test scores are averaged over all 6 subjects.

Two sets of LSTM-based models were trained for each of the three recommendation scenarios: a set of models were trained and evaluated on *inertial* examples and a set was trained and evaluated on *unrestricted* examples. For the carbohydrate and bolus given carbs scenarios, there were no inertial examples in subject 570's testing data. To make the results comparable, subject 570 is not used for computing the results in these scenarios.

5.1 Experimental Results

Table 5 shows the results for the two baselines and the LSTM-based models. Across all scenarios and for both example classes, the neural models outperform both baselines by a wide margin. There also is very little difference between the best model scores and the average model scores, which means that the model performance is stable with respect to the random initialization of the network parameters.

Of the results reported in Table 5, the most relevant for practical scenarios are the evaluations on inertial examples; unrestricted examples subsume examples that contain information about future events, which is difficult to have in practice. However, the set of unrestricted examples is larger; as such, it has the potential to improve performance on inertial examples through transfer learning. To determine if and to what extent transfer happens, in Table 6 we compare LSTM-based models trained on *inertial* versus *unrestricted* examples, in terms of their performance on inertial examples. For the carbohydrate and bolus given carbs recommendation scenarios, the results show that training on the extra non-inertial examples provided by the unrestricted dataset helps achieve better performance on the inertial examples. However, this type of positive transfer does not happen in the bolus recommendation scenario, for which the models trained solely on inertial examples performed better. This can be explained by the fact that there are two types of bolus events: boluses associated with meals, which are intended to *proactively* prevent spikes in blood glucose due to carbs in the meals, and boluses that are administered *reactively* to lower already high blood glucose levels. The bolus recommendation entry in the last column of Table 4

Table 5 Results for each recommendation scenario, for both classes of examples

	Inertial		Unrestricted	
Carbohydrate recommendation	RMSE	MAE	RMSE	MAE
Global average	16.58	13.66	16.54	13.65
ToD average	15.91	12.92	15.96	12.97
Model.mean	**9.61**	7.32	**9.37**	**7.00**
Model.best	9.68	**7.09**	9.88	7.24
Bolus recommendation	RMSE	MAE	RMSE	MAE
Global average	2.19	1.87	3.05	2.51
ToD average	2.28	1.82	2.97	2.38
Model.mean	**1.64**	1.22	**1.54**	**1.14**
Model.best	**1.64**	**1.20**	1.58	1.17
Bolus given carbs recommendation	RMSE	MAE	RMSE	MAE
Global average	2.64	2.23	2.67	2.25
ToD average	2.55	2.08	2.56	2.10
Model.mean	1.18	0.93	1.10	0.81
Model.best	**1.17**	**0.89**	**1.06**	**0.77**

Table 6 Comparison between models trained on Inertial versus Unrestricted examples, in terms of their performance on Inertial examples

		Trained on	RMSE	MAE
Carbohydrate recommendation	Model.mean	Inertial	9.61	7.32
		Unrestricted	**9.35**	**7.01**
	Model.best	Inertial	9.68	7.09
		Unrestricted	9.70	7.13
Bolus recommendation	Model.mean	Inertial	**1.64**	**1.22**
		Unrestricted	1.77	1.38
	Model.best	Inertial	**1.64**	**1.20**
		Unrestricted	1.85	1.46
Bolus given carbs recommendation	Model.mean	Inertial	1.18	0.93
		Unrestricted	**1.10**	**0.82**
	Model.best	Inertial	1.17	0.89
		Unrestricted	**1.07**	**0.78**

Table 7 Comparison between models trained on all prediction horizons versus one prediction horizon τ, when evaluated on the prediction horizon τ

		Carbohydrate recommendation											
		$\tau = 30$		$\tau = 45$		$\tau = 60$		$\tau = 75$		$\tau = 90$		Average	
	Trained on	RMSE	MAE	RMSE	MAE	RMSE	MAE	RMSE	MAE	RMSE	MAE	RMSE	MAE
Model.mean	One τ	11.43	8.40	12.04	8.96	11.69	8.57	11.90	9.01	11.96	9.25	11.80	8.84
	All τ	**10.79**	**8.08**	**10.56**	**7.77**	**10.44**	**7.69**	**10.84**	**7.96**	**10.69**	**7.93**	**10.66**	**7.89**
Model.best	One τ	11.17	8.34	11.83	8.57	11.46	8.28	11.77	8.63	11.58	8.80	11.56	8.52
	All τ	**10.87**	**8.15**	**10.79**	**7.75**	**10.44**	**7.54**	**10.71**	**7.83**	**10.66**	**7.84**	**10.69**	**7.82**
		Bolus recommendation											
Model.mean	One τ	1.70	1.21	1.65	1.18	1.58	1.18	1.59	1.17	1.64	1.20	1.63	1.19
	All τ	**1.53**	**1.11**	**1.49**	**1.10**	**1.52**	**1.12**	**1.56**	**1.15**	**1.56**	**1.16**	**1.53**	**1.13**
Model.best	One τ	1.69	1.19	1.64	1.17	**1.51**	1.14	1.57	1.16	1.58	1.15	1.60	1.16
	All τ	**1.54**	**1.09**	**1.50**	**1.09**	**1.51**	**1.11**	**1.54**	**1.13**	**1.53**	**1.14**	**1.52**	**1.11**
		Bolus given carbs recommendation											
Model.mean	One τ	**1.07**	**0.83**	**1.11**	**0.84**	**1.12**	**0.85**	1.17	0.90	**1.13**	0.87	**1.12**	0.86
	All τ	1.13	0.85	1.13	0.84	1.14	0.85	**1.15**	**0.86**	**1.13**	**0.86**	1.14	**0.85**
Model.best	One τ	**1.07**	**0.82**	1.13	0.85	**1.12**	0.84	1.15	0.90	1.15	0.90	**1.12**	0.86
	All τ	1.11	0.83	**1.12**	**0.83**	**1.12**	**0.82**	**1.12**	**0.82**	**1.10**	**0.83**	**1.12**	**0.83**

Table 8 Results with and without preprocessing of meals, for carbohydrate and bolus recommendation scenarios on unrestricted examples

	Carbohydrate recommendation		
	Preprocess	RMSE	MAE
Model.mean	No	22.45	12.52
	Yes	**9.37**	**7.00**
Model.best	No	23.86	13.08
	Yes	**9.88**	**7.24**
	Bolus recommendation		
Model.mean	No	1.93	1.42
	Yes	**1.54**	**1.14**
Model.best	No	1.97	1.43
	Yes	**1.58**	**1.17**

shows that the preprandial, proactive bolus examples represent the vast majority of unrestricted bolus examples: i.e., 13,667 out of 19,687, which is more than twice the 6,020 inertial, reactive bolus examples shown in Table 3. As such, a bolus recommendation model that is trained on unrestricted bolus examples is likely to be biased toward preprandial boluses for which the blood glucose behavior is different compared with the inertial, reactive boluses on which the model is evaluated.

In all experiments reported so far, one model was trained for all prediction horizons, using the value of $\tau \in \{30, 35, ..., 90\}$ as an additional input feature for the FCN component. This global mode was then tested on examples from all prediction horizons. To determine if transfer learning also happens among different prediction horizons, for each value of $\tau \in \{30, 45, 60, 75, 90\}$ at test time, we compare the performance of the globally trained model versus the performance of a model trained only on examples for that particular prediction horizon, using unrestricted examples for both. The results in Table 7 show transfer learning clearly happening for the carbohydrate and bolus recommendation scenarios, where the models trained on all prediction horizons outperform those trained only on a specific prediction horizon when evaluated on that prediction horizon. For the bolus given carbs prediction scenario, the results are roughly the same.

Finally, Table 8 shows the results of training models on unrestricted examples in the carbohydrate and bolus recommendation scenarios, with and without the preprocessing of meals described in Sect. 4. The results show substantial improvement when preprocessing is done, especially for the carbohydrate recommendation scenario. The fact that the models are able to perform much better when the meals are preprocessed in this way indicates that the timestamps recorded in the smartphone interface are very unreliable and meal times should instead be anchored to the bolus timestamps recorded by the Bolus Wizard in the insulin pump, as done by the preprocessing procedure.

6 Conclusion

We introduced a general neural architecture, composed of two chained LSTMs and a fully connected network, with the purpose of training models for making recommendations with respect to any type of quantitative events that may impact blood glucose levels, in particular, meal carbohydrate amounts and bolus insulin dosages. Experimental evaluations show that the proposed architecture substantially outperforms the baselines. The trained models are shown to benefit from transfer learning and from a preprocessing of meal events that anchors their timestamps shortly after their corresponding boluses. Overall, the results suggest that this novel approach could potentially be of significant use in easing the complex task of self-managing blood glucose levels for people with type 1 diabetes.

Acknowledgements This work was supported by grant 1R21EB022356 from National Institutes of Health (NIH). Conversations with Josep Vehi helped shape the research directions presented herein. The contributions of physician collaborators Frank Schwartz, MD, and Amber Healy, DO, are gratefully acknowledged. We would also like to thank the anonymous people with type 1 diabetes who provided their blood glucose, insulin, and meal data.

References

1. Bach, K., Bunescu, R., Farri, O., Guo, A., Hasan, S., Ibrahim, Z.M., Marling, C., Raffa, J., Rubin, J., Wu, H. (eds.): Proceedings of the 3rd International Workshop on Knowledge Discovery in Healthcare Data. CEUR-WS.org, Stockholm, Sweden (2018). http://ceur-ws.org/Vol-2148/
2. Bach, K., Bunescu, R., Marling, C., Wiratunga, N. (eds.): Proceedings of the 5th International Workshop on Knowledge Discovery in Healthcare Data. Santiago de Compostela, Spain (2020). In press
3. Beauchamp, J., Bunescu, R., Marling, C.: A general neural architecture for carbohydrate and bolus recommendations in type 1 diabetes management. In: The 5th International Workshop on Knowledge Discovery in Healthcare Data. Santiago de Compostela, Spain (2020). In press
4. Boutayeb, A., Chetouani, A.: A critical review of mathematical models and data used in diabetology. BioMed. Eng. OnLine **5**(43), (2006)
5. Bunescu, R., Struble, N., Marling, C., Shubrook, J., Schwartz, F.: Blood glucose level prediction using physiological models and support vector regression. In: Proceedings of the Twelfth International Conference on Machine Learning and Applications (ICMLA), pp. 135–140. IEEE Press (2013)
6. Cappon, G., Vettoretti, M., Marturano, F., Facchinetti, A., Sparacino, G.: A neural-network-based approach to personalize insulin bolus calculation using continuous glucose monitoring. J. Diabet. Sci. Technol. **12**(2), 265–272 (2018)
7. Hochreiter, S., Schmidhuber, J.: Long short-term memory. Neural Comput. **9**, 1735–1780 (1997). https://doi.org/10.1162/neco.1997.9.8.1735
8. Kingma, D.P., Ba, J.L.: Adam: a method for stochastic optimization. In: Third International Conference for Learning Representations (ICLR). San Diego, California (2015)
9. Marling, C., Bunescu, R.: The OhioT1DM dataset for blood glucose level prediction. In: The 3rd International Workshop on Knowledge Discovery in Healthcare Data. Stockholm, Sweden (2018). http://ceur-ws.org/Vol-2148/paper09.pdf

10. Marling, C., Bunescu, R.: The OhioT1DM dataset for blood glucose level prediction: Update 2020. In: The 5th International Workshop on Knowledge Discovery in Healthcare Data. Santiago de Compostela, Spain (2020). In press
11. Mirshekarian, S., Shen, H., Bunescu, R., Marling, C.: LSTMs and neural attention models for blood glucose prediction: Comparative experiments on real and synthetic data. In: Proceedings of the 41st International Conference of the IEEE Engineering in Medicine and Biology Society (EMBC 2019). Berlin, Germany (2019)
12. Mougiakakou, S.G., Nikita, K.S.: A neural network approach for insulin regime and dose adjustment in type 1 diabetes. Diabet. Technol. Ther. **2**(3), 381–389 (2000)
13. Plis, K., Bunescu, R., Marling, C., Shubrook, J., Schwartz, F.: A machine learning approach to predicting blood glucose levels for diabetes management. In: Modern Artificial Intelligence for Health Analytics: Papers Presented at the Twenty-Eighth AAAI Conference on Artificial Intelligence, pp. 35–39. AAAI Press (2014)
14. Sun, Q., Jankovic, M.V., Budzinski, J., Moore, B., Diem, P., Stettler, C., Mougiakakou, S.G.: A dual mode adaptive basal-bolus advisor based on reinforcement learning. IEEE J. Biomed. Health Inf. **23**(6), 2633–2641 (2019)
15. Walsh, J., Roberts, R., Bailey, T.S., Heinemann, L.: Bolus advisors: sources of error, targets for improvement. J. Diabet. Sci. Technol. **12**(1), 190–198 (2018)
16. Zisser, H.C., Robinson, L.T., Bevier, W., Dassau, E., Ellingsen, C.L., Doyle, F.J., Jovanovic, L.: Bolus calculator: a review of four "smart" insulin pumps. Diabet. Technol. Ther. **10**(6), 441–444 (2008)

Music Recommendation Systems: A Survey

Mariusz Kleć and Alicja Wieczorkowska

Abstract This introductory chapter presents an overview of music recommendation systems, supported by a comprehensive list of references. We pay special attention to user-centric systems which personalize their output by tracking the context of the user, including the user's emotions and personality. Besides, we emphasize the importance of social media, the usability of user interfaces and the application of deep learning techniques in the recent developments in music recommendation systems. We also outline inspirations for the future research in the field.

1 Introduction

The underlying purpose of Recommendation Systems (RS) is to help users to find appropriate items (such as books, news, products, websites, courses, music) from big repositories of data. Manual searching would be very ineffective. The music domain deserves special attention, as listening to short samples of songs to find an appropriate piece of music from thousands of titles is tiresome, frustrating and time-consuming. A great example is Spotify application, which has over 200 million active users monthly [61]. It gives access to more than 40 million tracks with the click of a button. That would give over 220 years of constant listening. Therefore, the process of searching musical content in a big data repository is a crucial concern for many researchers [39, 44].

A comprehensive study of currently existing Music RS (MRS) can be found in [58]. However, the heterogeneity and variety of approaches possible to implement in MRS continuously pose new challenges [69]. In this survey, we try to outline the diversity of these approaches and provide a survey and literature review through the recent advances in MRS and their applications. Since the music preferences can

M. Kleć (✉) · A. Wieczorkowska
Polish-Japanese Academy of Informtion Technology, Koszykowa 86, 02-008 Warsaw, Poland
e-mail: mklec@pjwstk.edu.pl

A. Wieczorkowska
e-mail: alicja@poljap.edu.pl

Z. W. Ras et al. (eds.), *Recommender Systems for Medicine and Music*,
Studies in Computational Intelligence 946,
https://doi.org/10.1007/978-3-030-66450-3_7

be inferred from a mood, time, activity, personality, place and other environmental factors [9, 71, 79], we decided to pay special attention to context-aware and user-centric MRS.

We performed the literature review by searching the ACM Digital Library, IEEE-explore and ScienceDirect databases. We also searched Google Scholar, as it provides results from a wide variety of other databases. We mainly choose Conference Proceedings and Journals published after 2016. The results of our bibliography search are shown in Table 1.

2 Music Recommendation Systems

Systems for automatic recommendation of music to users have become significant in the recent years, as we are facing the expansion of gigantic sets of music files. There-

Table 1 Literature review on Music Recommendation Systems with respect to keywords and search databases; 87% of these papers have been published after 2016

Keywords	ACM[a] (%)	IEEE[b] (%)	SD[c] (%)	Other[d] (%)	Literature
Review and current challenges	16	16	16	50	[11, 13, 41, 58, 68, 69]
Sequence modelling for playlists	38	44	0	16	[11, 13, 20, 27, 29, 35, 36, 44, 45, 60, 68, 69, 71, 74–76, 83, 84]
Deep learning	29	47	5	17	[2, 6, 12, 19, 21, 27–29, 34, 48, 57, 68, 71, 74, 76]
Cold start	40	10	10	40	[2, 12, 16, 25, 36, 57, 65, 69, 77, 83]
User interface	57	14	14	14	[5, 8, 16, 30, 37, 53]
Social context	50	33	0	16	[10, 14, 59, 60, 78, 79]
Personality context	53	6	0	40	[15, 16, 18, 25, 46, 49–51, 56, 59, 69, 73, 80]
Emotions context	20	40	10	30	[5, 6, 18, 21, 28, 48, 60, 69, 78, 79]
Physiological, activity, weather, time, text analysis and other contexts	29	41	11	17	[6, 7, 21, 26, 28, 35, 36, 42–44, 46, 50, 58, 69, 77, 79, 82]

[a]ACM Digital Library
[b]IEEEexplore
[c]ScienceDirect
[d]Google Scholar

fore, music recommender systems have been a topic of interest in the music information retrieval domain, starting approximately from the beginning of the twenty-first century, see [70] for a survey of early examples.

Music Recommendation Systems perform rating predictions for songs that suit the current music preference. They are closely related to content filtering and searching. An annual event called Music Information Retrieval (MIR) Evaluation eXchange (MIREX[1]) stimulates the development of MIR algorithms. These algorithms combine musicology, psychology, signal processing and machine learning. These areas are also reflected in the current development of MRS. Most of them rely on user-based Collaborative Filtering (CF), and Content-Based (CB) approaches.

The main advantage of CF is no need to store features and any metadata about recommended items. This approach is domain-independent and guarantees effective computation and easy maintenance [64]. However, it suffers some drawbacks. Namely, CF-based systems suffer from popularity bias. They tend to recommend popular music, and the effect of "surprise" is scarce [65]. Moreover, the small number of ratings produces poor predictions. The recommendation might not be even possible for a song that appears as a new item in the system and has not received ratings from others yet. This effect is known as Cold Start (CS) problem [64]. Many researchers try to overcome the CS problems by applying a variety of techniques [36, 57, 77]. However, the most popular approach to partially overcome these limitations is incorporating the CB approach. It compares the song features against a user's profile to calculate recommendations. These systems do not need ratings from others to start to operate. Therefore, the cold-start problem does not exist in this case. The most successful MRS systems in the market (Mufin,[2] Pandora,[3] Spotify,[4] Tidal,[5] Qobuz[6]) use hybrid approach, combining CF and CB approaches together. This strategy allows them to take advantage of the strengths of both approaches and eliminate their weaknesses which would occur when used separately.

The most common output from MRS is a playlist, defined as a finite set of songs, often in the form of an ordered list. People use different types of playlists for different activities such as driving, reading, working or working out [3, 82]. The main aim for which users create playlists is not only to satisfy their music expectations about the music itself but also about the order of songs [11]. The modelling of sequences of songs is an essential part of research [20, 27, 29, 45, 84].

The Automatic Playlist Continuation (APC) is a recent trend of research [13, 75, 76]. The goal of APC is to automatically generate a sequence of songs for an existing playlist so that they reflect the target characteristics of the original one. The user can enjoy a continuous and endless music session [60, 83]. The 2018 ACM

---

[1]http://www.music-ir.org/mirex/wiki/MIREX_HOME.

[2]https://www.mufin.com.

[3]https://www.pandora.com/.

[4]http://www.spotify.com.

[5]http://tidal.com.

[6]http://www.qobuz.com.

RecSys Challenge [13] evaluates and advances the current state-of-the-art in APC using a large-scale dataset released by Spotify [74, 76].

Recently, the Hidden Markov Model (HMM) also turned out to perform very well for sequence prediction [45]. The evaluation on a large-scale real-world dataset in a Kaggle[7] competition shows that the mixture model significantly outperforms traditional methods [45].

The paper [71] proposes a novel MRS, called MusicRecLSTM, which models the changes of music taste over time. They leverage modified LSTM network to learn the embeddings of both the user and the music (an embedding space is a low-dimensional space, in which similar items are close), based on the sequential data and the temporal context. The system also learns whether a user would tend to listen to a newly released piece of music at a specific time. Evaluations over three real-world datasets show that the system can provide high precision, compared to several state-of-the-art recommender systems.

Deep Learning (DL) is increasingly adopted in MRS. Researchers use DL for automatic feature learning from audio signals, or extracting metadata [27], finding latent factors from user-item rating data for CF models [2, 12], and for learning sequential patterns of songs from musical playlists [27, 74]. The latent factors are integrated into content-based and hybrid systems [19, 34, 68]. In [19], the authors propose the algorithm, Tunes Recommendation System (T-RECSYS), that uses CB and CF approaches as input to a deep classification model to produce an accurate recommendation with real-time prediction. They evaluate their approach with the data obtained from the ACM Recsys Challenge.

Convolutional Neural Networks (CNNs) have gained so much popularity after successful usage in image classification tasks that the authors of [12] applied a deep CNN to develop the emotion aware music recommendation system. To get correlation between the music and user data two approaches are combined: deep CNN, and weighted feature extraction. For the purpose of classification, latent features are extracted from audio by using deep CNN. Weighted feature extraction approach is used to get correlation between the music and the user data to finally generate user rating. User rating is generated by inverse document frequency and the term frequency weighted feature extraction approach. After that, emotion aware MRS recommends song based on user rating. The Million Song Dataset[8] is used for training in this paper. Based on the results, the system shows better performance than the content similarity based one.

Still, MRS are far from being perfect, due to a magnitude of factors that influence musical tastes and needs. To satisfy the users' musical need, the researchers need to take into account intrinsic, extrinsic and contextual aspects of the listener. Therefore, the next section focuses on the review of user-centric MRS, taking into account various types of contexts for personalizing the recommendations.

---

[7]https://www.kaggle.com/.

[8]http://millionsongdataset.com/.

3 Personalization of Music Recommendation Systems

The perception of music does not solely depend on the individual's listening history, but also on the user's context, such as emotional state [3], current activity [43], health (personal context) [7], location [3], time (physical context) [7], weather [42] or social activity (social context) [10, 78]. Therefore, recommendation strategies should go deeper into the very essence of the listener's needs, preferences and intentions of listening to music [9]. Furthermore, the musical taste might depend on gender, personality, education and the life experience of the listener [54]. Therefore, the subjective character of music enforces researchers to go beyond hybridizing CF and CB approaches with DL techniques [50]. The authors of [41] provide a comprehensive study of existing Context-Aware Music Recommendation Systems (CA-MRS). The article [69] highlights several promising newest trends in research, such as music recommendation inspired by the listener's personality and emotions [46, 59].

3.1 *Emotions*

Emotions play a crucial role in the motivation for listening to music and thus in MRS. Music helps people to improve their emotional regulation, achieve their self-awareness and express social relatedness [67]. In general, listeners use music to change emotions, or to sustain them [33]. Music can stimulate emotions in people; also, emotions can be identified in musical pieces [22, 23, 32, 62]. Tracking listener's emotions is one of the ways to improve the quality of recommendation [21]. It is usually achieved implicitly, by tracking the context (like keywords) from an extensive collection of documents written by users [26], or extracting the users' texts from social networks [48, 60]. Another approach is to derive emotions from the user's face using the mobile camera [21, 28], or from the signals obtained via wearable physiological sensors [6]. The authors of [21] identify the user's mood with an accuracy of 90.23%. They also classify the emotions perceived in music with 97.69% accuracy. Their system suggests songs to the user by mapping the user's emotions to the emotion type of the song, taking into consideration the preferences of the user.

3.2 *Personality*

The way people regulate their emotions depends not only on the current situation but also on their personality [81]. Users with different personalities tend to prefer different music [63]. Knowledge about the influence of personality traits on musical taste has been discussed in [38, 51, 63, 66].

Personality represents people's differences in their enduring emotional, interpersonal, experiential, attitudinal and motivational styles [31]. Most of the papers in this field focus on the Big-Five Factor Model [31, 55], which makes the results possible to interpret, and compare. This personality model defines personality as five factors: Openness to Experience, Conscientiousness, Extroversion, Agreeableness and Neuroticism. The discussion of the usability of this model in recommendation systems can be found in [73]. However, the main challenge is to identify the most efficient way of personality acquisition in MRS. In [16], the authors compared three personality acquisition variants and demonstrated that the explicit personality acquisition interface was preferred by most of the experiment participants in terms of satisfaction and ease of use. The most common and relatively short personality questionnaire is the Ten Item Personality Inventory (TIPI) [17]. The TIPI was also used in [46] to explore users' personality traits together with physiological signals recorded by a wearable, namely a wristband. Experiments with four regression algorithms show that personality features contributed significantly to the improvement of RS accuracy, while physiological features contributed less.

Knowledge on the influence of personality traits on musical taste was also exploited to improve the accuracy in the user similarity calculations and was used to address the cold-start problem [18, 24, 25]. In [25], the authors enhanced CF with personality information. They show that this approach can significantly improve the performance of the traditional rating-based CF in terms of the evaluation metrics Mean Absolute Error (MAE) and ROC (receiver operating characteristic curve, sensitivity vs. fall-out graph).

Since people's attitude towards new or diverse experiences varies considerably [72], the degree of diversity can also be personalized [80]. In [49], the authors proposed a system which incorporates the strategy of adjusting diversity of music recommendation, according to the user's personality. The authors of [56] implemented four MRSs and evaluated them on a sample of real users and real-world datasets. The experimental results show that MRSs which rely purely on users' personality information perform comparable or even better than state-of-the-art MRSs in terms of the diversity of recommendation.

3.3 Social Context

Nowadays, social media contain rich information about the user's frequent actions and may constitute a vast data mine for gathering information about similar interests between users. Users reveal much information about their lives during their interactions with others using mobile devices. This is an opportunity for researchers to gather contextual information instantly [10, 59, 60, 78].

In [14], the authors explore the effects of social influence on developing MRS. The experiments verify that this approach can outperform current state-of-the-art music recommendation methods substantially. Personality can also be derived from social media and utilized for music recommendation [59]. The article [79] utilizes social media context such as posts, comments and interactions for music recommendation to relax the user's mind, considering the current mood (happy, sad, calm and angry) extracted from the social media profile of the user. The songs are classified to moods based on the lyrics and audio of the songs.

3.4 New Interfaces

Recent work has unveiled the importance of recommendation explanation and transparency [40, 52, 53], especially regarding User Experience (UX) [4, 5, 8, 30, 37]. One of the most exciting trends is the rise of smart assistants from some of the world's largest technology companies, such as Apple's Siri,[9] Google Assistant[10] and Amazon Alexa [47]. The companies have integrated voice recognition technology into their products, as a way of interacting with users. Amazon's Alexa is a crucial feature for the company's music[11] and their smart speakers, the Amazon Echo [47]. Amazon Echo is, somewhat controversially, equipped with the functionality enabling this device to listen to contextual information in the user's environment, such as conversations and background music. However, this information is used to infer mood and music preferences which enable the device to recommend songs to the user. Additionally, voice recognition allows users to use a more intuitive way of music search. For example, the user may say that she or he wants to listen to happy funk from the 1980s. The user might not know the best tunes from that era, but the system will recommend her or him the song that suits the voice query and surroundings. With the context of this survey, the authors see an expressive potential of incorporating voice assistants, together with music recommendation, to help people to get therapeutic music in medical care places and users' homes.

3.5 Automatic Music Generation

Throughout history, the vast majority of music we consume was written by another human being. However, recently computers start to compose music that is difficult to distinguish from those composed by humans. The automatically generated music has started to be recommended by Spotify. Just like AiMi[12] generates electronic music for personal purposes and AIVA[13] which generates soundtrack for a podcast of short movies, it is not difficult to imagine a system that generates therapeutic musical compositions with the helpful impact on our health, and adjust the music for ongoing therapy. The example of such systems are ENDEL,[14] which provides

[9]https://www.apple.com/siri/.

[10]https://assistant.google.com/.

[11]https://www.amazon.com/music/.

[12]https://aimi.fm/.

[13]https://www.aiva.ai/.

[14]https://www.endel.io/.

personalized sound environments to help the user to focus, and Tinnitracks system that was designed to treat tinnitus with music [1].

4 Summary

Music recommendation systems are becoming more and more popular. The environmental factors that influence the perception of music are pervasive and varied. Including all of them in the music recommendation system is still a big challenge and difficult to evaluate. Nevertheless, the increasing amount of personal data left by users on social media, together with the recent development of deep learning techniques, contribute to more accurate inference of the user's musical preferences implicitly. The knowledge on this topic is still being expanded. Environmental factors that induce musical preferences and needs are wider utilized these days. Still, we see a significant potential for this kind of data. We hope that this survey will contribute to the future development of user-centric and context-aware music recommendation systems.

References

1. Tinnitracks: Treat Tinnitus with your favorite music! 6 July 2020. https://www.tinnitracks.com/en
2. Aljunid, M.F., Dh, M.: An efficient deep learning approach for collaborative filtering recommender system. Procedia Comput. Sci. **171**, 829–836 (2020)
3. Álvarez, P., Zarazaga-Soria, F., Baldassarri, S.: Mobile music recommendations for runners based on location and emotions: the DJ-running system. Pervasive Mob. Comput. **101242** (2020)
4. Alves, T., Natálio, J., Henriques-Calado, J., Gama, S.: Incorporating personality in user interface design: a review. Personal. Individ. Diff. **155**, 109709 (2020)
5. Andjelkovic, I., Parra, D., O'Donovan, J.: Moodplay: interactive music recommendation based on artists' mood similarity. Int. J. Hum.-Comput. Stud. **121**, 142–159 (2019)
6. Ayata, D., Yaslan, Y., Kamasak, M.E.: Emotion based music recommendation system using wearable physiological sensors. IEEE Trans. Consum. Electron. **64**(2), 196–203 (2018)
7. Bai, K., Kawagoe, K.: Background music recommendation system based on user's heart rate and elapsed time. In: Proceedings of the 2018 10th International Conference on Computer and Automation Engineering, pp. 49–52 (2018)
8. Baig, M.H., Varghese, J.R., Wang, Z.: Musicmapp: a deep learning based solution for music exploration and visual interaction. In: Proceedings of the 26th ACM International Conference on Multimedia, pp. 1253–1255 (2018)
9. Bauer, C., Novotny, A.: A consolidated view of context for intelligent systems. J. Amb. Intell. Smart Environ. **9**(4), 377–393 (2017)
10. Bauer, C., Schedl, M.: Cross-country user connections in an online social network for music. In: Extended Abstracts of the 2019 CHI Conference on Human Factors in Computing Systems, pp. 1–6 (2019)
11. Bonnin, G., Jannach, D.: Automated generation of music playlists: survey and experiments. ACM Comput. Surv. (CSUR) **47**(2), 1–35 (2014)

12. Chang, S.H., Abdul, A., Chen, J., Liao, H.Y.: A personalized music recommendation system using convolutional neural networks approach. In: 2018 IEEE International Conference on Applied System Invention (ICASI), pp. 47–49. IEEE (2018)
13. Chen, C.W., Lamere, P., Schedl, M., Zamani, H.: Recsys challenge 2018: automatic music playlist continuation. In: Proceedings of the 12th ACM Conference on Recommender Systems, pp. 527–528 (2018)
14. Chen, J., Ying, P., Zou, M.: Improving music recommendation by incorporating social influence. Multimed. Tools Appl. **78**(3), 2667–2687 (2019)
15. Cheng, R., Tang, B.: A music recommendation system based on acoustic features and user personalities. In: Pacific-Asia Conference on Knowledge Discovery and Data Mining, pp. 203–213. Springer (2016)
16. Dunn, G., Wiersema, J., Ham, J., Aroyo, L.: Evaluating interface variants on personality acquisition for recommender systems. In: International Conference on User Modeling, Adaptation, and Personalization, pp. 259–270. Springer (2009)
17. Ehrhart, M.G., Ehrhart, K.H., Roesch, S.C., Chung-Herrera, B.G., Nadler, K., Bradshaw, K.: Testing the latent factor structure and construct validity of the ten-item personality inventory. Personal. Individ. Diff. **47**(8), 900–905 (2009)
18. Ferwerda, B., Schedl, M.: Enhancing music recommender systems with personality information and emotional states: a proposal. In: Umap workshops (2014)
19. Fessahaye, F., Perez, L., Zhan, T., Zhang, R., Fossier, C., Markarian, R., Chiu, C., Zhan, J., Gewali, L., Oh, P.: T-recsys: a novel music recommendation system using deep learning. In: 2019 IEEE International Conference on Consumer Electronics (ICCE), pp. 1–6. IEEE (2019)
20. Furini, M., Martini, J., Montangero, M.: Automated generation of user-tailored and time-sensitive music playlists. In: 2019 16th IEEE Annual Consumer Communications & Networking Conference (CCNC), pp. 1–6. IEEE (2019)
21. Gilda, S., Zafar, H., Soni, C., Waghurdekar, K.: Smart music player integrating facial emotion recognition and music mood recommendation. In: 2017 International Conference on Wireless Communications, Signal Processing and Networking (WiSPNET), pp. 154–158. IEEE (2017)
22. Grekow, J.: From Content-based Music Emotion Recognition to Emotion Maps of Musical Pieces. Studies in Computational Intelligence, vol. 747. Springer (2018)
23. Grekow, J.: Musical performance analysis in terms of emotions it evokes. J. Intell. Inform. Syst. **51**(2), 415–437 (2018)
24. Hu, R., Pu, P.: A study on user perception of personality-based recommender systems. In: International conference on user modeling, adaptation, and personalization, pp. 291–302. Springer (2010)
25. Hu, R., Pu, P.: Enhancing collaborative filtering systems with personality information. In: Proceedings of the fifth ACM conference on Recommender systems, pp. 197–204 (2011)
26. Hyung, Z., Park, J.S., Lee, K.: Utilizing context-relevant keywords extracted from a large collection of user-generated documents for music discovery. Inform. Process. Manag. **53**(5), 1185–1200 (2017)
27. Irene, R.T., Borrelli, C., Zanoni, M., Buccoli, M., Sarti, A.: Automatic playlist generation using convolutional neural networks and recurrent neural networks. In: 2019 27th European Signal Processing Conference (EUSIPCO), pp. 1–5. IEEE (2019)
28. Iyer, A.V., Pasad, V., Sankhe, S.R., Prajapati, K.: Emotion based mood enhancing music recommendation. In: 2017 2nd IEEE International Conference on Recent Trends in Electronics, Information & Communication Technology (RTEICT), pp. 1573–1577. IEEE (2017)
29. Jiang, M., Yang, Z., Zhao, C.: What to play next? A RNN-based music recommendation system. In: 2017 51st Asilomar Conference on Signals, Systems, and Computers, pp. 356–358. IEEE (2017)
30. Jin, Y., Tintarev, N., Verbert, K.: Effects of individual traits on diversity-aware music recommender user interfaces. In: Proceedings of the 26th Conference on User Modeling, Adaptation and Personalization, pp. 291–299 (2018)
31. John, O.P., Srivastava, S.: The big five trait taxonomy: history, measurement, and theoretical perspectives. Handb. Personal.: Theory Res. **2**(1999), 102–138 (1999)

32. Juslin, P.N., Laukka, P.: Expression, perception, and induction of musical emotions: a review and a questionnaire study of everyday listening. J. New Music Res. **33**(3), 217–238 (2004)
33. Juslin, P.N., Sloboda, J.: Handbook of Music and Emotion: Theory, Research. Oxford University Press, Applications (2011)
34. Khoali, M., Tali, A., Laaziz, Y.: Advanced recommendation systems through deep learning. In: Proceedings of the 3rd International Conference on Networking, Information Systems & Security, pp. 1–8 (2020)
35. Kim, H.G., Kim, G.Y., Kim, J.Y.: Music recommendation system using human activity recognition from accelerometer data. IEEE Trans. Consum. Electron. **65**(3), 349–358 (2019)
36. Kim, J., Won, M., Liem, C.C., Hanjalic, A.: Towards seed-free music playlist generation: enhancing collaborative filtering with playlist title information. Proc. ACM Recommend. Syst. Challenge **2018**, 1–6 (2018)
37. Kittimathaveenan, K., Pongskul, C., Mahatanarat, S.: Music recommendation based on color. In: 2020 6th International Conference on Engineering, Applied Sciences and Technology (ICEAST), pp. 1–4. IEEE (2020)
38. Kleć, M.: The influence of listener personality on music choices. Comput. Sci. **18** (2017)
39. Kostek, B.: Wspomaganie procesu wyszukiwania nagrań w repozytoriach muzycznych. Przegląd Telekomunikacyjny+ Wiadomości Telekomunikacyjne (6), 200–205 (2011)
40. Kouki, P., Schaffer, J., Pujara, J., O'Donovan, J., Getoor, L.: Personalized explanations for hybrid recommender systems. In: Proceedings of the 24th International Conference on Intelligent User Interfaces, pp. 379–390 (2019)
41. Kulkarni, S., Rodd, S.F.: Context aware recommendation systems: a review of the state of the art techniques. Comput. Sci. Rev. **37**, 100255 (2020)
42. Lavanya, S., Saranya, G., Navin, K.: Weather based playlist generation in mobile devices using hash map. In: 2017 International Conference on IoT and Application (ICIOT), pp. 1–7. IEEE (2017)
43. Lee, W.P., Chen, C.T., Huang, J.Y., Liang, J.Y.: A smartphone-based activity-aware system for music streaming recommendation. Knowl.-Based Syst. **131**, 70–82 (2017)
44. Leung, C.K., Kajal, A., Won, Y., Choi, J.M.: Big data analytics for personalized recommendation systems. In: 2019 IEEE International Conference on Dependable, Autonomic and Secure Computing, International Conference on Pervasive Intelligence and Computing, International Conference on Cloud and Big Data Computing, International Conference on Cyber Science and Technology Congress (DASC/PiCom/CBDCom/CyberSciTech), pp. 1060–1065. IEEE (2019)
45. Li, T., Choi, M., Fu, K., Lin, L.: Music sequence prediction with mixture hidden markov models. In: 2019 IEEE International Conference on Big Data (Big Data), pp. 6128–6132. IEEE (2019)
46. Liu, R., Hu, X.: A multimodal music recommendation system with listeners' personality and physiological signals. Proceedings of the ACM/IEEE Joint Conference on Digital Libraries **2020**, 357–360 (2020)
47. Lopatovska, I., Rink, K., Knight, I., Raines, K., Cosenza, K., Williams, H., Sorsche, P., Hirsch, D., Li, Q., Martinez, A.: Talk to me: exploring user interactions with the Amazon Alexa. J. Librarianship Inform. Sci. **51**(4), 984–997 (2019)
48. Lopes, P.S., Lasmar, E.L., Rosa, R.L., Rodríguez, D.Z.: The use of the convolutional neural network as an emotion classifier in a music recommendation system. In: Proceedings of the XIV Brazilian Symposium on Information Systems, pp. 1–8 (2018)
49. Lu, F., Tintarev, N.: A diversity adjusting strategy with personality for music recommendation. In: IntRS@ RecSys, pp. 7–14 (2018)
50. Lytvyn, V., Vysotska, V., Shatskykh, V., Kohut, I., Petruchenko, O., Dzyubyk, L., Bobrivetc, V., Panasyuk, V., Sachenko, S., Komar, M.: Design of a recommendation system based on collaborative filtering and machine learning considering personal needs of the user. East. Eur. J. Adv. Technol. **4**(2), 6–28 (2019)
51. Melchiorre, A.B., Schedl, M.: Personality correlates of music audio preferences for modelling music listeners. In: Proceedings of the 28th ACM Conference on User Modeling, Adaptation and Personalization, pp. 313–317 (2020)

52. Millecamp, M., Htun, N.N., Conati, C., Verbert, K.: To explain or not to explain: the effects of personal characteristics when explaining music recommendations. In: Proceedings of the 24th International Conference on Intelligent User Interfaces, pp. 397–407 (2019)
53. Millecamp, M., Htun, N.N., Conati, C., Verbert, K.: What's in a user? Towards personalising transparency for music recommender interfaces. In: Proceedings of the 28th ACM Conference on User Modeling, Adaptation and Personalization, pp. 173–182 (2020)
54. North, A.C., Hargreaves, D.J.: Situational influences on reported musical preference. Psychomusicol.: J. Res. Music Cogn. **15**(1–2), 30 (1996)
55. Nunes, M.A.S.N.: Recommender systems based on personality traits. Ph.D. thesis (2008)
56. Onori, M., Micarelli, A., Sansonetti, G.: A comparative analysis of personality-based music recommender systems. In: Empire@ RecSys, pp. 55–59 (2016)
57. Oramas, S., Nieto, O., Sordo, M., Serra, X.: A deep multimodal approach for cold-start music recommendation. In: Proceedings of the 2nd Workshop on Deep Learning for Recommender Systems, pp. 32–37 (2017)
58. Patel, A., Wadhvani, R.: A comparative study of music recommendation systems. In: 2018 IEEE International Students' Conference on Electrical, Electronics and Computer Science (SCEECS), pp. 1–4. IEEE (2018)
59. Paudel, A., Bajracharya, B.R., Ghimire, M., Bhattarai, N., Baral, D.S.: Using personality traits information from social media for music recommendation. In: 2018 IEEE 3rd International Conference on Computing, Communication and Security (ICCCS), pp. 116–121. IEEE (2018)
60. Polignano, M., Basile, P., de Gemmis, M., Semeraro, G.: Social tags and emotions as main features for the next song to play in automatic playlist continuation. In: Adjunct Publication of the 27th Conference on User Modeling, Adaptation and Personalization, pp. 235–239 (2019)
61. Prey, R.: Nothing personal: algorithmic individuation on music streaming platforms. Media, Cult. Soc. **40**(7), 1086–1100 (2018)
62. Raś, Z.W., Wieczorkowska, A.A. (eds.): Advances in Music Information Retrieval. Studies in Computational Intelligence, vol. 274. Springer (2010)
63. Rentfrow, P.J., Gosling, S.D.: The do re mi's of everyday life: the structure and personality correlates of music preferences. J. Personal. Soc. Psychol. **84**(6), 1236 (2003)
64. Resnick, P., Varian, H.R.: Recommender systems. Commun. ACM **40**(3), 56–58 (1997)
65. Schafer, J.B., Frankowski, D., Herlocker, J., Sen, S.: Collaborative filtering recommender systems. In: The Adaptive Web, pp. 291–324. Springer (2007)
66. Schäfer, T., Mehlhorn, C.: Can personality traits predict musical style preferences? A meta-analysis. Personal. Individ. Diff. **116**, 265–273 (2017)
67. Schäfer, T., Sedlmeier, P., Städtler, C., Huron, D.: The psychological functions of music listening. Front. Psychol. **4**, 511 (2013)
68. Schedl, M.: Deep learning in music recommendation systems. Front. Appl. Math. Stat. **5**, 44 (2019)
69. Schedl, M., Zamani, H., Chen, C.W., Deldjoo, Y., Elahi, M.: Current challenges and visions in music recommender systems research. Int. J. Multimed. Inform. Retrieval **7**(2), 95–116 (2018)
70. Song, Y., Dixon, S., Pearce, M.: A survey of music recommendation systems and future perspectives. In: 9th International Symposium on Computer Music Modelling and Retrieval (CMMR 2012), pp. 395–410. Queen Mary University of London (2012)
71. Tao, Y., Zhang, Y., Bian, K.: Attentive context-aware music recommendation. In: 2019 IEEE Fourth International Conference on Data Science in Cyberspace (DSC), pp. 54–61. IEEE (2019)
72. Tintarev, N., Dennis, M., Masthoff, J.: Adapting recommendation diversity to openness to experience: a study of human behaviour. In: International Conference on User Modeling, Adaptation, and Personalization, pp. 190–202. Springer (2013)
73. Tkalcic, M., Chen, L.: Personality and recommender systems. In: Recommender Systems Handbook, pp. 715–739. Springer (2015)
74. Vagliano, I., Galke, L., Mai, F., Scherp, A.: Using adversarial autoencoders for multi-modal automatic playlist continuation. Proc. ACM Recommend. Syst. Challenge **2018**, 1–6 (2018)
75. Vall, A., Dorfer, M., Schedl, M., Widmer, G.: A hybrid approach to music playlist continuation based on playlist-song membership. In: Proceedings of the 33rd Annual ACM Symposium on Applied Computing, pp. 1374–1382 (2018)

76. Volkovs, M., Rai, H., Cheng, Z., Wu, G., Lu, Y., Sanner, S.: Two-stage model for automatic playlist continuation at scale. Proc. ACM Recommend. Syst. Challenge **2018**, 1–6 (2018)
77. Vystrčilová, M., Peška, L.: Lyrics or audio for music recommendation? In: Proceedings of the 10th International Conference on Web Intelligence, Mining and Semantics, pp. 190–194 (2020)
78. Wishwanath, C.H., Ahangama, S.: A personalized music recommendation system based on user moods. In: 2019 19th International Conference on Advances in ICT for Emerging Regions (ICTer), vol. 250, p. 1. IEEE (2019)
79. Wishwanath, C.H., Weerasinghe, S.N., Illandara, K.H., Kadigamuwa, A., Ahangama, S.: A personalized and context aware music recommendation system. In: International Conference on Human-Computer Interaction, pp. 616–627. Springer (2020)
80. Wu, W., Chen, L., He, L.: Using personality to adjust diversity in recommender systems. In: Proceedings of the 24th ACM Conference on Hypertext and Social Media, pp. 225–229 (2013)
81. Xu, L., Wen, X., Shi, J., Li, S., Xiao, Y., Wan, Q., Qian, X.: Effects of individual factors on perceived emotion and felt emotion of music: based on machine learning methods. Psychol. Music **0305735620928422** (2020)
82. Yakura, H., Nakano, T., Goto, M.: Focusmusicrecommender: a system for recommending music to listen to while working. In: 23rd International Conference on Intelligent User Interfaces, pp. 7–17 (2018)
83. Yang, H., Jeong, Y., Choi, M., Lee, J.: Mmcf: multimodal collaborative filtering for automatic playlist continuation. Proc. ACM Recommend. Syst. Challenge **2018**, 1–6 (2018)
84. Zhang, K., Zhang, Z., Bian, K., Xu, J., Gao, J.: A personalized next-song recommendation system using community detection and markov model. In: 2017 IEEE Second International Conference on Data Science in Cyberspace (DSC), pp. 118–123. IEEE (2017)

Repeated Listens in the Music Discovery Process

Brian Manolovitz and Mitsunori Ogihara

Abstract The long-tail problem for recommender systems is the phenomenon where few items in a system receive most of the interactions, while most items are unpopular and, therefore, are difficult to recommend. In the music domain, this problem is exacerbated by the fact that listeners revisit the songs and artists they enjoy, further widening the gap between popular and unpopular items. This chapter explores many avenues to address the long-tail problem, including a human-subjects study conducted by the authors, which tested the effects of repetition on retention rate. The results of the study indicate that with just one additional listen to a liked unfamiliar song, the listener is 10% more likely to revisit during normal listening.

Personalized music discovery systems can learn from their users' listening behaviors and recommend to them unexpected and interesting songs and artists. These serendipitous recommendations [1] increase the users' sense that the system knows them, while simultaneously assisting the users with the daunting task of music discovery. The expansive libraries on platforms such as Spotify[1] and Apple Music,[2] both containing over 45 million songs, are full of opportunities for users to broaden their tastes and, simultaneously, for lesser-known artists to reach a wider audience. Due to the nature of recommender systems, the most popular music is the easiest to recommend, but it is also usually the least interesting for the listeners. This is known

[1] www.spotify.com.
[2] www.apple.com/apple-music.

B. Manolovitz · M. Ogihara (✉)
University of Miami,1365 Memorial Drive, Coral Gables, FL 33146, USA
e-mail: mogi-hara@miami.edu

B. Manolovitz
e-mail: bmm157@miami.edu

Z. W. Ras et al. (eds.), *Recommender Systems for Medicine and Music*,
Studies in Computational Intelligence 946,
https://doi.org/10.1007/978-3-030-66450-3_8

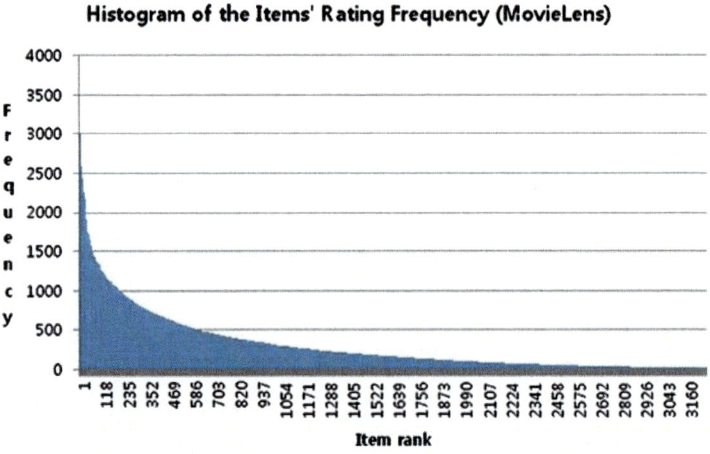

Fig. 1 Ordered histogram of rating counts for each movie in the MovieLens dataset [2]

as the long-tail problem for recommender systems (LTP) [2], and will be the first topic of discussion in this chapter.

The music domain is faced with a unique and interesting challenge that users are expected to revisit songs and thus, change their perception of the music over time. Therefore, it may be a mistake to conclude that a person's musical tastes have broadened after a single listen of a novel song. This chapter will present several studies which highlight the effects of repeated listens on liking and memory. Additionally, the relationship between familiarity and music listening behavior will be explored, highlighting studies from the psychology and neuroscience domains, among others. Finally, the authors share a recent experiment they conducted and analyze the results from that study.

1 The Long-Tail Problem

In recommender systems with a large volume of items to offer, there arises a phenomenon where few items are extremely popular (i.e., have the most ratings or most interactions), and the vast majority of items are relatively unpopular [2], thus creating a short head and a long tail in the popularity distribution. This is illustrated in Fig. 1, which shows the number of interactions between users and movies in the MovieLens dataset as a sorted histogram. The LTP is the result of this phenomenon, where the most interesting and unexpected items to recommend are in the long tail, but the lack of data prevents the system from confidently recommending those items. The long tail should be treated as a gold mine, rich with hidden gems waiting to be discovered by the users. This section will discuss the causes of the LTP as well as some potential solutions for extracting relevant items from the long tail.

2 Causes of the Long-Tail Problem

The radio has historically been the primary way people discover new music. The model of the radio is to play the most popular songs repeatedly until the newer popular songs are released. The distributions of the songs and the artists in terms of their play frequencies clearly resemble that in a recommender system with LTP. The most popular artists receive the benefit of radio play even before their newest songs have been vetted by the public. Online music streaming services have adopted the radio model to some extent [3] with the use of AI-curated radio stations and genre- and mood-based playlists.

While music streaming services have recommendation systems that are similar to radio stations, the chief attraction of their services is in their large catalogs, which have more songs than a person can listen to in a lifetime. The large catalogs give opportunities for the listeners to broaden their tastes and explore songs and artists they have not listened to before, including those from the long tail in the popularity distribution [4]. However, despite the existence of music streaming services for more than a decade, they still appear unable to exploit the long tail, due to the limitations of automated personalized recommendations.

The goal of a personalized recommender system is to suggest interesting and relevant items to its users. The quality of the system is typically measured on the reception or approval of those recommendations. Thus, it is logical for the system to recommend only the items in which it has the most confidence. To select the items to be recommended, a sense of similarity between items must be established. The most common approach for establishing similarity is the collaborative filtering (CF) method for recommendations. CF is a technique that finds a group of users whose tastes and activities show substantial similarity to each other. The CF mechanism uses k-nearest neighbors to find a group that is the most similar to the user at hand and makes recommendations based upon what the other members of the group liked. As a result, when limited amount of information is available about a user, CF may lean towards recommending popular items to compensate for the lack of adequate information.

3 Potential Solutions to the Long-Tail Problem

An alternative approach for establishing song or artist similarity is content-based filtering (CB), which bases its comparisons on the metadata and raw audio data. CB allows all items to be treated equally with respect to their popularity, making it an intriguing research topic [5]. Celma and Herrera [6] used the numerical representations of audio features, such as timbre, rhythm and tonality, to compute a distance metric between songs. They then found similar artists by comparing the songs between pairs of artists and finding the top-20 artists with a minimum distance between songs. In developing their Moodplay application, Andjelkovic et al. [7] used a similar approach but applied it to a visual space and factored in mood-based descriptive tags, ultimately representing songs in 2D space to show their similarity. Zheng et al. [8] built two deep neural networks, one learned hidden features from the music metadata and the other learned from the users' listening histories and their personal metadata. The outputs of these networks were fed into a recurrent neural network which dynamically learned the users' long-term and short-term preferences using their listening activities. Though the inputs were simple, the results were promising compared to state-of-the-art baselines.

Wang et al. [9] utilized the users' experience level to control the extent to which long-tail items are recommended, finding that more experienced users were more open to the items in the long tail. Hamedani et al. [10] used a multi-objective simulated annealing approach to adapt the diversification of recommendation lists based on the perceived preferences of the user towards diversity. Their method penalized the inclusion of popular items while simultaneously increasing accuracy. The resulting recommendation lists performed very well compared to existing methods.

A common solution to a lack of data is to cluster similar items, thus consolidating their data. Park [11] proposed an adaptive clustering method that clusters items based on their popularity but chose only the data objects in the long tail for clustering. Previous studies clustered all items, but the small increase in recommendation performance for items in the head did not justify the increase in runtime. The adaptive clustering method only clustered items in the tail, but it accounted for items moving between the head and the tail and adapted to those changes. This method performed better than prior approaches, both in terms of time performance and the system's ability to make effective recommendation of long-tail items.

An alternative to CF and CB approaches is a weighted graph model which connects users and items [12], where the weights of the edges are the user's ratings of the items. This model uses those weights and the network of edges to create a sense of separation from a user or item to another user or item. Recommending using this model involves a random walk through the graph. The longer the walk, though, the more likely it is to end up at a short head item. Luke et al. [13] proposed a tripartite graph structure which interconnects users, items and genres, as opposed to the typical bipartite graphs. Incorporating genre as an additional node type fills in additional connections where user-item data is sparse, which improves long-tail recommendation.

4 Effect of Repeated Listens on Memory and Liking

The potential solutions to the LTP that were discussed in the previous section focused on extracting relevant music from the long tail, which is an issue of what to recommend. However, merely exposing someone to an enjoyable novel song does not guarantee that they will revisit it in the future. Without additional listens, the data sparsity issue will continue to exist for those songs in the long tail, and they will never be able to break out. By exploiting the trait of the music domain where users are

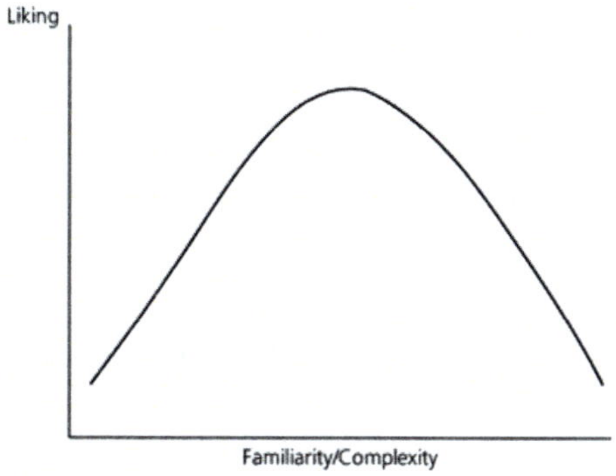

Fig. 2 The relationship between familiarity/complexity and liking, forming an inverted-U shape

expected to revisit items, music discovery systems can tackle the LTP on interactions beyond the first. This section will begin a discussion on how to recommend long-tail items by focusing on the effects of repetition of novel songs.

The root of this topic is the inverted-U theory coined by Berlyne [14], which states that as some collative variable (i.e., familiarity, complexity) increases, a person's preference increases to a point, then begins to decrease. This is shown in Fig. 2, where it is clear that this relationship takes the shape of an upside-down U. Chmiel and Schubert [15] examined the validity of this theory by performing a case study on 57 articles. They found that 50 of those 57 studies supported the inverted-U theory, at least to some extent. It is, therefore, safe to assume that the first time a person listens to a song will not be their most enjoyed listening experience. Vargas and Castells [16] point out that flaws exist in evaluating novel recommendations solely based on the accuracy of the selected songs. They offer an alternative strategy that accounts for the ranking of the chosen items and their relevance to the user. This section will highlight studies which tested the impact of repetition on memory and liking of novel music.

In his research, Hargreaves tested the validity and robustness of the inverted-U over the course of an experiment involving two types of repeated listens, continuous and at intervals [17]. The foundation research for this study showed that during continuous listening, the inverted-U shape held, but when listening at one-week intervals after the decline in preference had begun, there was a resurgence in liking, as if the time off had breathed new life into the music. Hargreaves tested this by first asking subjects to listen to two one-minute excerpts at three separate times each during a 3-hour class and rate their liking and familiarity with each after every listen. The liking rating for each piece did not change, but the familiarity ratings rose significantly. The second experiment involved three weekly meetings where subjects would listen to three musical excerpts four times each, providing liking and familiarity ratings between each listen. Again, the liking ratings remained static between listens, but the familiarity ratings show a clear start to the inverted-U shape.

Spuznar et al. conducted a series of user experiments to evaluate preference as a function of exposure [18]. The first experiment compared the effects of focused and unfocused listening on memory and preference. Focused listening yielded no significant change in preference with more exposures, though repeated exposure through unfocused listening had a positive, linear relationship with liking. In the second experiment, more complex excerpts were used, and the resulting liking curve showed an inverted-U shape for focused listening and a linearly increasing curve for unfocused listening. For both experiments, the graphs showing the subjects' ability to remember the instruments in the excerpts were very similar, with a linear increase for incidental listening and a sigmoid shape for focused listening. In general, for focused listening, the inverted-U shape relating familiarity to preference holds true, and memory relates to exposure such that a significant increase happens after the first few listens.

Madison and Schiölde hypothesized that increases in familiarity cause increases in liking, regardless of the complexity of the music [19]. The experiment they conducted involved a group of musical experts dividing a collection of songs into four levels of complexity, then presenting these songs to subjects several times over a four-week period. The results showed a linear increase in liking over the course of the study, no matter which complexity rating the songs had been assigned. Their conclusion was that familiarity is the single most important predictor for liking of music.

Since it is clear from these studies and others that the inverted-U relationship between preference and familiarity holds true, it is safe to assume that a person's first time hearing a piece of music will not yield the highest achievable preference toward that piece. Music discovery systems should aim to achieve optimal levels of preference by repeating novel songs during the discovery process, such that the likelihood of the listeners revisiting the song is maximized. The goal of any music discovery system should be to broaden the tastes of music listeners, which cannot happen unless the listeners remember to revisit the songs they enjoy.

5 Music Familiarity and Its Influence on Listening Behavior

Since repeated listens of novel songs will increase memory and, consequently, familiarity, the next logical step is to examine the relationship between familiarity and the behavior of the listener. Many factors contribute to the choices people make with their music listening, such as their context, mood, and current activity. Several studies have provided evidence that a person's familiarity with a piece of music is a strong indicator of whether that piece will be selected [19–21]. This is in contrast with the basic human desire for novelty [22], which is mirrored in many survey responses regarding people's interest in broadening their musical tastes [20]. Music discovery systems can resolve this dichotomy by extending the discovery process to the point of sufficient familiarity. This section will explore various aspects of music familiarity and highlight several research studies which analyzed the effect of familiarity on music listening behavior and emotions.

6 Aspects of Familiarity

Music familiarity is much more nuanced than simply the number of times one has listened to a song or artist. Musical qualities such as melody, rhythm, lyrics, instrumentation, and harmony are all partially responsible for one's overall familiarity with a piece of music, in addition to any nonmusical associations. A deeper understanding of music familiarity is valuable for prioritizing certain data points in a CB similarity algorithm.

Hébert and Peretz [23] compared the long-term memory of melody and rhythm to see which is more recognizable. They conducted three separate human-subject listening experiments involving popular song excerpts. The first divided the subjects into two groups, one heard arrhythmic melodies (all notes had the same duration and emphasis), while the other heard monotonic rhythms. The second paired melodies and rhythms from different songs. The third was similar to the first but included a song title in the presentation. The subjects in all cases were asked to identify the songs they were hearing. The results indicate that songs are more recognizable by their melody than by their rhythm, though melody alone is insufficient to perfectly recognize a song.

Crowder et al. [24] evaluated the extent to which one's familiarity with vocal melodies is dependent on the lyrics, and vice-versa. The authors conducted three experiments on this topic, all of which were based on the general premise of playing old, unfamiliar folk songs, then either presenting the same songs again or the same melody with different, equally familiar words. The first experiment translated the lyrics of each song into nonsense text, then it asked the subjects to indicate whether they had already heard the exact melodies of the songs presented (correct and with nonsense lyrics). The second experiment was like the first, but the exact representations of the songs were never presented to the subjects. In the third experiment, subjects were divided into two groups: one received spoken text recorded on top of melodies, and the other received sung words. The results of all three experiments led the authors to conclude that melody recognition is stronger in the presence of text and vice-versa.

Halpern researched the extent to which similarity between songs affects familiarity. She hypothesized that songs are not remembered in isolation, but rather, they are part of a network of musically and nonmusically similar songs [25]. Her approach involved two human-subject experiments. The first asked subjects to group songs in two different ways: one based on musical similarity and the other based on nonmusical similarity. The results showed strong nonmusical groupings and weak musical groupings. These results were used for the second experiment, in which subjects were asked to indicate whether the title of a song matched the tune being played. More similar songs were more often confused for one another, as was expected. Finally, Halpern analyzed the results relative to the subjects' musical backgrounds and found no significant distinctions in either experiment, which, she explained, was likely due to the subjects' familiarity with the songs.

Another facet to consider is whether frequency or recency of listening events has a stronger influence on familiarity. This is important in evaluating listening behavior, especially when attempting to establish a sense of a listener's familiarity with a song without receiving explicit feedback. McAuley et al. conducted a two-day human-subject listening experiment which asked subjects to listen to songs and estimate how many times and on what day they heard each song [26]. The songs were played either the first or the second day once or three times, and the subjects were given a survey at the end of the second day. Those played once on the first day and three times on the second were consistently identified correctly, whereas the songs played three times on the first day were commonly identified as having been played on the second day. These results suggest that frequency has a much stronger influence on memory than does recency. Extrapolating this to familiarity, it is fair to assume that songs heard several times in the past are more familiar to a person than a song heard once recently.

7 Familiarity and Emotions

The relationship between familiarity and emotional responses to auditory stimuli has become a popular research topic, particularly in the field of neuroscience. Van den Bosch et al. investigated the role that familiarity plays in the connection between self-reported pleasure and emotional arousal, hypothesizing that as familiarity increases, so too does this connection [27]. They conducted two experiments, both involved psychophysiological scans to measure electrodermal activity and a report on their overall liking of the music: the first asked the subjects to listen to completely unfamiliar music, while the second involved repeating songs from the first experiment to establish familiarity. In the first experiment, no connection was found between reported pleasure and the measurements from the scan, whereas, in the second, these connections began to form as the subjects became more familiar with the music.

The field of neuroscience has become interested in music familiarity, specifically the way it affects emotional responses and memory [28–31]. Freitas et al. [32] performed a case study of 11 journal articles which sought to distinguish between familiar and unfamiliar listening using neural scans. The selected studies utilized electroencephalography (EEG), positron emission tomography (PET), and functional magnetic resonance imaging (fMRI). The consensus of these studies was that familiar listening typically activates regions of the brain associated with motor functions, suggesting anticipation of melodies and a higher level of engagement, especially with the rhythm. The authors concluded that higher powered studies are necessary, specifically ones which emphasize the nature of the audio and the musical backgrounds of the participants.

Pereira et al. conducted a study using fMRI to determine if there is a difference in the way the brain responds to familiar and unfamiliar music with respect to emotions [33]. Prior studies found that emotional responses to music activate the limbic and paralimbic structures of the brain. The results of this study showed that familiar songs (whether they were liked or disliked) mirrored those emotional responses much more closely than liked songs (whether they were familiar or unfamiliar). In other words, familiarity has a greater influence on emotional reactions to music than does preference toward the song.

8 How Familiarity Influences Listening Behavior

It should be apparent by now that familiarity strongly influences the liking of a song, so it is important now to assess its influence on listening behavior. Ward et al. [20] tested the effects of familiarity on music choice by asking subjects to rate songs in terms of familiarity and preference. After the initial rating, the songs were partitioned into pairs, each pair consisting of one familiar and one unfamiliar, and the subjects were asked which they would rather hear. They found that the subjects tended to select the songs with which they were more familiar, regardless of their liking ratings. This led the authors to conclude that people generally prefer to hear familiar music, despite claiming they would like to hear more novel songs. Alternatively, their results indicate a greater need to boost familiarity during the discovery process, so that novel songs are more likely to be chosen.

Repetition within the songs themselves, specifically in the lyrics, can influence popularity. Nunes et al. [21] examined the lyrical content of songs which reached #1 on Billboard's Hot 100 singles chart, as well as songs that made it onto the chart but never placed higher than #90. They found that the repetition of the chorus from the song was a positive indicator of reaching #1, as well as an indicator of the speed at which the song would reach the top spot. However, excessive repetition would negate this effect, which mirrors the inverted-U with respect to familiarity or novelty.

The goal of any music discovery system should be to broaden the tastes of music listeners, and that only happens if the listeners incorporate novel songs into their repertoires. This section provided evidence that familiarity is the key to achieving this goal, most notably by extending the music discovery process up to the point of familiarity. By recommending novel songs additional times, listeners will likely achieve a deeper emotional connection, higher preference, and stronger memory of those songs. The next section will present a recent study conducted by the authors which tests the effects of repeated recommendations of novel songs in a real-world listening setting.

9 Music Listening Study

When discovering new music, listeners need to remember to revisit the songs they enjoy, usually by saving them or adding them to a playlist. If they forget to do this, or if they prefer to listen to new music in the background [34], missed opportunities to expand the listeners' repertoires arise. Additionally, since repeated listens to unfamiliar songs have been shown to increase liking, the first listen is likely not the most enjoyable. Therefore, additional missed opportunities occur when a song would have increased in favor with additional plays.

The authors recently conducted a six-week music listening study involving 19 Spotify users [35]. The goal of the study was to introduce 'retention rate' as an additional parameter for evaluating music discovery systems. Retention rate examines the rate at which the listener revisits the novel songs during his/her normal listening. The study was designed to answer the research question: is the retention rate higher for songs which are presented to the listeners more times? The following section will provide a detailed summary of the methodology and findings of the study.

10 Experiment Methodology

Initially, the subjects were asked to provide their most recent Spotify Discovery Weekly playlist, which contains 30 songs which are novel and interesting to the user. Each week of the six-week study, subjects were provided with a playlist comprised of 10 songs from their Discover Weekly playlist. These songs were presented to the subject for the first, second, or third time, such that by the end of the study, there was an even distribution between the play counts. The subjects were asked to listen to the playlist once before filling out a survey. The survey asked them to rate the playlist in terms of their liking and again in terms of its effectiveness for discovery. They were also asked to place each of the 10 songs in one of three categories: I like this song, Neutral/Not sure yet, or I do not like this song (*like*, *neutral*, *dislike*, for short).

The selection of songs to be repeated preserved an even distribution of liking ratings across the three play counts. Figure 3 illustrates this procedure, which involves sorting the songs by their rating and selecting half of the songs in an alternating fashion. The repeated songs were evenly distributed throughout the playlist to increase the perception of diversity [36]. The playlists for weeks 1 and 2 contained entirely new songs; weeks 3 and 4 contained 5 new songs and 5 repeated songs; weeks 5 and 6 contained 5 songs being presented for the second time and 5 being presented for the third time.

At the end of the 6-week listening portion of the study, the subjects were asked to fill out a survey where they rated their likelihood to revisit each of the 30 songs. They were asked to complete this without listening to the songs again, relying on their memory of the song and artist names from filling out the earlier surveys. If they forgot the song, they were asked to place an asterisk. We use these results to compute the forgetting rate, which is the proportion of songs that were forgotten. If they had heard the song prior to the experiment, which was possible since Spotify is only aware of listens on the Spotify platform, they were asked to leave that response blank.

One month after the conclusion of the listening portion, the subjects received another survey asking them to state whether, for each of the 30 songs, they had gone out of their way to listen to the song in that month. This meant that, for example,

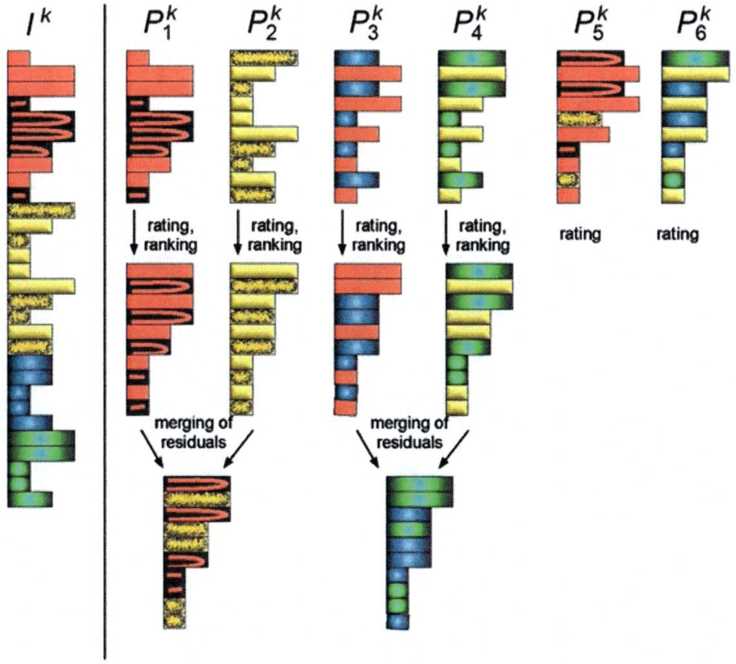

Fig. 3 The playlist construction process. The boxes in red are the first ten songs of Discover Weekly, those in yellow are the next ten, those in blue are the next five, and those in green are the last five

they searched for the song, added it to a playlist, or saved it in their library. These results were used to compute the retention rate, R, which is simply the proportion of songs that were revisited.

11 Results and Discussion

Of the 570 songs (30 for each of 19 subjects), 26 were omitted because they were heard prior to the experiment. Additionally, one subject failed to provide the follow-up survey with the retention data. To evaluate the preference and discovery ratings of the playlists, they were grouped according to their makeup (1 + 2, 3 + 4, 5 + 6). The preference ratings remained fairly constant throughout, while the discovery ratings significantly dropped as fewer new songs were presented, as shown in Fig. 4. This was to be expected, and it was outside of the scope of the experiment to test the optimal proportions of new and repeated songs.

The individual song ratings tended to remain the same with increased plays, though if the rating changed, it increased almost twice as often as it decreased (73 increased, 43 decreased). Specifically, for the 116 songs with an initial rating of neutral and

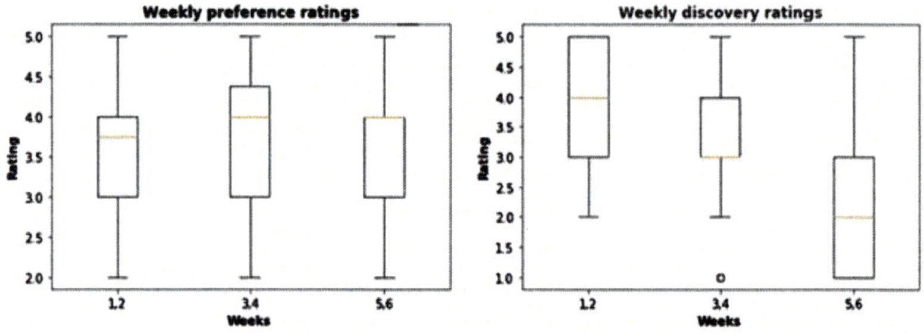

Fig. 4 Boxplots of the grouped weekly preference (left) and discovery (right) ratings for all subjects

more than one presentation, 43 had a final rating of like, whereas 20 had a final rating of dislike. An initial rating of neutral is not likely to inspire the listener to revisit the song, yet 37% of the time, the listener would enjoy the song more with subsequent listens. Therefore, had the songs only been presented once, there would have been a substantial number of missed opportunities.

The forgetting rate, F, for songs can be grouped according to the initial rating of the songs, F_r, as well as the play count, F_c. In total, 105 of the 544 songs were forgotten. The results show that F_r is more or less constant, indicating that initial rating does not influence memory significantly. However, for F_c, there is a major decline as play count increases, as shown in Fig. 5. When isolating the songs with a like initial rating, the number of forgotten songs shows a similar pattern, indicating that play count influences memory regardless of preference.

Finally, the retention rate can be grouped by the initial rating of the songs, R_i, final rating, R_f, and by play count, R_c. As shown in Fig. 6, there is a significant increase in R_c from 1 to 2 plays, but there is little change from 2 to 3 plays. Additionally, R_i is significantly higher for higher preference ratings. Figure 7 shows the number of retained songs grouped by play count with respect to both initial and final rating. In terms of the initial rating, the retention rate only showed a significant increase for liked songs, specifically between those with one play versus those with two. Still, this increase indicates that there are potential missed opportunities when only recommending novel songs once. Even if the listener enjoys a song after the first listen, she will benefit from an additional presentation of that song, assuming she truly wishes to broaden her tastes.

The behavior of the neutral songs is fairly erratic, but it can be explained by looking at R_f, shown in Fig. 7. Since neutral songs saw their ratings increase to like 37% of the time, it is clear from this graph that songs with a final rating of neutral did not entice the listeners to listen again. On the other hand, there is now a clear increase in retention rate between liked songs with 2 versus 3 plays. Perhaps the most interesting result is that the retention rate is almost identical for neutral and liked songs with only one play. This could be because there is still some curiosity about the neutral songs, or simply because, as has been shown, one listen is insufficient to properly evaluate a person's liking of a song.

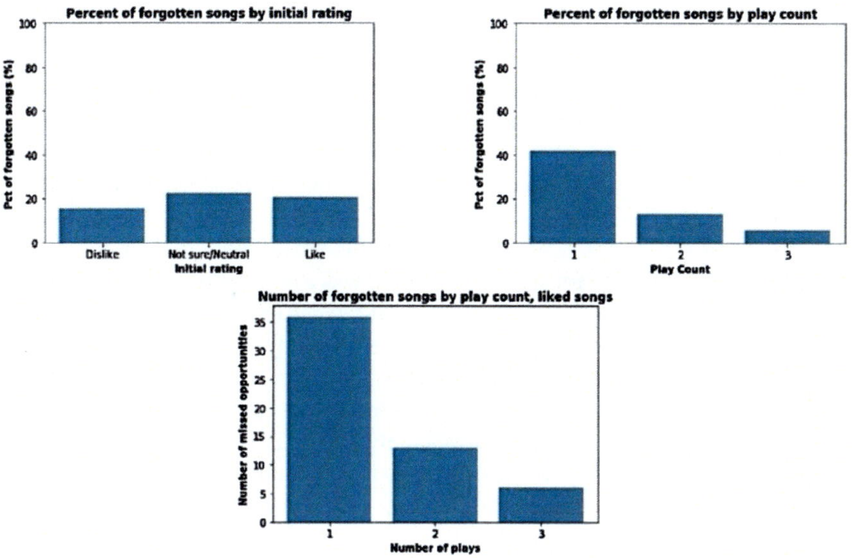

Fig. 5 The percentage of forgotten songs by initial rating (top left) and play count (top right), as well as the number of forgotten *liked* songs by play count (bottom)

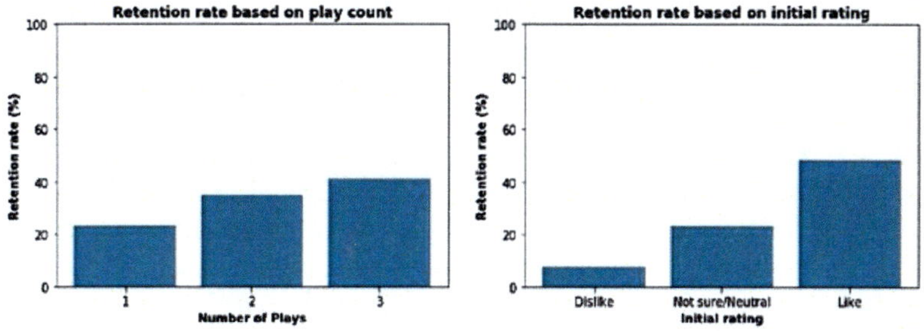

Fig. 6 The retention rate with respect to play count (left), initial rating (right)

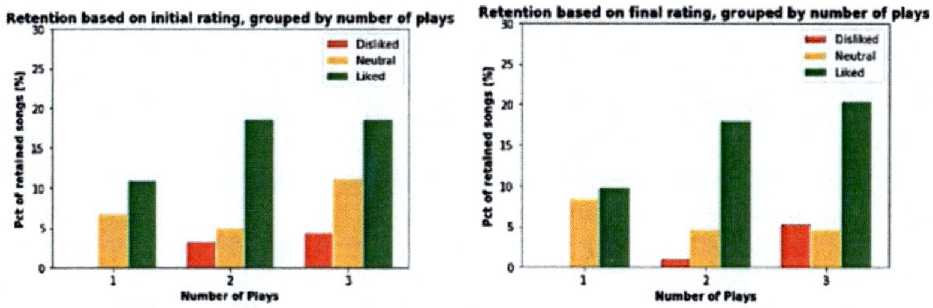

Fig. 7 The number of retained songs, grouped by number of plays, with respect to initial (left) and final (right) ratings

12 Conclusions and Future Work

This chapter proposed incorporating repetition in the music discovery process as a potential solution to the long-tail problem. First, studies which addressed the extraction of interesting and relevant items from the long tail were discussed as a baseline. Next, the authors analyzed the results of several studies which tested the effects of repetition on the listener's response. These studies showed that repetition of novel songs increases memory and liking for as long as those songs remain novel. The psychological background for this phenomenon was extracted from various studies on music familiarity with respect to musical qualities and emotional and neurological responses. Ultimately, the authors presented a recent study of theirs which tested the effects of repeated presentations of novel songs to human subjects on the likelihood of the subjects to revisit the novel songs. The results of the study indicate that even one additional presentation yields a substantial increase in retention rate.

The next step for the authors is to investigate the neurological response to repeated listens of novel music using EEG. Ideally, the responses can be used to train a model which can predict whether the listener is familiar with the associated piece of music. Another avenue to be explored is cognitive load during a sustained period of novel music listening. This will be coupled with a data mining experiment to determine if the amount of new music a person can reasonably consume each week should be scaled based on recent listening patterns. Finally, additional user listening studies will be conducted in the realm of repetition of novel music.

As for the long-tail problem in the music domain, there is plenty of work to be done with regards to efficiently and effectively extracting songs and artists from the long tail. There have been numerous studies which explored the impact of a user interface on music discovery and long-tail recommendation [7, 37, 38]. A visual association with the novel recommendations creates a transparency which builds trust between the user and system. Another area worth investigating is the trajectory of artists who have broken out of the long tail with respect to their song consumption patterns. These patterns could prove insightful when designing a music discovery system which aims to move artists out of the long tail.

References

1. Kotkov, D., Wang, S., Veijalainen, J.: A survey of serendipity in recommender systems. Knowl.-Based Syst. **111**, 180–192 (2016)
2. Park, Y.-J., Tuzhilin, A.: The long tail of recommender systems and how to leverage it. In: Proceedings of the 2008 ACM Conference on Recommender systems, pp. 11–18 (2008)
3. Glantz, M.: Internet radio adopts a human touch: a study of 12 streaming music services. J. Radio Audio Media **23**(1), 36–49 (2016)
4. Datta, H., Knox, G., Bronnenberg, B.J.: Changing their tune: How consumers' adoption of online streaming affects music consumption and discovery. Mark. Sci. **37**(1), 5–21 (2018)

5. De Gemmis, M., Lops, P., Musto, C., Narducci,F., Semeraro, G.: Semantics-aware content-based recommender systems. In: Recommender Systems Handbook, pp. 119–159. Springer (2015)
6. Celma, Ò., Herrera, P.: A new approach to evaluating novel recommendations. In: Proceedings of the 2008 ACM Conference on Recommender Systems, pp. 179–186 (2008)
7. Andjelkovic, I., Parra, D., O'Donovan, J.: Moodplay: interactive mood-based music discovery and recommendation. In: Proceedings of the 2016 Conference on User Modeling Adaptation and Personalization, pp. 275–279 (2016)
8. Zheng, H.-T., Chen, J.-Y., Liang, N., Kumar Sangaiah, A., Jiang, Y., Zhao., C.-Z.: A deep temporal neural music recommendation model utilizing music and user metadata. Appl. Sci. **9**(4), 703 (2019)
9. Wang, Y., Wang, J., Li, L.: Enhancing long tail recommendation based on user's experience evolution. In: 2018 IEEE 22nd International Conference on Computer Supported Cooperative Work in Design (CSCWD), pp. 25–30. IEEE (2018)
10. Hamedani, E.M. Kaedi, M.: Recommending the long tail items through personalized diversification. Knowl.-Based Syst. **164**, 348–357 (2019)
11. Park, Y.-J.: The adaptive clustering method for the long tail problem of recommender systems. IEEE Trans. Knowl. Data Eng. **25**(8), 1904–1915 (2012)
12. Yin, H., Cui, B., Li, J.. Yao, J., Chen, C.: Challenging the long tail recommendation (2012). arXiv preprint arXiv:1205.6700
13. Luke, A., Johnson, J., Ng, Y.-K.: Recommending long-tail items using extended tripartite graphs. In: 2018 IEEE International Conference on Big Knowledge (ICBK), pp. 123–130. IEEE (2018)
14. Berlyne, D.E.: Aesthetics and Psychobiology. Appleton-Century-Crofts, New York, NY (1971)
15. Chmiel, A., Schubert, E.: Back to the inverted-u for music preference: a review of the literature. Psychol. Music **45**(6), 886–909 (2017)
16. Vargas, S., Castells, P.: Rank and relevance in novelty and diversity metrics for recommender systems. In: Proceedings of the Fifth ACM Conference on Recommender Systems, pp. 109–116 (2011)
17. Hargreaves, D.J.: The effects of repetition on liking for music. J. Res. Music Educ. **32**(1), 35–47 (1984)
18. Szpunar, K.K., Schellenberg, E.G., Pliner, P.: Liking and memory for musical stimuli as a function of exposure. J. Experimental Psychol.: Learn. Memory Cogn. **30**(2), 370 (2004)
19. Madison, G., Schiölde, G.: Repeated listening increases the liking for music regardless of its complexity: implications for the appreciation and aesthetics of music. Front. Neurosci. **11**, 147 (2017)
20. Ward, M.K., Goodman, J.K., Irwin, J.R.: The same old song: the power of familiarity in music choice. Mark. Lett. **25**(1), 1–11 (2014)
21. Nunes, J.C., Ordanini, A., Valsesia, F.: The power of repetition: repetitive lyrics in a song increase processing fluency and drive market success. J. Consum. Psychol. **25**(2), 187–199 (2015)
22. González-Cutre, D., Sicilia, Á., Sierra, A.C., Ferriz, R., Hagger, M.S.: Understanding the need for novelty from the perspective of self-determination theory. Person. Individ. Diff. **102**, 159–169 (2016)
23. Hébert, S., Peretz, I.: Recognition of music in long-term memory: are melodic and temporal patterns equal partners? Memory Cogn. **25**(4), 518–533 (1997)
24. Crowder, R.G., Louise Serafine, M., Repp, B.: Physical interaction and association by contiguity in memory for the words and melodies of songs. Memory Cogn. **18**(5), 469–476 (1990)
25. Halpern, A.R.: Organization in memory for familiar songs. J. Exp. Psychol.: Learn. Memory Cogn. **10**(3), 496 (1984)
26. McAuley, J.D., Stevens, C., Humphreys, M.S.: Play it again: did this melody occur more frequently or was it heard more recently? The role of stimulus familiarity in episodic recognition of music. Acta Psychologica **116**(1), 93–108 (2004)

27. Van Den Bosch, I., Salimpoor, V., Zatorre, R.J.: Familiarity mediates the relationship between emotional arousal and pleasure during music listening. Front. Hum. Neurosci. **7**, 53 (2013)
28. Hadjidimitriou, S.K., Hadjileontiadis, L.J.: EEG-based classification of music appraisal responses using time-frequency analysis and familiarity ratings. IEEE Trans. Affect. Comput. **4**(2), 161–172 (2013)
29. Jagiello, R., Pomper, U., Yoneya, M., Zhao, S., Chait, M.: Rapid brain responses to familiar vs. unfamiliar music–an eeg and pupillometry study. Scie. Rep. **9**(1), 1–13 (2019)
30. Kumagai, Y., Arvaneh, M., Tanaka, T.: Familiarity affects entrainment of EEG in music listening. Front. Hum. Neurosci. **11**, 384 (2017)
31. Madsen, J., Hellmuth Margulis, E., Simchy-Gross, R., Parra, L.C.: Music synchronizes brainwaves across listeners with strong effects of repetition, familiarity and training. Sci. Rep. **9**(1), 1–8 (2019)
32. Freitas, C., Manzato, E., Burini, A., Taylor, M.J., Lerch, J.P., Anagnostou, E.: Neural correlates of familiarity in music listening: a systematic review and a neuroimaging meta-analysis. Front. Neurosci. **12**, 686 (2018)
33. Pereira, C.S, Teixeira, J., Figueiredo, P., Xavier, J., Luís Castro, S., Brattico, E.: Music and emotions in the brain: familiarity matters. PloS One **6**(11) (2011)
34. Garcia-Gathright, J., Thomas, B.S., Hosey, C., Nazari, Z., Diaz, F.: Understanding and evaluating user satisfaction with music discovery. In: The 41st International ACM SIGIR Conference on Research & Development in Information Retrieval, pp. 55–64 (2018)
35. Manolovitz, B., Ogihara, M.: Practical evaluation of repeated listens in personalized music discovery. Unpublished paper (2020)
36. Karakaya, M., Aytekin, T.: Effective methods for increasing aggregate diversity in recommender systems. Knowl. Inform. Syst. **56**(2), 355–372 (2018)
37. Bountouridis, D., Van Balen, J., Rodríguez-López, M., Aljanaki, A., Wiering, F., Veltkamp, R.C.: Tonic: combining ranking and clustering dynamics for music discovery. In: Proceedings of the Audio Mostly 2015 on Interaction With Sound, pp. 1–6 (2015)
38. Schedl, M.: Intelligent user interfaces for social music discovery and exploration of large-scale music repositories. In: Proceedings of the 2017 ACM Workshop on Theory-Informed User Modeling for Tailoring and Personalizing Interfaces, pp. 7–11 (2017)

What Songs We Listen to Together: Automatic Music Selection for Groups

Jun'ichi Suzuki and Tetsuro Kitahara

Abstract *Group music recommendation* aims to find songs that could potentially please everyone (or most persons) who is present at a particular place. Although there are many situations, such as carpooling and parties, where more than one person listen to the same music together at the same time and place, there have been relatively few works to recommend songs that are appropriate to play in such situations. In this chapter, we describe some attempts, including ours, to develop a system that recommends songs for a group of persons.

1 Introduction

As many people know, the research on music recommendation has a long history. The typical focus of this research is to model, learn, and/or predict users' musical preferences. In other words, one of its objectives is to optimize the music selection process for individual users because different users have different musical preferences.

Obviously, we do not always listen to music alone. There are many situations, such as carpooling and parties, where a group of people (e.g., family, friends, colleagues, party participants) listen to the same Background Music (BGM) at the same time and place. In such a situation, the BGM should satisfy the musical preferences of most (ideally, all) persons who are present there. However, it is not easy. When a particular member in the group selects songs based on his/her musical preferences, this may result in that the other members' preferences are ignored. If they make agreeable decisions about BGM selection through discussions, the selected songs will satisfy all members' preferences. But few people would prefer to spend time for BGM selection.

In this chapter, we review some attempts to improve such group music selection. First, we discuss issues for computing technologies to help group members select BGM that satisfies their preferences. Then, we mention existing works aiming at

J. Suzuki · T. Kitahara (✉)
Nihon University, 3-25-40 Sakurajosui, Setagaya-ku, Tokyo, Japan
e-mail: kitahara@kthrlab.jp

Z. W. Ras et al. (eds.), *Recommender Systems for Medicine and Music*,
Studies in Computational Intelligence 946,
https://doi.org/10.1007/978-3-030-66450-3_9

this goal. Even though there have been relatively few works, some systems have been developed. We here review four systems: MusicFX [1], Flytrap [2], GroupFun [3], and BlueMusic [4]. After that, we describe our own research [5], in which we developed an Android application that enables users to select and play songs that could please most members in the group. We show here its system design, music selection algorithm, and evaluations.

2 Issues in Group Music Selection

Outside the music domain, some researchers have dealt with group recommendation. Jameson discussed issues and challenges for group recommendation with the Travel Decision Forum, which helps a group of users agree on the desired attributes of a vacation they are planning to take together [6]. He pointed out that group recommendation consists of the following four phases:

Phase 1: Members specify their preferences.
Phase 2: The system generates recommendations.
Phase 3: The system presents recommendations to the members.
Phase 4: Members decide which recommendation (if any) to accept.

At Phase 1, he pointed out that each member may have interest in other members' preferences. He then proposed a user interface that enables users to know each other's preferences when specifying their own preferences.

At Phase 2, the system aggregates the preferences given by multiple users. He pointed out the importance of aggregation algorithms that are difficult to manipulate. For example, if aggregation takes the least misery strategy, someone can "remove" a particular option by giving it the worst rate.

At Phase 3, many recommendation systems present not only a recommendation but also its acceptability, sometimes with complex visualization. For group recommendation, the acceptability of a recommendation can be analyzed for each individual member, for the whole group, and for subsets of the group. He introduced two approaches, one of which is to present the acceptability of each recommendation evaluated through the members' preferences. The other is to provide the representatives of the members as animated characters, which explain unacceptable points of a recommendation (that is, what are deviated in the recommendation from their preferences), such as "the proposal for Massage is much too low for me."

At Phase 4, he introduced a feature that supports the process of arriving at a final decision in a non-face-to-face situation. Given a proposal by the mediator, a real user interacts with the system about its acceptability. At the same time, the animated representatives of other members respond whether this real user's interaction is agreeable, based on the parameter settings specified by those members. Through such interaction by one real user and multiple representatives, decision-making will help in avoiding synchronous communication.

This attempt is very interesting, but there is a clear difference between song selection for BGM and vacation planning: it is not acceptable to spend time to arrive at a final decision for BGM. For song selection for BGM, the following points are important to consider:

- **No time consumption for specifying musical preferences**
  For most users, manually specifying their musical preferences (e.g., how much they prefer each of the target songs/artists/genres) is too troublesome. It would be better to extract their musical preferences automatically from a certain information such as listening histories on their music players.
- **Possibility of disjoint preference data**
  Especially when the users' preferences are extracted from their listening histories, each user's preference data easily become disjoint. Suppose that the user u_i prefers and frequently listens to the song m_k while the user u_j has not listened to this song on his/her own music player. If this is the case, the system cannot evaluate how much u_j prefers m_k because of the missing preference data, even if it is potentially very preferable. To solve this problem, the system has to estimate the preference for this song from other information. A typical approach is to estimate it from the preferences for other songs similar to m_k.
- **Access to the content**
  To estimate the preference for a song from those for songs similar to it, the system has to measure the similarity between songs. There are two different approaches for measuring the similarity: content-based and social-filtering-based. To adopt the content-based approach, the content (i.e., the waveforms) of the target songs should be accessible.
- **Copy-free playback**
  In almost all situations, song selection is not a final goal. Once songs are selected, they need to be played. The technical issue depends on how users listen to music. If they use a web-based on-demand streaming music service, the music selection system has to access to the API of the streaming service to start playing the selected songs. If they store songs on their own devices (such as smartphones and portable music players), the system needs to start playing the songs stored on their devices. Note that the selected songs may be stored on separate devices, that is, the first song may be stored on the user u_i's device while the second song may be stored on the user u_j's device. Such a series of songs stored separately should be seamlessly played because manually switching the device for playback is too troublesome. One approach may be to collect all songs into one device but it is usually unsuitable due to the copyright matter.

In the rest of this chapter, we investigate how to tackle these issues in existing studies (including ours) for group music selection.

3 Existing Works

In this section, we introduce four systems that aim at group music recommendation.

3.1 MusicFX [1]

MusicFX, developed by McCarthy and Anagnost, is probably the earliest system that aims at group music selection. This system is supposed to be used in a fitness center. In the target fitness center, BGM provided through 91 digital music stations, each of which corresponds to one musical genre, is played while many members work out there. The music stations were selected manually by the fitness center's staff. MusicFX aims to offload this task from the staff. Additionally, MusicFX also aims to democratize the music selection process and to increase the variety of music played.

When a member joins the fitness center, he/she specifies the preference for each of the 91 genres on a five-point scale (ranging from −2 to +2). These preference data can be updated at any time. When entering the fitness center, a member logs in MusicFX by swiping the electronic badge. Through this, MusicFX identifies who is present there.

When the members present change (someone enters or exits) or someone's preference data are updated, the music selection process runs. This process is performed based on the $M \times N$ table of integer-valued preferences ranging from −2 to +2, where M is the number of the genres (= 91) and N is the number of the members present. When the member j's individual preference for the genre i is denoted by IP_{ij}, the group preference for this genre is defined by

$$GP_i = \sum_j (IP_{ij} + 2)^2.$$

The music stations are selected according to a weighted random selection policy with weights given by the group preferences.

This work is impressive as the earliest attempt and also a 6-week evaluation with 71 participants in the real fitness center is suggestive. However, this system seems to assume that every member specifies his/her preference for every genre. This assumption is sometimes unrealistic because it may burden the members a lot. As we pointed out above, dealing with missing preference data is important.

3.2 *Flytrap [2]*

The concept of *Flytrap* is a sort of "Virtual DJ," which automatically constructs a soundtrack that tries to please everyone in the room. Similarly to MusicFX, Flytrap is installed in a public space and identifies who is present there by detecting his/her electronic badge. This system consists of four components: Track Information Recorder, Genre Network, Voting Mechanism, and Vote Visualizer.

Track Information Recorder: The RealJukebox music player installed on each user's machine gathers information about what tracks the user is listening to and records it in Flytrap's database. The tracks themselves are uploaded to the server. Unlike MusicFX, the user's musical preferences are learned through the acts of listening.

Genre Network: The genre network is used to determine the similarity between artists. A map from artists to genres is identified via metadata in MP3 files (i.e., ID3 tags). The similarity network of genre is hand-crafted.

Voting Mechanism: An agent representing each user present in the room gives a numerical vote to each track in the system's database. The agent gives a high vote to a song if it is an artist he/she has listened to previously. Votes for songs that he/she has not listened to are given based on the songs he/she has listened to with the same or similar genre. The agents' votes are combined and normalized into a probability distribution; however, the agents' votes are partly overridden by a DJ agent based on some rules such as not playing two tracks by the same artist in a row.

Voting Visualizer: The voting process is graphically visualized in real time. Different text colors in track titles represent different users while the brightness represents the strength of the voting.

This system estimates users' musical preferences based on their listening behaviors instead of asking them to manually specify the preferences. Missing preferences (due to no listening experience) are estimated from listening behaviors of the same or similar genre. These approaches would be effective to reduce the users' burden. However, the similarity network of genres is hand-crafted, so it does not consider acoustic similarities. Also, a method for playing the selected songs is not mentioned in the paper.

3.3 *GroupFun [3]*

GroupFun is a web application, implemented as a Facebook plug-in, that helps a group of friends to agree on a common music playlist for an event they will attend (e.g., a graduation ceremony). It allows a user to manage and share his/her favorite songs with friends so that they can enjoy listening together to the shared music collection in which different music tastes are integrated. The application has the rating for each song given by each user. This rating is aggregated with four algorithms: a deterministic weighted sum, a probabilistic weighted sum, the least misery (evaluating each song using the minimum of all users' ratings for that song), and probabilistic selection with equal probability. These algorithms were evaluated through a user study with 16 participants.

3.4 *BlueMusic [4]*

BlueMusic aims at personalization of BGM in a public environment. Each user specifies musical preferences by checking their favorite artists chosen from different genres on a web form. These checked/unchecked statuses are encoded such as "Bm+A1R3E5T3" and then it is set to the Bluetooth name for the user's mobile phone. Because these Bluetooth names are broadcasted, the music player can scan them to analyze the musical preferences of the persons present there.

3.5 *Other Works*

Apart from the above, Dias and Magalhães proposed a group music recommendation algorithm [7]. However, this algorithm discovers clusters of users with similar musical preferences with the k-means algorithm in order to apply group-based music recommendation. It seems different from music recommendation for a group of persons present in the same place.

There have been developed several commercial applications for smartphones. Examples include *FESS*, developed by Kayac (http://fess.kayac.com/). This application enables users present in the same place to share songs via Bluetooth. Songs stored separately on multiple devices are collected into a master device and songs with different musical tastes owned by different users can be easily played. Another application, called *Listen with* (https://www.listenwith.jp/), enables users to join a virtual music event, in which an artist selects and plays songs via the network. Users can enjoy listening to the songs together as well as chatting with the artist. This is one approach for sharing musical experience but is different from group music selection.

4 Case Study: A Bluetooth-Based Music Selection Application

In this section, we describe our Android application that tries to select songs that potentially please most of the persons present in the same place.[1] Our target is a small

[1]This research has been presented at [5].

group of three or four persons who know each other well. When they enjoy doing something together, such as driving, conversation, meals, and casual parties, at the same time and place, they may listen to the same BGM. The aim of this application is to automatically select and play the BGM in which all members' musical preferences are equally reflected.

4.1 Concept

Here, we assume that each user owns his/her song waveforms (such as MP3 files) on his/her Android device and listens to them daily on this device. When they gather with their devices, selecting and playing BGM should be easily startable without any special equipment nor time-consuming processes. We therefore resolve the four issues described above with the following approaches:

- **No time consumption for specifying musical preferences**
  Our application has a single-user music playback mode. We assume that users listen to music using this daily to collect their listening histories. From these listening histories, their musical preferences are estimated.
- **Possibility of disjoint preference data**
  Similarly to some existing systems such as Flytrap and GroupFun, the potential preference for songs with no listening histories is estimated from the preferences for songs similar to them.
- **Access to the content**
  Because the user u_i's favorite songs are stored on the user u_i's device, the acoustic features of those songs are analyzed by this device. The acoustic features (not waveforms themselves) are then transmitted to the master device to calculate the similarity between songs stored on separate devices.
- **Copy-free playback**
  Although a generated playlist may consist of songs stored on separate devices, no waveforms should be copied to any server or devices. Instead, the connection to a Bluetooth speaker is automatically switched from device to device. If the first song is stored on the device d_i, the master device commands d_i to connect itself directly to the Bluetooth speaker. If the second song is stored on a different device d_j, the master device commands d_i to disconnect itself then d_j to connect itself to the speaker.

4.2 System Design

This application aims to select songs from a collection separately stored on different devices and to play the songs seamlessly. We designed the application based on the following policies:

- Every device communicates information about songs (not the waveforms themselves) to the master device.
- After the song selection process occurs, the master device commands the device storing the selected song to connect itself directly to the Bluetooth speaker to avoid copying the waveform somewhere.
- Each user's preferences for songs stored on other users' devices are estimated based on the similarity between these songs and the songs stored on his/her device.

The application has two different modes. One is the normal playback mode, in which the user listens to songs in a normal way. This mode provides basically the same functionalities as a typical music player and is used to store the playback history, particularly the number of plays (i.e., how many times the user has listened to each song). The other mode is a networked playback mode, which is the primary mode of this application. Once users gather and launch the application on their devices, the devices start to communicate with one other via Bluetooth, and one of the devices (selected randomly) is set to be the master device. After establishing a Bluetooth connection, the master device collects information about the list of songs stored on each device and the number of plays (how many times each song has been played back) from the other devices. Then, the master device generates a playlist and commands the device storing each song in the playlist to play back the song.

We illustrate the procedure of the networked playback mode in Fig. 1.

4.2.1 Launching the Application

Let $\mathcal{U} = \{u_1, \ldots, u_n\}$ and $\mathcal{D} = \{d_1, \ldots, d_n\}$ be a group of users and a set of the users' devices, respectively, where d_1 is the master device. Each device d_i communicates the list of songs $M_{(d_i)} = \{m_{(d_i,1)}, \ldots, m_{(d_i,n(d_i))}\}$ and the number of plays for every song $F(m_{(d_i,k)})$ $(k = 1, \ldots, n(d_i))$ to the master device d_1.

4.2.2 Calculating the Degree of Preference

For each user u_i, the degree of preference for every song is calculated. Let $W(u_i, m_{(d_j,k)})$ be the degree of preference of user u_i for song $m_{(d_j,k)}$. We formulate the degree of preference based on the following assumptions:

(1) If a user listens to a song frequently, his/her preference for that song should be high.
(2) If Song A is similar to Song B, which is highly favored, Song A should also be highly favored.

Based on the first assumption, we can calculate the degree of a user's preference for songs stored on his/her own device using the number of plays. On the other hand, the degree of preference for songs stored on others' devices cannot be calculated based on the number of plays because such information is not available. Based on

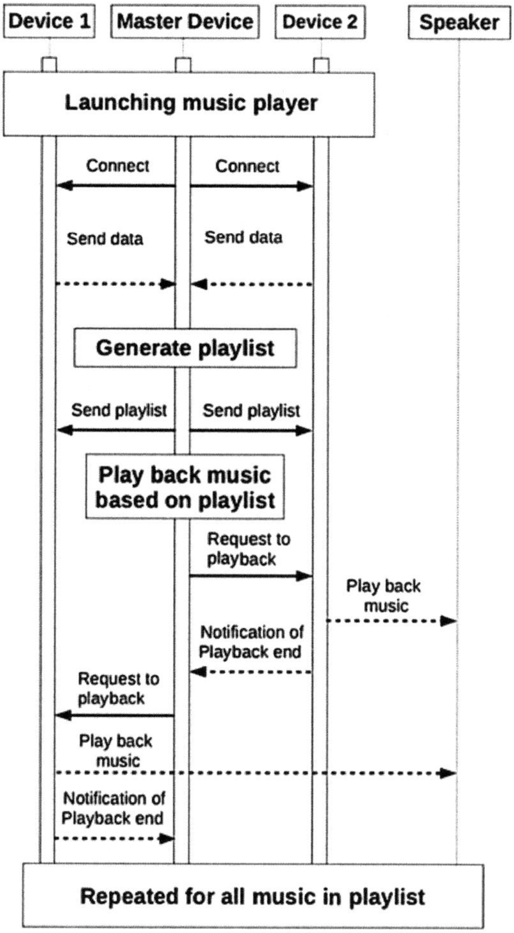

Fig. 1 Overview of system flow in the networked playback mode

the second assumption, we calculate the degree of preference for such songs using that for similar songs owned by oneself.

Preference for Owned Songs

The degree of preference for songs stored on a user's own device is calculated based on the number of plays. Here, we prepare two different definitions:

$$W(u_i, m_{(d_i,k)}) = 1 - \frac{1}{\{F(m_{(d_i,k)}) + 1\}^{\alpha}} \tag{1}$$

and

$$W(u_i, m_{(d_i,k)}) = \cosh \beta F(m_{(d_i,k)}), \tag{2}$$

where α and β are parameters.

Preference for Unowned Songs

Here, we calculate the degree of preference for songs stored on other users' devices $W(u_i, m_{(d_j,k)})$ $(i \neq j)$.

First of all, the similarity of $m_{(d_j,k)}$ to every song stored on d_i is calculated. Musical similarity is a very difficult concept and its calculation is still an open problem. However, various similarity measures have been developed from different points of view (e.g., [8]). Here, we combine two different similarity measures: acoustic similarity and (socially obtained) artist similarity.

To calculate acoustic similarity between two songs, $m_{(d_j,k)}$ and $m_{(d_i,l)}$, a sequence of 20-dimensional mel-frequency cepstral coefficient (MFCC) vectors is calculated from each song by adopting a shift by 160 samples after the waveform is resampled to 16 kHz. The Earth mover's distance between the two sequences, denoted by $D(m_{(d_j,k)}, m_{(d_i,l)})$, is calculated. The similarity $\mathrm{sim}_{\mathrm{MFCC}}(m_{(d_j,k)}, m_{(d_i,l)})$ is then calculated by using

$$\mathop{\mathrm{sim}}_{\mathrm{MFCC}}(m_{(d_j,k)}, m_{(d_i,l)}) = \frac{1}{1 + D(m_{(d_j,k)}, m_{(d_i,l)})}.$$

The artist similarity between $m_{(d_j,k)}$ and $m_{(d_i,l)}$ is calculated based on the Last.fm API.[2] The Last.fm API has a function, *artist.getSimilar*, which returns up to 100 similar artists to a specified artist, along with similarity values on a scale of 0 to 1. Let $a_{(d_j,k)}$ be the artist of the song $m_{(d_j,k)}$. The list of artists similar to $a_{(d_j,k)}$, denoted by $\mathcal{A}_{(d_j,k)}$, and their similarities $\mathrm{sim}_{\mathrm{last.fm}}(a_{(d_j,k)}, a')$ $(a' \in \mathcal{A}_{(d_j,k)})$ are obtained using Last.fm. In general, $\mathrm{sim}_{\mathrm{last.fm}}(\cdot, \cdot)$ is not symmetric. We therefore define the artist similarity as follows:

(i) When $a_{(d_j,k)} = a_{(d_i,l)}$,

$$\mathop{\mathrm{sim}}_{\mathrm{artist}}(m_{(d_j,k)}, m_{(d_i,l)}) = 1.0.$$

(ii) When $a_{(d_j,k)} \in \mathcal{A}_{(d_i,l)}$ and $a_{(d_i,l)} \in \mathcal{A}_{(d_j,k)}$,

$$\mathop{\mathrm{sim}}_{\mathrm{artist}}(m_{(d_j,k)}, m_{(d_i,l)}) = \frac{1}{2}\left\{\mathop{\mathrm{sim}}_{\mathrm{last.fm}}(a_{(d_j,k)}, a_{(d_i,l)}) + \mathop{\mathrm{sim}}_{\mathrm{last.fm}}(a_{(d_i,l)}, a_{(d_j,m)})\right\}$$

(iii) When $a_{(d_j,k)} \in \mathcal{A}_{(d_i,l)}$ and $a_{(d_i,l)} \notin \mathcal{A}_{(d_j,k)}$,

$$\mathop{\mathrm{sim}}_{\mathrm{artist}}(m_{(d_j,k)}, m_{(d_i,l)}) = \mathop{\mathrm{sim}}_{\mathrm{last.fm}}(a_{(d_j,k)}, a_{(d_i,l)})$$

(iv) When $a_{(d_j,k)} \notin \mathcal{A}_{(d_i,l)}$ and $a_{(d_i,l)} \in \mathcal{A}_{(d_j,k)}$,

$$\mathop{\mathrm{sim}}_{\mathrm{artist}}(m_{(d_j,k)}, m_{(d_i,l)}) = \mathop{\mathrm{sim}}_{\mathrm{last.fm}}(a_{(d_i,l)}, a_{(d_j,k)})$$

[2] http://www.last.fm/api.

(v) When $a_{(d_j,k)} \notin \mathcal{A}_{(d_i,l)}$ and $a_{(d_i,l)} \notin \mathcal{A}_{(d_j,k)}$,

$$\underset{\text{artist}}{\text{sim}}(m_{(d_j,k)}, m_{(d_i,l)}) = \varepsilon,$$

where ε is basically zero but can be set to a very small positive value to take into account the possibility of sparseness in similar artist responses ($\varepsilon = 0.01$ in the current implementation).

The similarity between two songs, denoted by $\text{sim}(m_{(d_j,k)}, m_{(d_i,l)})$, can be calculated as

$$\text{sim}(m_{(d_j,k)}, m_{(d_i,l)}) = \underset{\text{MFCC}}{\text{sim}}(m_{(d_j,k)}, m_{(d_i,l)}) \cdot \underset{\text{artist}}{\text{sim}}(m_{(d_j,k)}, m_{(d_i,l)}).$$

Using this similarity measure, the degree of preference can be calculated as follows:

$$W(u_i, m_{(d_j,k)}) = \frac{\text{sum}_l\ \text{sim}(m_{(d_j,k)}, m_{(d_i,l)}) W(u_i, m_{(d_i,l)})}{\text{sum}_l\ \text{sim}(m_{(d_j,k)}, m_{(d_i,l)})}.$$

4.2.3 Integration of Degrees of Preference

The degree of every user's preference is integrated as follows:

$$W_{\text{all}}(m_{(d_j,k)}) = \prod_{q=1}^{n} W(u_q, m_{(d_j,k)})$$

4.2.4 Generating a Playlist

After the integrated degrees of preference $W_{\text{all}}(m_{(d_j,k)})$ for all songs stored on all of the devices are calculated, a necessary number of songs are selected in order of the integrated degree of preference.

4.2.5 Playing Songs

Let $L = \{m_1, \ldots, m_c\}$ be the list of the selected songs and let $d(m_i)$ be the device storing the song m_i. For each song m_i, the following steps are executed:

(1) The master device d_1 commands $d(m_i)$ to connect itself to the Bluetooth speaker.
(2) The device $d(m_i)$ starts to play m_i.
(3) The master device d_1 broadcasts the information (title, artist name, etc.) of the song being played to all devices to alert users about which song is being played.
(4) Once the playback ends, the device $d(m_i)$ disconnects from the Bluetooth speaker and sends the master device d_1 a message representing the end of playback.

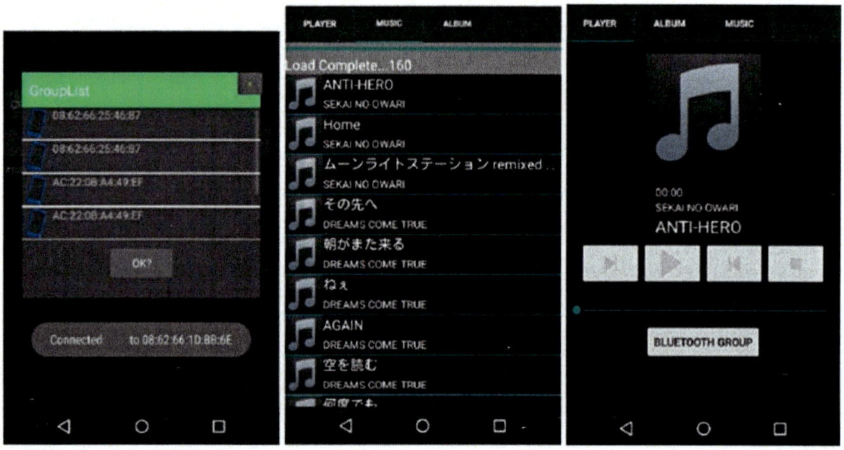

Fig. 2 Screenshot of our Android music player. Left: search of other devices via Bluetooh, Center: playlist display, Right: music playback

(5) Return to (1) for the next song.

Advanced Audio Distribution Profile (A2DP) is used for the connection between each device and the speaker. For communication between devices, Serial Port Profile (SPP) is used.

4.3 Implementation

We implemented this music player on Android 5.0 smartphones. Screenshots are shown in Fig. 2. A demo video of this application is available at https://www.youtube.com/watch?v=gcOWjkBcEA. For roughly one hour, we confirmed that this application successfully selected songs, switched the connection to the Bluetooth speaker, and played the selected songs without any troubles.

4.4 Evaluation of Preferences for Owned Songs

We confirmed the appropriateness of the calculation of the degrees of preference for a user's own songs by checking how these degrees calculated with our method matched the actual level of preference reported by the users.

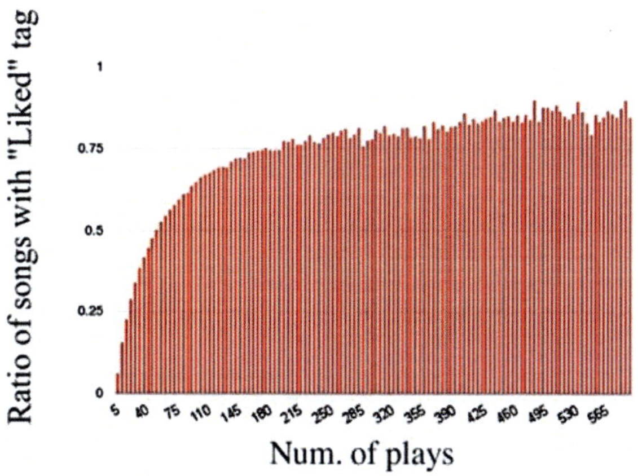

Fig. 3 The ratio of songs with the "Liked" tag with respect to the numbers of plays

4.4.1 Dataset

Data of playback histories and preferences were obtained from Last.fm. Using the Last.fm API, we obtained a user profile containing playback histories and evaluations (the "Liked" tag or no tag) for various songs. We collected user profiles for 45,745 users, who were specified by choosing one user at random and then traversing "Friend" links recursively. However, many users did not apply the "Liked" tag to any songs, we therefore chose to focus on the 11,074 users who gave "Liked" tags to 20–5000 songs. The total number of playback histories is 98,504,128.

4.4.2 Results

We analyzed the ratio of songs with the "Liked" tag with respect to the numbers of plays binned by 5 (Fig. 3). From this figure, one can see that as the number of plays increases, the ratio of songs with the "Liked" tag increases. Regarding this ratio as the ground truth of the degree of preference, we evaluated the degree of preference calculated with Eqs. (1) and (2). The results are shown in Fig. 4. One can see that using Eq. (1) with $\alpha = 0.01$ approximates the ground truth well. For songs with <20 times of plays, Eq. (1) with $\alpha = 0.10$ and Eq. (2) with $\beta = 0.005$ approximate better.

4.5 Evaluation of Preferences for Unowned Songs

Next, we confirmed the appropriateness of the calculation of the degree of preferences for songs not owned by a user.

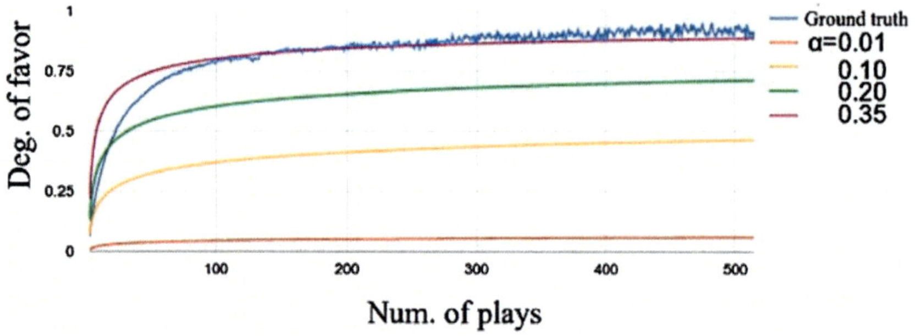

(a) With Equation (1)

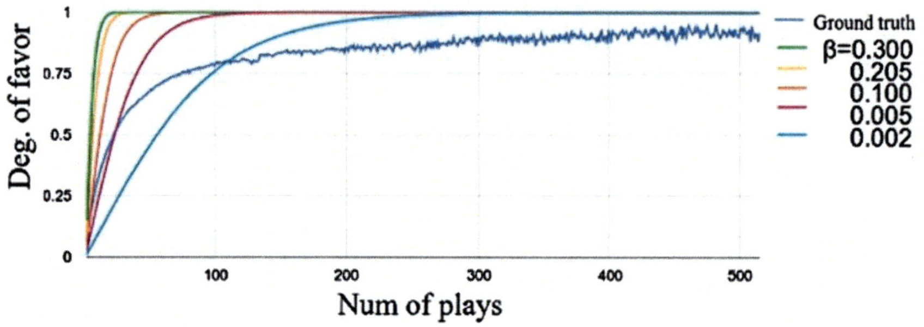

(b) With Equation (2)

Fig. 4 Estimation of degree of preference for owned songs

4.5.1 Dataset

We used the Last.fm Dataset,[3] which consists of playback histories of 1000 users. Of the songs contained in this database, some songs were regarded as owned songs and other songs were regarded as unowned songs and their playback histories were accordingly hidden. From the playback histories of the songs regarded as unowned, the degrees of preference were estimated. Ideally, the estimated degrees should be compared with real favor values (e.g., from questionnaires), but such data were not available from this database. We therefore regarded the degrees of preference calculated from the playback histories as the quasi-ground truth. Because this database does not include the waveforms themselves, a 30 s version of every song is downloaded via 7digital API[4] for feature extraction for calculating acoustic similarity.

[3] http://ocelma.net/.

[4] https://www.7digital.com/.

Table 1 Estimation of degree of preference for unowned songs

(a) With Eq. (1) for owned songs					
α	0.01	0.1	0.2	0.3	0.4
Corr.	0.60548	0.60419	0.60217	0.5960	0.59658
(b) With Eq. (2) for owned songs					
β	0.002	0.005	0.100	0.205	0.300
Corr.	0.56625	0.56708	0.60060	0.60132	0.59658

4.5.2 Procedure

We extracted 118 three-user groups such that the number of songs listened to by three users of every group exceeded 300. For each group, we divided the songs listened to by the group members into three sets; each set was regarded as being owned by each member. We calculated the degrees of preference for unowned songs of each member using the proposed method. At the same time, the degrees of preference for the same songs were calculated using Eqs. (1) and (2) and were regarded to be the quasi-ground truth.

4.5.3 Results

The correlations between the degrees of preference calculated using our method and the quasi-ground truth are listed in Table 1. These data show that the correlation is approximately 0.6 with almost any parameters and therefore that the degree of preference is fairly appropriately estimated. Figure 5 shows the correlations for each user, in which the quasi-ground truth is calculated using Eq. (1) with $\alpha = 0.01$. The correlations were higher than 0.5 for roughly half of the users.

5 Discussion

We developed an application that tries to find songs that are expected to be commonly favored by multiple users present together. Here, we discuss how successfully we dealt with the four issues mentioned above.

- **No time consumption for specifying musical preferences**
  We reduced the users' burden by collecting their listening histories instead of directly asking them their musical preferences. Exploiting listening histories is a widely used approach to estimate their musical preferences. One negative point is that users have to listen to music daily using our application. This is a non-negligible disadvantage because it takes away the freedom of choosing a music player. To solve this problem, listening histories on external music players have to

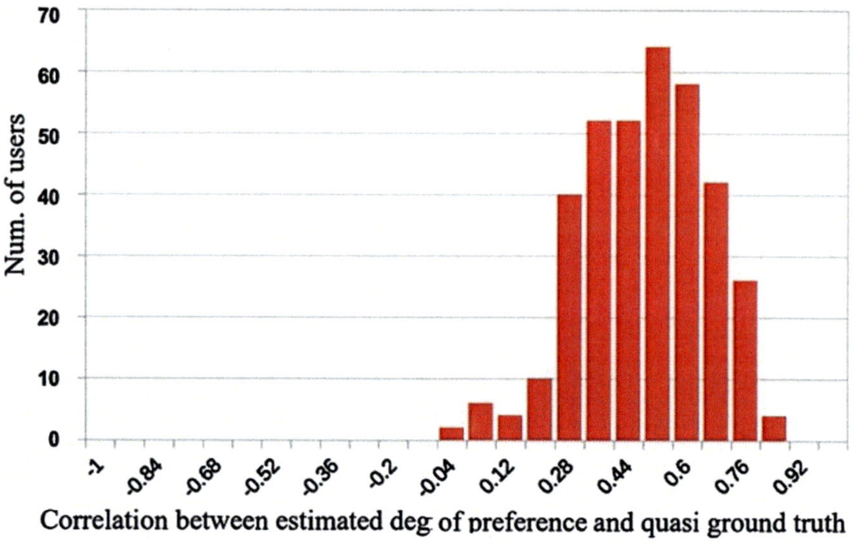

Fig. 5 Histogram of per-user correlations between the estimated degree of preference and the quasi-ground truth

be accessible from our application, but most players do not permit to access their listening histories from external applications. Use of the #nowlistening hashtag on Twitter, etc., could be one option to solve this problem, but it is not common enough.

- **Possibility of disjoint preference data**
  We assumed that there were many missing preference data because only each user's listening histories for songs that he/she owns himself/herself are available. The preference for songs that other members own is therefore estimated based on the principle that similar songs should have similar preferences. The similarity between songs is calculated by combining a song-level acoustic similarity and an artist-level social-based similarity. Developing a musical similarity measure is one of the central issues in the field of music information retrieval, so we would be able to use more sophisticated similarity measure. On the other hand, we did not deal with a situation where the members' musical preferences are truly disjoint; for example, one member listens to classical music only, whereas another member listens to rock music only. This situation is essentially difficult to reach an agreement on what songs are good as BGM.
- **Access to the content and copy-free playback**
  The access to the content (waveforms) of each song was possible because we assumed that the waveform of every target song was stored on some of the members' devices. In addition, by assuming the use of a Bluetooth speaker, we achieved the automatic switching of the devices to be connected to the speaker. However, in recent years, the mainstream music listening environment has been shifting to

on-demand music streaming services. To adapt our application to such streaming services, we have to resolve some technical issues such as the availability of the API for controlling playback and obtaining waveforms.

In addition, there are remaining issues as follows:

- **Playlist generation**
  The current application just places songs in order of the degree of the estimated preference. This is too naive. We have to improve this process to maintain the users' satisfaction from the beginning to the end of the playlist. Also, some rules used in Flytrap, such as not playing two songs by the same artist in a row, may be necessary to introduce.
- **Suitability of group listening**
  Not all songs are considered suitable for group listening. Some users may prefer listening to particular songs alone to listening to them together with friends. From a privacy point of view, each user should be able to control whether each of his/her songs is allowed to be included in candidates of group listening.
- **User study**
  Our application has not been evaluated in realistic situations. We should investigate how well our application works through a long-term user study with a large number of participants.

6 Conclusion

In this chapter, we described attempts to music selection in a situation where some people listen to the same music together. Listening to music together with friends, family, and/or someone else is an enjoyable experience, but due to the variability of people's musical preferences, it is difficult to select music acceptable for everyone. The attempts mentioned above, including ours, tried to tackle this problem by developing a system that analyzes and aggregates individual users' musical preferences.

The number of attempts for group music selection/recommendation is obviously fewer than non-group (individual users) music selection/recommendation. However, we believe that group music selection/recommendation has a great demand. We hope that the number of such attempts will increase and thus the enjoyment of listening to music together with someone will be further enriched.

Acknowledgments This work was supported by JSPS KAKENHI Grant Numbers 26240025, 26280089, 16K16180, 16H01744, 16KT0136, and 17H00749. We appreciate Prof. Tomonobu Ozaki for his fruitful comments.

References

1. McCarthy, J.F., Anagnost, T.D.: MusicFX: an arbiter of group preferences for computer supported collaborative workouts. In: Proceedings of the 1998 ACM Conference on Computer Supported Cooperative Work (CSCW '98), pp. 363–372 (1998)
2. Crossen, A., Budzik, J., Hammond, K.J.: Flytrap: intelligent group music recommendation. In: Proceedings of International Conference on Intelligent User Interfaces (IUI '02), pp. 184–185 (2002)
3. Popescu, G., Pu, P.: What's the best music you have? Designing music recommendation for group enjoyment in GroupFun. In: Works-in-Progress of the ACM SIGCHI Conference on Human Factors in Computing Systems (CHI '12), pp. 1673–1678 (2012)
4. Mahato, H., Kern, D., Holleis, P., Schmidt, A.: Implicit personalization of public environments using Bluetooth. In: Proceedings of CHI EA '08 Extended Abstracts on Human Factors in Computing Systems, pp. 3093–3098 (2008)
5. Suzuki, J., Kitahara, T.: A music player with song selection function for a group of people. In: Proceedings of the 18th International Society for Music Information Retrieval Conference (ISMIR 2017), pp. 229–234, October 2017
6. Jameson, A.: More than the sum of its members: challenges for group recommender systems. In: Proceedings of the Working Conference on Adanced Visual Interfacec (AVI 2004), pp. 48–54 (2004)
7. Dias, P., Magalhães, J.: Music recommendations for groups of users. In: Proceedings of the 2013 ACM International Workshop on Immersive Media Experiences, pp. 21–24. ACM (2013)
8. Aucouturier, J.-J., Pachet, F.: Tools and architecture for the evaluation of similarity measures: case study of timbre similarity. In: Proceedings of the 5th International Conference on Music Information Retrieval (ISMIR 2004), pp. 198–203 (2004)

Body Data for Music Information Retrieval Tasks

Tejaswinee Kelkar

Abstract This chapter deals with the question of how can different technologies for gathering information from the body— such as motion capture, gestural interfaces, EEG, and so on—be used for music information retrieval applications. Music information retrieval (MIR) is an interdisciplinary domain that draws from signal processing, electrical engineering, machine learning, and music cognition, among other fields, to build a computational understanding of musical content. Historically, the methods of MIR have relied on metadata and information processing, but as technology for non-traditional capture of body data becomes more accessible, more and more research aims to map different aspects of the body to the musical responses of a person. This chapter is a review of systems and algorithms that use data from the body for the purpose of retrieving music. I aim to provide a theoretical background for these tasks as well as a review of current literature on the subject.

1 Music and the Body

Music moves the body—as has been suggested by research in musicology, psychology, and cross-disciplinary fields. In the recent past, we have seen a surge in the use of commercially available, ready-to-use devices that enable us to use data from our bodies for various kinds of insights related to sports, health, and general well-being. The availability of computer vision-enabled tools to map and also to enhance our immediate physical environment—measuring and augmenting it—is also unprecedented compared to the technology of the first-generation consumer electronics. As one might expect, these technologies find creative and information retrieval contexts also for music use. Commercially available highly successful applications and interactive platforms also exploit this potential specially related to music listening. This chapter will explore academic and commercial works in progress that relate to the information retrieval paradigm of music, in context of data from the body.

T. Kelkar (✉)
Forskningsveien 3A, 0373 Oslo, Norway
e-mail: tejaswinee.kelkar@imv.uio.no

Z. W. Ras et al. (eds.), *Recommender Systems for Medicine and Music*,
Studies in Computational Intelligence 946,
https://doi.org/10.1007/978-3-030-66450-3_10

By data from the body, I firstly mean motion data in various forms, such as accelerometers, gyroscopes, object tracking, and optical flow tracking; secondly, I am also including the use of data as complex as EEG, electromyography, electrodermal activity, for retrieval tasks that approach music content retrieval. I will review research pertaining to these data types, mapped to music. The aim of some of these developments is to create interactive music applications of the future.

Non-traditional music applications fall into two broad categories: creation, or compositional or interactive technology on the one hand, and multimodally mapped, music content retrieval on the other. At first glance, it may seem that these two are vastly separate: interactive technology has only to do with sound mapping, synthesis, and generative models while retrieval is about music databases. However, upon closer look, we can learn that multimodal mapping techniques are used in various ways in both contexts. The usage scenario for developing the technology for multimodal input interfaces for music is comparable in both these contexts.

2 Music Content Retrieval

The storage and consumption of music have undergone a radical change since the time of digital music distribution through content services. This has created very large databases that are primarily served on the basis of metadata—such as looking for other music from the same artist, or the same label, and recommendation based on learning typical user profiles and preferences. Other systems of finding music, simply locating the right label for a user-generated query, are becoming both in demand, and are very popular. The success of the *audio fingerprinting* application Shazam can be seen as an example of this. Historically, MIR has focused on the use of metadata and tagging for a variety of tasks.

However, this has been changing for some time. Some examples of the use of MIR techniques include studies on emotional affect using mood detection algorithms [25], where the MIR toolbox [34] is used to enumerate the acoustic characteristics of the stimulus set, which are evaluated against listeners' ratings of affect. Knox et al. [30] analyzed pain-relieving music using MIR techniques to study acoustic characteristics. Malandrakis et al. [38] used MIR techniques for emotion tracking in film music. MIR-based methods and tools are used on both symbolic and signal-based datasets.

2.1 Audio Content-Based Music Retrieval

There are three levels of sound representations in computing applications: *physical*, *digital*, and *perceptual*. Physical representations of sound are included in the data from direct recordings. Digital representations of sound include transcriptions of melodies and transformation of contour data into the symbolic domain. Perceptual descriptors of sound and motion include computational models that mimic perceptual qualities, such as "smoothness" of movement and "loudness" of sound.

Research deals with human body motion, or the "response" material for the perceived qualities in melody, as the data that could be purely *physical* or *perceptual*. Analysis of these data involves, for example, the notion of an *effector*, which refers to any body part that might be involved carrying out a movement (hands, legs, the head), or an object held by or attached to the body, such as a wand. Whether body movement is measured using cameras, motion capture, and so on, also dictates how the data are obtained, and what these data can show us.

More specifically, for auditory descriptors, I refer to three different levels of concepts: the *acoustic*, *psychoacoustic*, and *musical*. Acoustic analysis includes features that are calculated mathematically, for example, the energy of a sound signal or its spectral features. Psychoacoustic features can also be approximated through computational methods, such as perceptual loudness of a sound signal. Musical features of a sound stimulus are different from these, and may be embedded within a musical culture, for instance, cadence or specific intervals. They may also be psychoacoustic approximations that are understood as having a "musical" quality, such as melody or intervals.

Audio content-based retrieval occurs in an interaction of various combinations of these. Here, I would also like the reader to note a disambiguation for the word "cross-modal" or cross-modality. While cross-modality in the context of psychology, or perception refers to an interaction, or interactions of different sensory modalities, in computing, cross-modality may simply mean different types of data. For example, score and audio for the same musical piece are two different computing modalities, whereas audition and motion are two different perceptual modalities.

2.2 *Content Retrieval Using Melody*

Audio content retrieval tasks can often be thought of as tasks regarding melodic retrieval. A class of these problems have high specificity, for example, cover song detection tasks.

Several projects on melodic content retrieval using intuitive and multimodal representations of musical data have been developed for use on different datasets. The oldest example of this is the 1975 project, "Directory of Tunes and Musical Themes," in which the author used a simplified contour notation method involving letters to denote contour directions to create a dictionary of musical themes, from which one may look up a tune they remember [48]. The aim of this book was for people to be able to look up a tune stuck in their head as long as they could describe the contour direction of the melody.

Parsons' model has been adopted for melodic contour retrieval by Musipedia [20]. Another system has been proposed in the recent project called SoundTracer, in which the motion of a user's mobile phone is used to retrieve tunes from a music archive [33]. A critical difference between these approaches is how they handle contour and musical mappings, especially variations in time scales and time representations. Most of these methods do not have ground truth models of contours, and instead use one of several ways of mappings, each with its own assumptions.

Interactive systems to generate music that fill in the gaps as it were, from skeletal notions of melodic contour are popular. Typically, the interface involves a way for a user to generate a contour, onto which generative models are mapped, to give a possible musical solution. Several studies on embodied music cognition investigate the idea of drawing or tracing as a method of understanding the mappings of shapes and lines to musical material.

3 Body Data

3.1 Body Data and Music Creation

Another question is, how can these interfaces be used to create music—or—how can music creation become a goal of a system that is otherwise created for music retrieval? Common modes of interaction for explicitly melodic interfaces include tracing, drawing, sketching, and hand-waving for contour depiction. Mappings from these contour depictions take various forms. Generated melodies are usually harder to evaluate for goodness and fit in music generation, than, for example, harmonic adherence to a particular style or time period in music. Depending on the task at hand, melodic generation tasks may or may not require continuity and development, and some idea of self-similarity—creating a thematic identity through a notion of repetition. Although melodic generation spans a large range of mathematical, parametric, and learning methods, generally melodic generation is constrained to the symbolic domain. A majority of the systems for generation are thus in the symbolic domain, and inapplicable to musical cultures and styles where either datasets for symbolic music do not exist, or symbolic generation is insufficient to capture the musical style.

Typically, gesture–music interfaces start with some assumption of musical grammars, goals, strategies, and styles; gestural interfaces start with some baseline measurements of user actions. There is a mid-level representation of the input and output, at which point mapping might be carried out. The goals of some of these instruments might either be the real-time generation of melodies or complete songs based on one or a few factors mapped from the gesture. A proof-of-concept for exploring this was recently published as part of Google's Magenta project offshoot, titled Piano Genie [10]. Here, contour enumeration happens through a series of press buttons, reducing the 88 piano keys to four, and mapping improvisation using generation on top of these contours. A system of sketching melodies on paper is also described in [29], where people use a tablet to draw melodic contours on a grid that resembles the piano roll format. TrAP uses a tablet-based interface to map four types of contour profiles by segmentation [51]. The MicroJam application by Martin et al. includes a sketch-based interface to input melodies and rhythm; the application can also be used for collaborative performances and modeling [39]. *He* is an interface for generating melodic material based on brush calligraphy [27]. The system uses computer vision techniques to analyze brush stroke features and ink thickness and map them onto a pentatonic scale. The Melodic Brush interface by Lo et al. [40] is another example of the use of calligraphy inputs, with the specific intention of generating Chinese music, using a kinect depth camera [40].

Several recent research articles suggest that a growing number of researchers are interested in using body movement in music information retrieval [37, 41, 44, 59]. Other researchers have also explored this area. Müller's book titled "Information Retrieval for Music and Motion" [41] deals specifically with retrieval techniques for music as well as retrieval techniques for movement. However, development of datasets and methods for music retrieval through motion is still an open task, even though in the following paragraphs I will describe various works that try to address this.

3.2 Body Data for Music Retrieval

Understanding the close relationship between music and motion is vital to understand subjective experiences of performers and listeners, [8, 13, 14]. Many empirical experiments aimed at investigating music–motion correspondences deal with stimulus data that is made to explicitly observe certain mappings, for example, pitched and non-pitched sound, vertical dimension and pitch, or player expertise [5, 32, 46]. This means that the music examples themselves are sorted into types of sound (or types of motion). Kelkar and Jensenius [28] use melodies from musical styles from various parts of the world, including those that contain microtonal inflections, which can find representation through contour and shape, as opposed to rely on Western notation as the main representational language, in order to observe how sound tracings of melodies represent their contour content.

Masahiro et al. [57] provide a dance dataset in the context of music information retrieval. The authors provide a large dataset of several people dancing to specific styles of music and dance. This work was published in a music information retrieval context. They also present research for querying music by video, or in other words, a method to retrieve dance motion by a video query. The authors rely on rhythm extraction and matching the obtained tempo to the user's movements [56]. This approach is based on calculating several angles of the body in order to get different dimensions of rhythm. Using this mapping, the system generates music as its output, the rhythm of which is used for retrieval through comparing with extracted rhythm from a number of pieces. This could be considered to be the state of the art for this family of ideas at the time of writing this chapter. However, not all music is a dance music. Systems to retrieve melodic or timbral content from music using body movement or movement-like data are even rarer. Lee et al. [35] have developed a system for automatic generation of dance, given a music query. Huang et al. [18] provide a machine-informed identification of expressive semantics in orchestral conducting. Hu et al. [17] analyze user interactions with MIR Systems using eye-tracking data.

4 Search and Retrieval Algorithms

4.1 Multimodal Retrieval

There seems to be a growing interest in the field of music and multimodality, in its meeting with music information retrieval. Multimodal retrieval is the paradigm of information retrieval used to handle different types of data together. The objective is to learn a set of mapping functions that project the different modalities into a common metric space, to be able to retrieve relevant information in one modality through a query in another. We see that this paradigm is used often in the retrieval of image from text and text from image. Canonical Correlation Analysis (CCA) is a common tool for investigating linear relationships of two sets of variables. In the review paper by Wang et al. for cross-modal retrieval [58], several implementations and models are analyzed. CCA has also been used to explore cross-relationships between music and brain imaging [42].

4.2 EEG Data for Music Information Retrieval

Recent papers that discuss mapping EEG signals to music data try to use the intermediate domain of affective tagging. Through this method, personalized physiological signals can be classified into one of a few possible tags in a mid-level representation space, and then using this space to map several music instances onto. Stober and others [52] refer to this as Musical Imagery Information Retrieval or MIIR. In their work, they hope to capture imagining a musical stimulus, by mapping it to EEG data from 14 participants. This is an open dataset for incorporating EEG signals in a music retrieval paradigm. There have later been many related research articles trying to map EEG signals, and also using openMIIR dataset.

Other research in the EEG domain is also for mapping affective states while music listening, and using this as a form of music retrieval. Koelstra et al. [31] write about the recognition of the affective states of users, and gathering this to conduct classification of affective states using EEG, and then using them for music recommendation. Kaneshiro and Dmochowski [26] surveyed neuroimaging techniques that can be used in MIR research, and highlighted a number of potential research topics spanning the two fields.

4.3 Motion Capture

Motion capture, often shortened as *MoCap*, is a general term referring to a group of methods used to measure motion. There are a number of techniques that can be thought of as motion capture, and a recent overview can be found at [23]. Verbal descriptions and annotations of movement are the simplest ways to capture motion; codes for describing gestures are often used in annotating gestures accompanying speech [50]. Photography, video analysis, and light-sensing have also been used to capture motion [22]. The following methods for motion tracking are most important, and have been detailed by [43]

1. Acoustical tracking: The use of phase differences to measure reflections of sound, and hence the changing distance of a moving object [3].
2. Mechanical tracking: Tracking or measuring the angles between two mechanical parts that are changing the length of a resistor to infer the distance or angle of the tracked object, for example, as used by [9]. A joystick is a good example of this.
3. Magnetic tracking: Tracking the magnetic field of a moving electromagnet, measuring its distance from a stationary electromagnet [3].
4. Inertial tracking: Using accelerometers and gyroscopes to track the position of an object based on its interaction with gravity [3]. Inertial Motion Units (IMU) are example of this type of tracking [53] as are, for example, Xsens suits.
5. Optical tracking: Using infrared (IR), regular video, stereo video, thermal, or depth cameras to estimate an object's position in space. Using optical tracking requires post-processing using computer vision algorithms.

Several works have described retrieval paradigms based on motion capture. Kelkar and Jensenius [28] describe work done on melodic sound tracings using IR motion capture systems. This work is for macro-music samples that could be described as melodic phrases, whereas [43] describes methods to retrieve small sound samples. In [21], the authors provide a well-rounded overview of what such a system of the future might look like.

5 Methods for Multimodal Retrieval

5.1 Time Series Analysis

A simple way to analyze sound-tracing-related movement data would be to compare different time series. Several tasks in this family of problems involve measuring the distance between two time series. In essence, time series are matrices. Several methods have been proposed for time series distance matching, which can be imagined as the extent of the variance between two different time series. Broadly, the methods can be classified as follows:

1. Reduced dimensionality measures: These are useful when time series are large or tightly sampled, and therefore time series distance cannot be measured by sample-to-sample distances. Reduced dimensionality measures can include, for example, discrete Fourier transform, and then a comparison between the transforms. Discrete Cosine Transform (DCT) to time series (e.g., sound samples in the time domain) to frequency domain, approximating data through Chebyshev polynomials, are some ways to measure time series distance using reduced dynamics.
2. Distance measures: The easiest way to think about distance measures is to calculate the Euclidean or edit distance, which would be the distance per sample between the two series. Edit distance measures can also be improved by introducing edit distance penalties, or using a weighted alignment before distance is calculated.
3. Longest common subsequence (LCS): LCS is a set of problems to detect the longest common subsequences in any two sequences of data. This problem can be adapted to string commonalities and continuous time series.
4. Data adaptive measures: Data adaptive measures try to fit first to the series data before computing distance, for example, polynomial interpolation or regression using piecewise polynomials or splines. In these methods, the approximated functions are then compared to find distances. For symbolic data, such methods can include substrings, case modification, or other kinds of approximation.
5. Non-data adaptive measures: Wavelet transforms, spectral measures such as Discrete Fourier Transform (DFT), DCT, and piecewise aggregation approximation methods can be used.

We can also take another approach, i.e., instead of trying to find the distance between two time series in a hyperspace, we can measure their similarities. Broad classifications of similarity measures are as follows:

1. Lock step measures: Distance measures such as L1 and L2 norms.
2. Elastic measures: DTW, LCS, edit distance, and sequence weighted alignment can be thought of as elastic distance measures because they aim to match subsequences or subsections of data.
3. Threshold-based measures: TQuEST or the Threshold Query Execution for Large Sets of Time Series [2].
4. Pattern-based measures: Spatial Assembling Distance, also called SpADe [7].

5.2 Canonical Correlation Analysis

CCA is a statistical method to find a linear combination of two variables $X = (x_1, x_2, \ldots, x_n)$ and $Y = (y_1, y_2, \ldots, y_m)$ with n and m lengths of sets of variables as vectors a and b such that the linear correlation $\rho = corr(aX, bY)$ of the transformed variables is maximized. Linear vectors a' and b' can be found such that $a', b' = \underset{a,b}{\operatorname{argmax}} \ \operatorname{corr}(a^T X, b^T Y)$. We can then find the second set of coefficients which maximize the correlation of the variables $X' = aX$ and $Y' = bY$ with the additional constraint to keep (X, X') and (Y, Y') uncorrelated. This process can be repeated till $d = \min(m, n)$ dimensions.

The CCA can be extended to include non-linearity by using a neural network to transform the X and Y variables as in the case of Deep CCA [1]. θ_1 and θ_2, the objective is to maximize the correlation $corr(f(X, \theta_1), f(Y, \theta_2))$. The network is trained by following the gradient of the correlation objective as estimated from the training data.

In a review paper, Wang et al. analyze several models for cross-modal retrieval [58]. Firstly, CCA allows us to approach the data through real-value-based methods. The method also allows us to approach the data in a pairwise retrieval paradigm. Just like unsupervised methods, the CCA method uses similar pairs to learn meaningful distance metrics between different modalities. CCA has also been used previously to show music and brain imaging inter-relationships.

CCA has also been used in research related to the analysis and retrieval of music–motion [5, 6, 44, 45]. The biggest reservations in analyzing music–motion data using CCA are that non-linearity cannot be represented, and that the method is highly dependent on time synchronization. The temporal evolution of motion and sound remains linear over time [6]. To get around this, kernel-based methods can be used to introduce non-linearity. Ohkushi et al. [47] present a study that used kernel-based CCA methods to analyze motion and music features together using video sequences from classical ballet, and optical-flow-based clustering. Bozkurt et al. present a CCA-based system to analyze and generate speech and arm motion for a prosody-driven synthesis of the "beat gesture," which is used to emphasize prosodically salient points in speech [4]. CCA is used to explore the datasets due to the previous successes associated with using this family of methods. The same data are also analyzed using deep CCA, a neural network approximation of CCA, to better understand the non-linear mappings.

A previous paper analyzing tracings to pitched and non-pitched sounds also used CCA to understand music–motion relationships [44], where the authors describe inherent non-linearity in the mappings, despite finding intrinsic sound–action relationships. This work was extended in [45], in which CCA was used to interpret how different features correlate with each other. Pitch and vertical motion have linear relationships in this analysis, although it is important to note that the sound samples used for this study were short and synthetic.

6 Structures of Multimodal Retrieval

6.1 Granularity and Specificity

In [15], the authors explore the notion of mapping content-based music retrieval onto the dimensions of **granularity** and **specificity**. For problems with high specificity, exact musical pieces often lie in the database, that is to say, that a query should ideally be able to correctly retrieve an exact version of a particular audio sample. High specificity, on the other hand, refers to category-based retrieval that might have a label set for both music and movement. This intermediate domain is often descriptive and dependent on several variables.

6.2 Intermediate Domain Representation

Movements related to the production and interpretation of music have been studied in various types of detail using experimental and empirical methods. Most significantly, recent research in neuroscience and psychology has shown that *action* plays an important role in perception [16, 22]. In phonology and linguistics, the co-articulation of action and sound is also well understood. Theories from embodied music cognition [36] have been critical to this exploration of multimodal correspondences.

Contour perception is a coarse-level musical ability that we acquire early during childhood [49, 54, 55]. Research suggests that our memory for contour is enhanced when melodies are tonal, and when tonal accent points of melodies co-occur with strong beats [24], making melodic memory a salient feature in musical perception. More generally, it is easier for people to remember the general shape of melody rather than precise intervals [19], especially if they are not musical experts. Coarse representations of melodic contour, such as with drawing or moving hands in the air, may be intuitive to capturing musical moments of short time scales [11, 44].

Representation in an intermediate domain can be of various types. For example, an affective retrieval EEG system may map both the brain signals to one of many possibilities in a genre cloud, or an affective tag cloud, to which in turn music samples may also be mapped. A problem such as this is a low specificity problem, in that the ground truth is often subjectively mapped to a pre-test containing subjective evaluations.

Intermediate domain representation may also be used to retrieve music from motion data, as seen in Tsuchida et al. [56]. Here, the motion domain is transferred to an intermediate domain, for example, to map to beat analysis. This ensures that a relevant intermediate modality accurately represents the similarities that are relevant to the dance in both modalities. Goto [12] also describes a system for active listening interfaces based on music signal processing.

7 Conclusions

In this chapter, we have seen a range of multimodal and cross-modal music retrieval methods that help to bring the ideas for music retrieval and music information retrieval, to incorporate data from the body.

Treating sound tracings as annotation material provides a new way of thinking about music analysis and studies on segmentation and phrasing. Through the experiments conducted, I have shown that people demonstrate a remarkable amount of consistency in their spatial and motor representations of music and sonic objects. Experiments akin to these could inform our understanding of musical phrasing, and the differences in people's phrasing boundaries in various contexts. This could help us build a more sophisticated understanding of music perception and create interesting interfaces for music retrieval.

We also see how both music creation and retrieval systems show parallels in their use of multimodal data. This chapter also summarizes a number of motion capture methods, time series comparison, and multimodal analysis methods.

Several of these interfaces are built upon medical applications—such as the EEG and EMG systems—which were first used for medicine and not music, thus illuminating use cases of this data much beyond their intended use, in a new and exciting domain.

References

1. Andrew, G., Arora, R., Bilmes, J., Livescu, K.: Deep canonical correlation analysis. In: International Conference on Machine Learning, pp. 1247–1255 (2013)
2. Aßfalg, J., Kriegel, H.-P., Kröger, P., Kunath, P., Pryakhin, A., Renz, M.: Tquest: threshold query execution for large sets of time series. In: International Conference on Extending Database Technology, pp. 1147–1150. Springer (2006)
3. Bishop, G., Welch, G., Danette Allen, B.: Tracking: beyond 15 minutes of thought. SIGGRAPH Course Pack **11**, (2001)
4. Bozkurt, E., Yücel, Y., Erzin, E.: Multimodal analysis of speech and arm motion for prosody-driven synthesis of beat gestures. Speech Commun. **85**, 29–42 (2016)
5. Caramiaux, B., Bevilacqua, F., Schnell, N.: Towards a gesture-sound cross-modal analysis. In: International Gesture Workshop, pp. 158–170. Springer (2009)
6. Caramiaux, B., Tanaka, A.: Machine learning of musical gestures. In: Proceedings of the 13th International Conference on New Interfaces for Musical Expression, pp. 513–518 (2013)
7. Chen, Y., Nascimento, M.A., Ooi, B.C., Tung, A.K.H.: Spade: on shape-based pattern detection in streaming time series. In: 2007 IEEE 23rd International Conference on Data Engineering, pp. 786–795 (2007)
8. Clayton, M., Leante, L.: Embodiment in music performance (2013)
9. De Laubier, S.: The meta-instrument. Comput. Music J. **22**(1), 25–29 (1998)
10. Donahue, C., Simon, I., Dieleman, S.: Piano genie (2018). arXiv preprint arXiv:1810.05246
11. Godøy, R.I., Haga, E., Jensenius, A.R.: Exploring music-related gestures by sound-tracing: a preliminary study. In: Kia, N. (ed.) Proceedings of the COST287-ConGAS 2nd International Symposium on Gesture Interfaces for Multimedia Systems (GIMS2006), pp. 27–33. Leeds, UK (2006)
12. Goto, M.: Active music listening interfaces based on signal processing. In: 2007 IEEE International Conference on Acoustics, Speech and Signal Processing-ICASSP'07, vol. 4, pp. IV–1441. IEEE (2007)
13. Gritten, A., King, E.: Music and Gesture. Ashgate Publishing Ltd. (2006)
14. Gritten, A., King, E.: New Perspectives on Music and Gesture. Ashgate Publishing, Ltd (2011)
15. Grosche, P., Müller, M., Serra, J.: Audio content-based music retrieval. In: Dagstuhl Follow-Ups, vol. 3. Schloss Dagstuhl-Leibniz-Zentrum für Informatik (2012)

16. Hari, R.: Action-perception connection and the cortical mu rhythm. Progr. Brain Res. **159**, 253–260 (2006)
17. Hu, X., Que, Y., Kando, N., Lian, W.: Analyzing user interactions with music information retrieval system: An eye tracking approach. In: Proceedings of the 20th International Society for Music Information Retrieval Conference (ISMIR), Delft, Netherlands (2019)
18. Huang, Y.-F., Chen, T.-P., Moran, N., Coleman, S., Su, L.: Identifying Expressive Semantics in Orchestral Conducting Kinematics, pp. 115–122 (2019)
19. Huron, D.: The melodic arch in western folksongs. Comput. Musicol. **10**, 3–23 (1996)
20. Irwin, K.: Musipedia: The open music encyclopedia. Ref. Rev. **22**(4), 45–46 (2008)
21. Jensenius, A.R., Kvifte, T., Godøy, R.I.: Towards a gesture description interchange format. In: Proceedings of the 2006 Conference on New Interfaces for Musical Expression, pp. 176–179. IRCAM–Centre Pompidou (2006)
22. Jensenius, A.R.: Action-sound: developing methods and tools to study music-related body movement (2007)
23. Jensenius, A.R.: Methods for Studying Music-Related Body Motion, pp. 805–818. Springer, Berlin, Heidelberg (2018)
24. Jones, M.R., Pfordresher, P.Q.: Tracking musical patterns using joint accent structure. Can. J. Exp. Psychol./Revue canadienne de psychologie expérimentale **51**(4), 271 (1997)
25. Juslin, P.N., Harmat, L., Eerola, T.: What makes music emotionally significant? exploring the underlying mechanisms. Psychol. Music **42**(4), 599–623 (2014)
26. Kaneshiro, B., Dmochowski, J.P.: Neuroimaging methods for music information retrieval: current findings and future prospects. In: ISMIR, pp. 538–544 (2015)
27. Kang, L., Chien, H.Y.: Hé: Calligraphy as a musical interface. In: NIME, pp. 352–355 (2010)
28. Kelkar, T., Jensenius, A.R.: Analyzing free-hand sound-tracings of melodic phrases. Appl. Sci. **8**(1), 135 (2018)
29. Kitahara, T., Giraldo, S.I., Ramírez, R.: Jamsketch: a drawing-based real-time evolutionary improvisation support system. In: Proceedings of the 17th International Conference on New Interfaces for Musical Expression, pp. 505–506 (2017)
30. Knox, D., Beveridge, S., Mitchell, L.A., MacDonald, R.A.R.: Acoustic analysis and mood classification of pain-relieving music. J. Acoust. Soc. America **130**(3), 1673–1682 (2011)
31. Koelstra, S., Yazdani, A., Soleymani, M., Mühl, C., Lee, J.-S., Nijholt, A., Pun, T., Ebrahimi, T., Patras, I.: Single trial classification of EEG and peripheral physiological signals for recognition of emotions induced by music videos. In: International Conference on Brain Informatics, pp. 89–100. Springer (2010)
32. Kussner, M.: Creating shapes: musicians' and non-musicians' visual representations of sound. In: Seifert, U., Wewers, J. (eds.) Proceedings of 4th International Conference of Students of Systematic Musicology. epOs-Music, Osnabrück (2012)
33. Wallace, B., Jensenius, A.R.: SoundTracer: A brief project summary (2018)
34. Lartillot, O., Toiviainen, P.: A matlab toolbox for musical feature extraction from audio. In: International Conference on Digital Audio Effects, pp. 237–244. Bordeaux (2007)
35. Lee, J., Kim, S., Lee, K.: Automatic choreography generation with convolutional encoder-decoder network. ISMIR (2019)
36. Leman, M.: Embodied Music Cognition and Mediation Technology. MIT Press (2008)
37. Liem, C., Müller, M., Eck, D., Tzanetakis, G., Hanjalic, A.: The need for music information retrieval with user-centered and multimodal strategies. In: Proceedings of the 1st International Association for Computing Machinery Workshop on Music Information Retrieval with User-Centered and Multimodal Strategies, pp. 1–6. Association for Computing Machinery (2011)
38. Malandrakis, N., Potamianos, A., Evangelopoulos, G., Zlatintsi, A.: A supervised approach to movie emotion tracking. In: 2011 IEEE International Conference on Acoustics, Speech and Signal Processing (ICASSP), pp. 2376–2379. IEEE (2011)
39. Martin, C.P., Tørresen, J.: Microjam: an app for sharing tiny touch-screen performances. In: Proceedings of the International Conference on New Interfaces for Musical Expression, pp. 495–496. Aalborg University Copenhagen (2017)

40. Lo, K.W.K., Lau, C.K., Ngai, G., Chan, S.C.F., Huang, M.X., Tang, W.: MelodicBrush: a cross-modal link between ancient and digital art forms. In: Proceedings of the Designing Interactive Systems Conference on—DIS '12, p. 418, July 2012
41. Müller, M.: Information retrieval for music and motion, vol. 2. Springer (2007)
42. Berger, J., Dmochowski, J.P., Gang, N., Kaneshiro, B.: Decoding neurally relevant musical features using canonical correlation analysis. In: Proceedings of the 18th International Society for Music Information Retrieval Conference, Souzhou, China (2017)
43. Nymoen, K.: Methods and technologies for analysing links between musical sound and body motion. Ph.D. thesis, University of Oslo (2013)
44. Nymoen, K., Caramiaux, B., Kozak, M., Torresen, J.: Analyzing sound tracings: A multimodal approach to music information retrieval. In: Proceedings of the 1st International Association for Computing Machinery Workshop on Music Information Retrieval with User-centered and Multimodal Strategies, MIRUM '11, pp. 39–44. Association for Computing Machinery, New York, NY, USA (2011)
45. Nymoen, K., Godøy, R.I., Jensenius, A.R., Torresen, J.: Analyzing correspondence between sound objects and body motion. Assoc. Comput. Machin. Trans. Appl. Percept. **10**(2), 9:1–9:22 (2013)
46. Nymoen, K., Torresen, J., Godøy, R., Jensenius, A.: A statistical approach to analyzing sound tracings. In: Speech, Sound and Music Processing: Embracing Research in India, pp. 120–145 (2012)
47. Ohkushi, H., Ogawa, T., Haseyama, M.: Music recommendation according to human motion based on kernel CCA-based relationship. EURASIP J. Adv. Signal Process. **2011**(1), 121 (2011)
48. Parsons, D.: The Directory of Tunes and Musical Themes. S. Brown, Cambridge, Eng (1975)
49. Patel, A.D.: Music, Language, and the Brain. Oxford University Press (2010)
50. Poggi, I.: Towards the alphabet and the lexicon of gesture, gaze and touch. In: Virtual Symposium on Multimodality of Human Communication (2002). http://www.semioticon.com/virtuals/index.html
51. Roy, U., Kelkar, T., Indurkhya, B.: Trap: an interactive system to generate valid raga phrases from sound-tracings. In: Proceedings of the 14th International Conference on New Interfaces of Musical Expression Conference, pp. 243–246 (2014)
52. Stober, S., Sternin, A., Owen, A.M., Grahn, J.A.: Towards music imagery information retrieval: introducing the openmiir dataset of EEG recordings from music perception and imagination. In: ISMIR, pp. 763–769 (2015)
53. Tanenhaus, M.E., Lipeles, J.L.: Miniaturized inertial measurement unit and associated methods. US Patent 7,526,402 (2009)
54. Trehub, S.E., Becker, J., Morley, I.: Cross-cultural perspectives on music and musicality. Philosophical Trans. Royal Soc. Lond. B: Biol. Sci. **370**(1664), 20140096 (2015)
55. Trehub, S.E., Bull, D., Thorpe, L.A.: Infants' perception of melodies: the role of melodic contour. Child Dev. **821–830**, (1984)
56. Tsuchida, S., Fukayama, S., Goto, M.: Query-by-dancing: a dance music retrieval system based on body-motion similarity. In: International Conference on Multimedia Modeling, pp. 251–263. Springer (2019)
57. Masahiro, H., Shuhei, T., Satoru, F., Goto, M.: Aist dance video database: multi-genre, multi-dancer, and multi-camera database for dance information processing, pp. 501–510 (2019)
58. Wang, K., Yin, Q., Wang, W., Wu, S., Wang, L.: A comprehensive survey on cross-modal retrieval (2016). arXiv preprint arXiv:1607.06215
59. Xiao, Q., Song, R.: Motion retrieval based on motion semantic dictionary and hmm inference. Soft Comput. **21**(1), 255–265 (2017)

Music Recommendation Based on Emotion Tracking of Musical Performances

Jacek Grekow

Abstract This chapter presents a content-based music recommendation approach, in which perceived emotions extracted from audio signals were used to compare different performances of the same composition. Recommendations were based on suggesting recordings that were the most similar to the performance specified by the user. Different metrics for similarities between emotion trajectories were evaluated, and the results obtained from the presented approach were evaluated using the opinions of music experts. The obtained results confirmed that the detected values of emotions in music files can be used to recommend performances similar to those selected by the user and be used to build a music recommendation system.

1 Introduction

The emergence of Internet music databases, online music stores, and music streaming services (Spotify, Apple Music) have enabled access to enormous music resources. Music recommender systems help users find the music that interests them. This chapter presents a somewhat unusual recommender, which looks for similar performances of the same composition. Among the searched songs, we have one composition but different performances.

The problem of searching different performances of the same composition mostly pertains to classical music, where the compositions of the greatest old masters, such as J.S. Bach, W.A. Mozart, L.v. Beethoven, R. Schumann, or F. Chopin, have many interpretations played by known and less known performers. Just as human speech has its emotional content, in addition to verbal [7], the same composition, based on one musical notation, can be performed differently with each performance differing in the emotional content. Performing a piece written by a composer, performer, musician, artist gives it its own shape—interpretation. We may enjoy some performances more

J. Grekow (✉)
Faculty of Computer Science, Bialystok University of Technology, Bialystok, Poland
e-mail: j.grekow@pb.edu.pl

Z. W. Ras et al. (eds.), *Recommender Systems for Medicine and Music*,
Studies in Computational Intelligence 946,
https://doi.org/10.1007/978-3-030-66450-3_11

than others. Some performances are more known, others less, some more liked, others less.

The aim of this work was to present a music recommender system that helps to find similar or different performances of the same composition. The presented system could be helpful for music lovers, musicologists, and students to find new, interesting performances that match their tastes.

2 Related Work

The presented approach can be included in the group of content-based music recommendation solutions, where semantic information from music recordings is extracted. Content-based music recommender systems use information that describes music files in the form of meta data (e.g., song name, album cover, etc.) or information extracted from the audio signal [18]. The aim of audio signal processing is to extract meaningful features describing the music files, which will then be used to calculate item similarity by calculating the distance between the vectors of the extracted features. The advantage of music recommender systems based on audio content is that they are not affected by a song's popularity among users, as is the case with collaborative filtering methods [1].

In music recommender systems that use audio content analysis, the data used for comparisons can be divided into two groups. The first is acoustic and musical features computed directly from the audio. The second is automatic semantic annotations predicted from these acoustic features by machine learning techniques. Machine learning techniques can foresee such labels as genre, emotion, and instrumentation.

An example of a solution using acoustic and musical features computed directly from audio was presented by Celma and Herrera in [5]. Audio analysis considered not only timbral features (MFCC) but also musical descriptors related to rhythm and tonality. An approach based on Euclidean distance and acoustic and musical features was compared to item-based collaborative filtering. Luand and Tseng [14] proposed a hybrid music recommendation system by combining content-based, collaboration-based, and emotion-based methods by computing the weights of the methods according to the users' interests. In the proposed system, they used manual emotion annotations.

An example of a solution using semantic annotations obtained by machine learning techniques was presented by Barrington et al. in [2]. The authors used semantic concepts like genres, moods, instrumentation, vocals, and rhythm to measure music similarity in a music recommendation system. These concepts were computed on the basis of MFCC features and were used as annotations of tracks to assess similarity. Bogdanov et al. [3] used timbral, temporal, and tonal features obtained from classifier annotations (genre, mood, instrumentation, rhythm) to build a similarity-based music recommendation approach.

In [13], Kuo et al. proposed a generic emotion-based music recommendation model to recommend music by association discovery from film music. They used feature extraction and an affinity graph to discover the relationships between music features and emotions from film music.

This work presents the concept of using perceived emotion changing over time to compare compositions. The use of emotion tracking in music recommendation was defined as the main future directions in music recommender systems research [19]. The approach presented in this work uses information extracted from audio signals as well as machine learning techniques (automatic emotion detection) to build a music recommender system that searches for performances of the same composition. In this work, the recommendations are based on suggesting the most similar performance of the composition to the one selected by the user. The user may also be interested in the most distant interpretation for a composition. The presented recommendation system enables the user to ask: "Which performance is most similar to performance *X*" or "Which performance is least similar to performance *X*?" where *X* is the initial performance selected by the user.

The rest of this chapter is organized as follows. Section 3 describes the preparatory activities for building a content-based music recommender system, such as regressor training for emotion detection or the automatic alignment of audio recordings. Section 4 presents the intermediate results in the form of emotion tracking of different performances of the same composition. Different metrics for counting distance between recordings and the results of calculating similarity matrices are presented in Sect. 5. Section 6 describes the evaluation of the results obtained by a recommender system and Sect. 7 summarizes the main findings.

3 Preparatory Activities for Finding Similarities

To build a music recommender system, which recommends the most similar performances of the same composition for a given musical piece, preparatory activities were done. First, a module for automatic emotion detection was built to track emotions throughout a song's duration. The next module performs automatic alignment of different performances, which allows to align the songs so that the comparisons apply to the same segments of music.

3.1 Annotation of Music Data for Regressor Training

Emotion recognition was treated as a regression problem. The dataset for regressor training consisted of 324 6-second fragments, where tracks were 22050 Hz mono 16-bit audio files in .wav format. The training data were taken from the generally accessible data collection project Marsyas.[1] The author selected samples and shortened them to the first 6 s. This is the shortest possible length at which experts could

[1] http://marsyas.info/downloads/datasets.html.

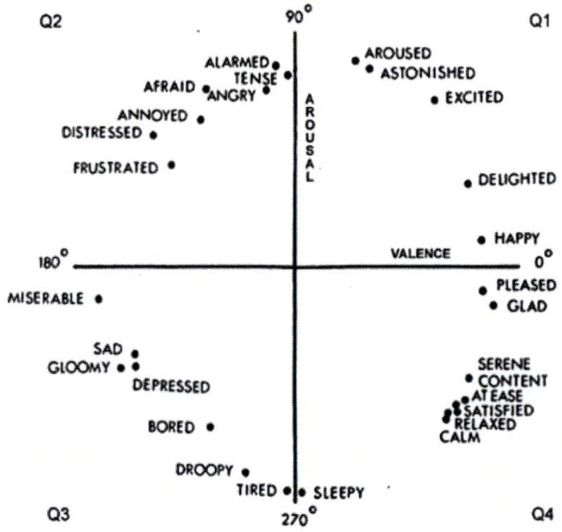

Fig. 1 Russell's circumplex model [17]

detect emotions for a given segment. On the other hand, a short segment ensures that emotional homogeneity of a segment is much more probable.

Data annotation of perceived emotion was done by five music experts with a university musical education and each annotator annotated all records in the dataset. During annotation of music samples, the two-dimensional arousal-valence (A-V) model [17] to measure emotions in music was used. The model (Fig. 1) consists of two independent dimensions of arousal (vertical axis) and valence (horizontal axis).

Each expert making annotations, after listening to a music sample, had to specify values on the arousal and valence axes in a range from -10 to 10 with step 1. On the arousal axis, a value of -10 meant low while 10 high arousal. On the valence axis, -10 meant negative while 10 positive valence. The data collected from the five music experts was averaged.

The amount of examples in the quarters on the A-V emotion plane: Q1 (A:high, V:high): 93, Q2 (A:high, V:low): 70; Q3 (A:low, V:low): 80; Q4 (A:low, V:high): 81. Pearson correlation coefficient was calculated to check if valence and arousal dimensions are correlated in our music data. The obtained value $r = -0.03$ indicates that arousal and valence values are not correlated, and the music data are a well spread in the quarters on the A-V emotion plane. Considering the internal reliability of the collected data, arousal and valence both showed high mutual consistency, with a Cronbach's α of 0.98 and 0.90, respectively.

The previously prepared, labeled by A-V values, music dataset served as input data for the tool used for feature extraction. For feature extraction, a tool for audio analysis, Essentia, was used [4]. The obtained length of feature vector was 529.

3.2 Training Regressors for Emotion Prediction

Regressors for predicting arousal and valence were built. For training and testing, the following regression algorithms were used: SMOreg [20], REPTree [22], and M5P [15, 21]. Before constructing regressors arousal and valence annotations were scaled between $[-0.5, 0.5]$, thus the MAE value also corresponds to the average error percentage. The regression performance using the tenfold cross-validation technique (CV-10) was evaluated.

Table 1 presents the results obtained for the tested algorithms. The highest values for coefficient of determination (R^2) were obtained using SMOreg (implementation of the support vector machine for regression). After applying attribute selection (attribute evaluator: WrapperSubsetEval [12], search method: BestFirst), $R^2 = 0.79$ for arousal and $R^2 = 0.58$ for valence were obtained. Mean absolute error reached values $MAE = 0.09$ for arousal and $MAE = 0.10$ for valence.

Before attribute selection, the best results were obtained using algorithm M5P ($MAE = 0.12$ for arousal, $MAE = 0.14$ for valence). As can be seen, it can handle even a greater number of attributes. Using attribute selection makes sense, since after applying it the results of all algorithms improved and SMOreg turned out to be the winner. One could conclude that a large number of attributes has a negative effect on SMOreg algorithm effectiveness and that using attribute selection clearly improves its effectiveness.

When comparing algorithm accuracy in predicting arousal and valence, one can notice that predicting arousal is a much easier task for regressors than valence and the values predicted for arousal are more precise. The process of building regressors and discovering what combination of audio features gives the best results with music emotion detection was presented in detail in a previous paper [10].

Table 1 R^2 and MAE obtained for regression algorithms

Algorithm	Attribute selection (AS)	Arousal		Valence	
		R^2	MAE	R^2	MAE
M5P	Before AS	0.63	0.12	0.26	0.14
M5P	After AS	0.70	0.11	0.53	0.11
REPTree	Before AS	0.43	0.15	0.15	0.15
REPTree	After AS	0.58	0.12	0.19	0.15
SMOreg	Before AS	0.48	0.18	0.27	0.17
SMOreg	After AS	**0.79**	**0.09**	**0.58**	**0.10**

3.3 Automatic Alignment of Different Performances

The task was to compare different performances of the same composition using emotional distribution. Because the musical performances are played at varying tempos, with various accelerations and decelerations, an alignment of audio recordings is necessary to compare two performances. This enables comparing the same fragments of different renditions. Without doing an alignment to compare performances second to second, we would be comparing fragments of varying content. Just adjusting the time of different renditions, for example, through stretching or compression of time, will not synchronize the performances in terms of music content. Only an exact alignment of the recordings guarantees that we are comparing the same fragments.

MATCH [8], a toolkit for accurate automatic alignment of different renditions of the same piece of music, was used. MATCH is based on a dynamic time warping algorithm (DTW), which is a technique for aligning time series and has been well known and used in the speech recognition community [16]. Frames of audio input data are represented by positive spectral difference vectors, which emphasize note onsets in the alignment process. They are used in the DTW algorithm's match cost function, which uses an Euclidean metric. The path returned by the DTW algorithm, as result of alignment of two audio files, is used to find the location of the same musical fragment in both files.

4 Results of Emotion Tracking

To build a music recommendation system for different performances of the same composition, the experiments were carried out on a collection of the following compositions by Frédéric Chopin (1810–1849): Prelude in C major, Op.28, No.1; Prelude in D major, Op.28, No.5; Prelude in F minor, Op.28, No.18; Prelude in C minor, Op.28, No.20 (the first 8 bars). Five different audio recordings were collected for each composition, played by five famous pianists: Artur Rubinstein recorded in 1946; Emil Gilels recorded in 1953; Grigory Sokolov recorded in 1990; Martha Argerich recorded in 1997; Rafał Blechacz recorded in 2007.

The best obtained regression models (Sect. 3.2) for predicting arousal and valence of the musical performances were used. The collected performances were divided into 6-second segments with a 3/4 overlap. For each segment, features were extracted and models for arousal and valence were used. As a result, arousal and valence values for every 1.5 s of a musical piece were obtained. Details of creating the emotional trajectories on the arousal-valence plane were described in my previous work [9, 11]. The detailed analysis and presentation of the results were restricted to five different performances of Prelude in C major, Op.28, No.1 by Frédéric Chopin.

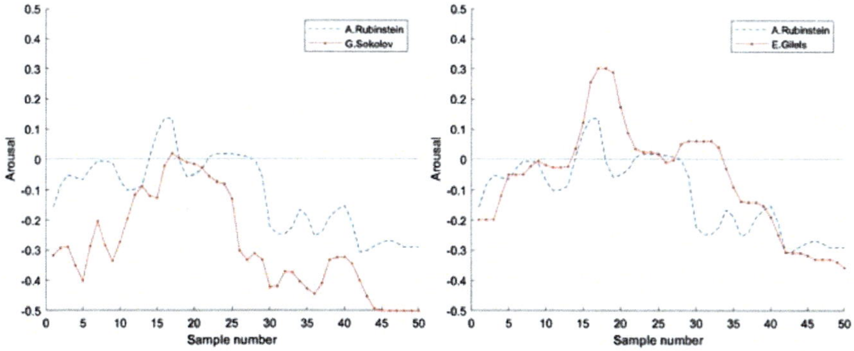

(a) (b)

Fig. 2 Arousal over time for performances by A. Rubinstein—G. Sokolov (**a**) and A. Rubinstein—E. Gilels (**b**) of Prelude in C major, Op. 28, No. 1

4.1 Arousal and Valence Trajectories

The first results after performing emotion detection and alignment of performances are the sequences of arousal and valence values from which emotion trajectories were created. The values of arousal, recognized during emotion tracking of Prelude in C major, Op.28, No.1, are presented in Fig. 2. To keep the charts readable, only three trajectories were selected for the graph presentation (A. Rubinstein, E. Gilels, G. Sokolov). In Fig. 2a, we can notice quite similar fragments, correlated between two performances by A. Rubinstein and G. Sokolov (samples 30–50). In Fig. 2b, which presents performances by A. Rubinstein and E. Gilels, there are also fragments where arousal values move in the same directions (samples 10–15, 40–50). From observing the graphs, however, it is difficult to say which performance (E. Gilels or G. Sokolov) is closer to the performance by A. Rubinstein.

We have a similar situation in the case of the values of valence recognized during emotion tracking in Fig. 3. Comparing the lines of change in emotion, we see similar (Fig. 3a, samples 35–50) and different fragments (Fig. 3b, samples 25–35). Ultimately, however, it is hard to say which performance (E. Gilels or G. Sokolov) is closer to the performance by A. Rubinstein. This will be settled later in the chapter (Sect. 5.3) after finding the right metrics for testing similarities between performances.

4.2 Visual Emotion Tracking on the A-V Plane

After using automatic emotion detection for subsequent fragments of the studied composition, a sequence of arousal and valence values was obtained. The resulting values can be used to create trajectories on the arousal-valence (A-V) emotion plane. From the sequence of arousal and valence values

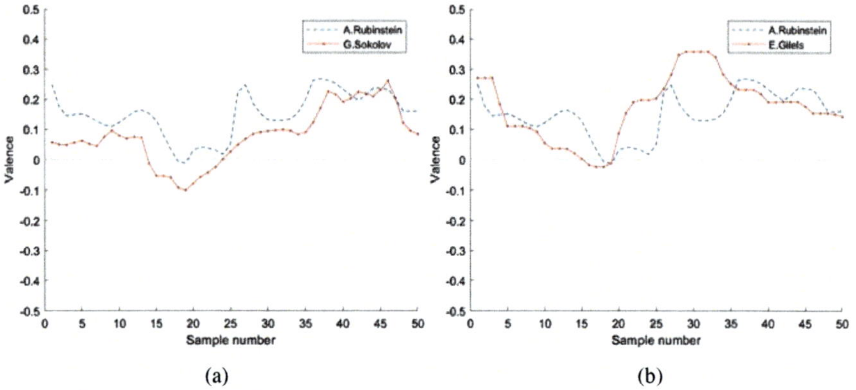

Fig. 3 Valence over time for performances by A. Rubinstein—G. Sokolov (**a**) and A. Rubinstein—E. Gilels (**b**) of Prelude in C major, Op. 28, No. 1

$$A_i = (a_1, a_2, ..., a_i, ..., a_n) \tag{1}$$

$$V_i = (v_1, v_2, ..., v_i, ..., v_n) \tag{2}$$

we can compile a sequence of point coordinates,

$$P_i = (p_1(a_1, v_1), p_2(a_2, v_2), ..., p_i(a_i, v_i), ..., p_n(a_n, v_n)), \tag{3}$$

where n is the sample number in the sequence. The $p(a, v)$ points in sequence P_i determine the trajectory of the course of emotions in the musical piece on the A-V plane.

Exemplary emotion trajectories obtained from a sequence of points described by arousal and valence values are presented in Fig. 4. A square marker on the trajectory indicates the beginning of a piece and corresponds to point $p_1(a_1, v_1)$ from the sequence of points P_i. Figure 4 presents the trajectories of three different performances (A. Rubinstein, G. Sokolov, E. Gilels) of Prelude in C major, Op.28, No.1 by Frédéric Chopin on the A-V emotion plane. The trajectories (Fig. 4a) illustrate how the artist moved in the four quarters on the arousal-valence emotion plane. Both performances begin and end in quarter Q4 (arousal low—valence high). The course of the middle part of these two performances varies. G. Sokolov's trajectory moves through quarter Q3 (arousal low—valence low), and A. Rubinstein's through quarter Q1 (arousal high—valence high). Both trajectories end in quarter Q4. Figure 4b compares two other performances. We can note that the performance by E. Gilels has more straight sections compared with the curved line for the performance by A. Rubinstein, which suggests that these performances are quite distant.

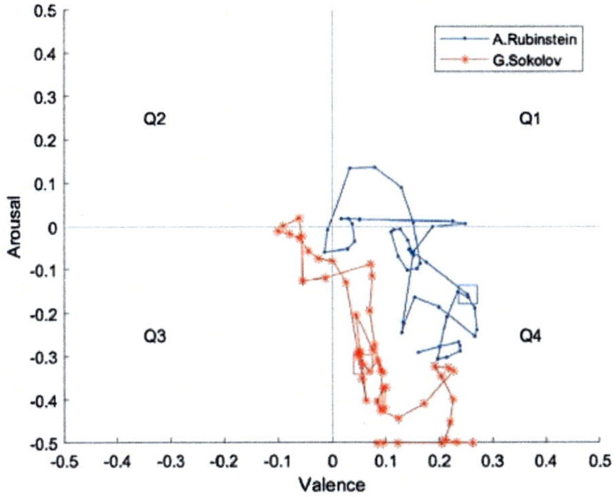

(a)

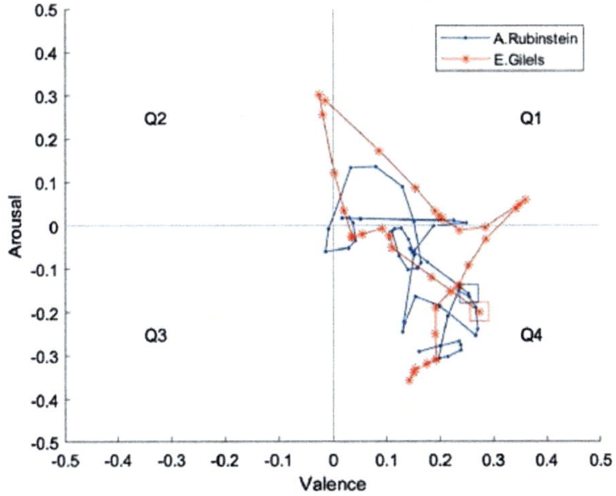

(b)

Fig. 4 Performances by A. Rubinstein—G. Sokolov (**a**) and by A. Rubinstein—E. Gilels (**b**) of Prelude in C major, Op. 28, No. 1 on the A-V emotion plane

4.3 *Visual Emotion Tracking on the A-V Plane After Ranking*

Another method of looking at the trajectories of emotions in a musical piece is ranking the arousal and valence values. Ranking consists of swapping the real values in a given sequence with an index of a given value after sorting the sequence in an ascending order. Thus, in our case, the smallest sequence value will get a new value of 1 and the highest a value of 50, because we have 50 samples in the sequence.

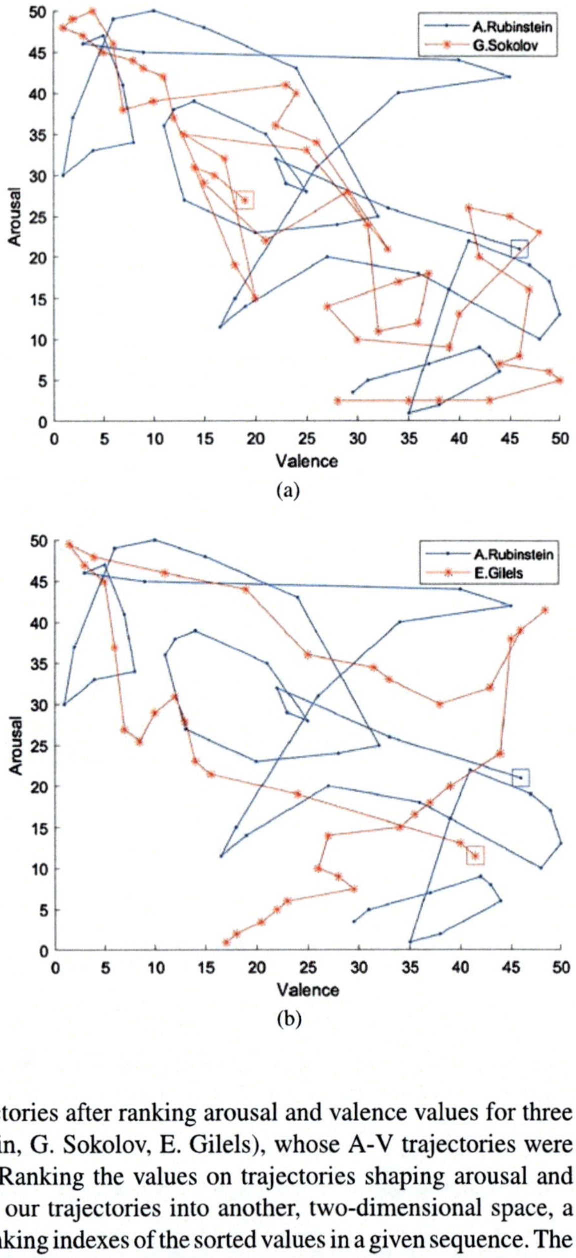

Fig. 5 Performances by A. Rubinstein—G. Sokolov (**a**) and by A. Rubinstein—E. Gilels (**b**) of Prelude in C major, Op. 28, No. 1 after ranking

Figure 5 shows the trajectories after ranking arousal and valence values for three performances (A. Rubinstein, G. Sokolov, E. Gilels), whose A-V trajectories were presented earlier in Fig. 4. Ranking the values on trajectories shaping arousal and valence over time transfers our trajectories into another, two-dimensional space, a space associated with the ranking indexes of the sorted values in a given sequence. The new space is no longer a linear plane in the range of $[-0.5, 0.5]$ on the arousal-valence axes; quarters Q1–Q4 can no longer be marked on it. The vertical and horizontal axes of the new space are, however, associated with the arousal and valence axes.

Observing Figs. 4 and 5, we see very different interpretations of the same trajectories of emotions on the A-V plane. Ranking introduced great changes in the visualization; it unified the increase in subsequent samples. Figure 5a shows the rather winding lines of both trajectories, which are difficult to compare visually. In Fig. 5b, we can notice a clearly different nature of the line of the performance by E. Gilels compared with the one by A. Rubinstein. The trajectory by E. Gilels almost does not intersect and turns in a clockwise circle. The trajectory by A. Rubinstein has more intersections and loops, which expresses the completely different nature of the performance.

5 Similarity Findings

Our goal is to find similarities between the two sequences containing the values of emotions from the performed compositions. The output data is two sequences X_i and Y_i of the same length n, between which we must measure similarity:

$$X_i = x_1, x_2, ..., x_i, ..., x_n, \tag{4}$$

$$Y_i = y_1, y_2, ..., y_i, ..., y_n. \tag{5}$$

5.1 *Metrics of Similarity*

To compare the musical performances, the following metrics were selected to describe the relationships between two sequences:

- Euclidean distance;
- Pearson correlation coefficient;
- Spearman's rank correlation coefficient.

5.1.1 Euclidean Distance

Euclidean distance between two sequences X_i and Y_i is defined as

$$ED(X_i, Y_i) = \sqrt{\sum_{i=1}^{n} (x_i - y_i)^2}, \tag{6}$$

where x_i and y_i are values of elements in sequences.

5.1.2 Pearson Correlation Coefficient

Pearson's correlation coefficient r between two sequences X_i and Y_i is defined as

$$r(X_i, Y_i) = \frac{\sum_{i=1}^{n} (x_i - \overline{x})(y_i - \overline{y})}{\sqrt{\sum_{i=1}^{n} (x_i - \overline{x})^2 \sum_{i=1}^{n} (y_i - \overline{y})^2}}, \tag{7}$$

where x_i and y_i are values of elements in sequences, $\overline{x}$ and $\overline{y}$ are mean values of each sequence. The correlation coefficient ranges from 1 to -1. Value 1 means perfectly correlated sequences, 0 there is no correlation, and -1 that the sequences are perfectly correlated negatively. A correlation coefficient between two of the same performances is at maximum equal to 1.

5.1.3 Spearman's Rank Correlation Coefficient

Spearman's rank correlation coefficient (Spearman's ρ) [6], which is the Pearson correlation coefficient between ranked variables. Before calculating correlations, variables are converted to ranks. The rank correlation coefficient ranges from 1 to -1. A positive ρ indicates a positive relationship between the two variables, while a negative ρ expresses a negative relationship.

The following formula (Eq. 8) is used to calculate the Spearman rank correlation between n values of two sequences X_i , Y_i:

$$\rho(X_i, Y_i) = 1 - \frac{6 \sum_{i=1}^{n} d_i^2}{n(n^2 - 1)}, \tag{8}$$

where $d_i = rg(X_i) - rg(Y_i)$ are the differences between ranks.

5.2 *Joining Arousal and Valence Sequences*

To calculate similarities between two trajectories in the A-V plane, each trajectory should be represented by one sequence of values. In our case, each trajectory is represented by two value sequences (arousal and valence). To compare performances described by two sequences of values (arousal and valence), these sequences should be joined. In order to join the two sequences of arousal (Eq. 9) and valence (Eq. 10) values of one performance, standard deviation and the mean of the two sequences of data should be equivalent. We decided to leave arousal values without change and convert valence values (Eq. 12) although we could have converted arousal and left valence without a change and this would not have affected the correlation results. During joining, the sequences of each feature are interleaved (Eq. 11).

Sequences for arousal and valence:

$$A_i = (a_1, a_2, a_3, ..., a_n) \tag{9}$$

$$V_i = (v_1, v_2, v_3, ..., v_n). \tag{10}$$

Result of joining arousal and valence sequence into one sequence AV:

$$AV_i = (a_1, vnew_1, a_2, vnew_2, a_3, vnew_3, ..., a_n, vnew_n). \tag{11}$$

Formula for calculating new valence sequence values:

$$vnew_n = \overline{a} + sd_a \frac{v_n - \overline{v}}{sd_v}, \tag{12}$$

where sd_a stands for standard deviation of sequence A, sd_v—standard deviation of sequence V, $\overline{a}$—mean value of sequence A, and $\overline{v}$—mean value of sequence V.

5.3 Results of Calculating Similarity Matrices

For each performance of the musical composition, an AV_i sequence was obtained that represented the emotions in a given performance. The distances between these sequences were then calculated using the following metrics:

- Euclidean distance;
- Pearson correlation coefficient;
- Spearman's rank correlation coefficient.

As a result, three similarity matrices were obtained for each analyzed composition. The obtained detailed results will be presented for only one composition: Prelude in C major, Op. 28, No.1 by F. Chopin.

To compare the results obtained with the Euclidean distance (ED) metric and the correlation coefficient metric, the Euclidean distance matrix was subjected to a small transformation: one minus the Euclidean distance ($1 - ED$). In this way, on the diagonal representing the distance between the same performances, we obtained a value of 1, i.e., the maximum similarity.

Table 2 presents the matrix obtained using Euclidean distance calculated for each pair of performances. In each column, i.e., for each subsequent performer, bold indicates the highest similarity value, i.e., bold indicates which performances are the most similar to each other. For example, according to the results from Table 2, the most similar performance by A. Rubinstein is R. Blechacz ($1 - ED = 0.17$).

A slightly different matrix was obtained using Pearson's correlation coefficients r, calculated for each pair of performances (Table 3), as a similarity metric. We see that the most similar performances are by R. Blechacz and G. Sokolov (r = 0.82), and the most different by A. Rubinstein and E. Gilels ($r = 0.58$).

Table 2 Similarity matrix obtained using Euclidean distance $(1 - ED)$, calculated for each pair of performances of Prelude in C major, Op. 28, No. 1

	A. Rubinstein	E. Gilels	G. Sokolov	M. Argerich	R. Blechacz
A. Rubinstein	1.00	−0.53	−0.96	−0.13	**0.17**
E. Gilels	−0.53	1.00	−1.70	−0.26	−0.44
G. Sokolov	−0.96	−1.69	1.00	−1.68	−0.93
M. Argerich	−0.13	**-0.26**	−1.69	1.00	−0.09
R. Blechacz	**0.17**	−0.44	**−0.93**	**−0.09**	1.00

Table 3 Similarity matrix obtained using Pearson's correlation coefficient r, calculated for each pair of performances of Prelude in C major, Op. 28, No. 1

	A. Rubinstein	E. Gilels	G. Sokolov	M. Argerich	R. Blechacz
A. Rubinstein	1.00	0.58	**0.81**	0.67	0.77
E. Gilels	0.58	1.00	0.60	**0.72**	0.64
G. Sokolov	**0.81**	0.60	1.00	0.64	**0.82**
M. Argerich	0.67	**0.72**	0.64	1.00	0.72
R. Blechacz	0.77	0.64	**0.82**	0.72	1.00

Table 4 Similarity matrix obtained by using Spearman's ρ, calculated for each pair of performances of Prelude in C major, Op. 28, No. 1

	A. Rubinstein	E. Gilels	G. Sokolov	M. Argerich	R. Blechacz
A. Rubinstein	1.00	0.56	0.79	0.64	0.74
E. Gilels	0.56	1.00	0.56	**0.78**	0.58
G. Sokolov	**0.79**	0.56	1.00	0.64	**0.83**
M. Argerich	0.67	**0.78**	0.64	1.00	0.67
R. Blechacz	0.74	0.58	**0.83**	0.67	1.00

Table 4 presents the matrix obtained using Spearman's ρ coefficient calculated for each pair of performances. Observing Tables 3 and 4, we can notice similar winners in the columns, even though we have different correlation values. Comparing these two tables, the winners in the given columns remain the same, but the correlations between performances have changed slightly. The value ranking operation did not affect the selection of the winners much, although ranking may reveal other relationships of shaping the emotions between the performances.

Based on Tables 3 and 4, it can be stated that we have two groups in which we have similar performances. The first group consists of performances by R. Blechacz, G. Sokolov, and A. Rubinstein, and the second group by E. Gilels and M. Argerich.

6 Evaluation

6.1 Ground Truth Similarity Matrix

Three music experts (Expert 1–3) with a university musical education participated in the experiment. A similarity matrix form [5 × 5], presented in Table 5, was used to collect expert opinions, which is a symmetric matrix, with the main diagonal values equal to 10.

The experts' task was to determine which performances to a given performance are most similar and which are the least. Each expert (Expert 1–3) had to determine these values in the similarity matrix form. Each value described the degree of similarity between performances. The filled values were subsequent natural numbers in the range of $[1, 9]$, where 9 meant a very similar performance, and 1 very different. A value of 10 on the diagonal meant that the given performance is maximally similar. Information on the performer of a given rendition was kept from the evaluators. Sample answers from Expert 1, for Prelude in C major, Op. 28, No. 1, are presented in Table 6.

After collecting data from the experts, the data was ranked. In this way, different individual opinions on the similarity scale were obtained and the sequence of degree of similarity was maintained. Finally, the obtained values were averaged and rescaled to the range of [0, 1]. Thus, a *similarity matrix obtained from all experts* was built. It constituted the ground truth for similarities for a given composition and was used

Table 5 Form for similarity matrix between performances

	Performance 1	Performance 2	Performance 3	Performance 4	Performance 5
Performance 1	10	?	?	?	?
Performance 2	?	10	?	?	?
Performance 3	?	?	10	?	?
Performance 4	?	?	?	10	?
Performance 5	?	?	?	?	10

Table 6 Similarity matrix obtained from Expert 1 for performances of Prelude in C major, Op.28, No.1

	A. Rubinstein	E. Gilels	G. Sokolov	M. Argerich	R. Blechacz
A. Rubinstein	10	1	**6**	4	3
E. Gilels	1	10	2	**8**	4
G. Sokolov	**6**	2	10	2	**6**
M. Argerich	4	**8**	2	10	2
R. Blechacz	3	4	6	2	10

Table 7 Similarity matrix obtained from experts' opinions for performances of Prelude in C major, Op. 28, No. 1

	A. Rubinstein	E. Gilels	G. Sokolov	M. Argerich	R. Blechacz
A. Rubinstein	1.00	0.25	**0.90**	0.18	0.48
E. Gilels	0.25	1.00	0.27	**0.90**	**0.60**
G. Sokolov	**0.90**	0.27	1.00	0.10	0.42
M. Argerich	0.18	**0.90**	0.10	1.00	0.52
R. Blechacz	0.48	0.60	0.42	0.52	1.00

Table 8 Agreement between three experts' opinions

Composition	Cronbach's α
Prelude No. 1	0.76
Prelude No. 5	0.73
Prelude No. 18	0.77
Prelude No. 20	0.68
Averages	0.74

to compare with the *matrices of similarity between performances obtained by a recommender system.*

Table 7 presents the final similarity matrix obtained from all experts for Prelude in C major, Op. 28, No. 1 after ranking, averaging, and rescaling to the range of [0, 1]. This is our ground truth matrix for this composition. In this way, we made ground truth matrices for all analyzed compositions.

To check the agreement between three experts' opinions, Cronbach's α [24] was calculated (Table 8), and the obtained averaged value turned out to be acceptable ($\alpha = 0.74$).

6.2 *Evaluation Results*

6.2.1 Visual Comparison of Matrices

To demonstrate similarities between the results obtained from the experts and the results obtained from the recommender system, a visual comparison was first used. The visual comparison of matrices is presented only for performances of Prelude in C major, Op. 28, No. 1 by Frédéric Chopin. Figure 6 compares the results obtained from experts (Table 7) with the results obtained using Euclidean distance (Table 2) rescaled to the interval [0, 1], the results obtained from a computer using Pearson's correlation coefficient (Table 3), and the results from the matrix obtained using Spearman's rank correlation coefficient (Table 4).

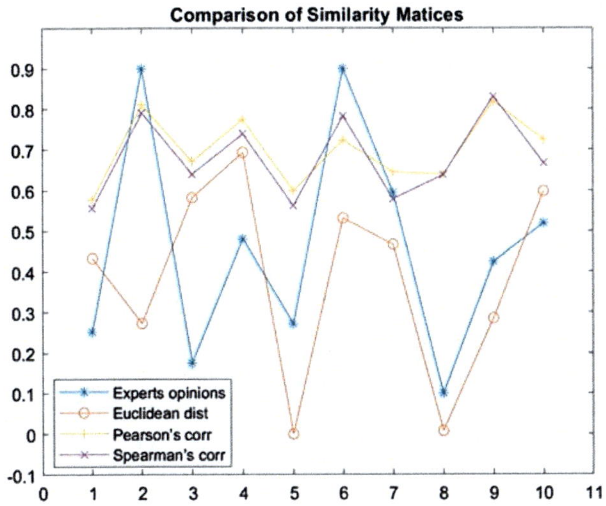

Fig. 6 Comparison of matrices obtained from the experts and from the recommender system for Prelude in C major, Op.28, No.1

Because the compared matrices [5 × 5] are symmetrical, only 10 values were taken for comparisons (the lower triangle matrix, the values on the diagonal, and the upper triangle are insignificant). Although the data are in different scales, there are clearly correlations between the values of both results. The high values obtained from experts' opinions often coincide with the results obtained using Pearson's and Spearman's correlation (sample 2, 6); it is similar at low values (sample 1, 3, 5). A worse correlation can be seen between the experts' opinions and the results obtained using Euclidean distance (sample 1, 2, 3).

6.2.2 Correlation Between Similarity Matrices

Due to the fact that the results obtained from the music experts and those from the recommender system are in different scales, and we are most interested in the order in these matrices, Spearman's ρ, which is Pearson's correlation coefficient between ranked variables, was used to study the correlations between these results.

In our case, Spearman's ρ measures how much the similarity values provided by the recommender system and experts have a similar rank. While calculating Spearman's ρ between the *similarity matrix obtained from the experts* and the *similarity matrices obtained from the recommender system*, only elements below the main diagonal from the matrix were taken into account. The matrices are symmetric; diagonal and upper diagonal elements are irrelevant. The greater the obtained Spearman's rank correlation coefficient, the closer the system's results were to the experts' opinions.

Table 9 Spearman's ρ between the similarity matrix obtained from the experts and the different similarity matrices obtained from the recommender system

Composition	Random matrix	Similarity matrix A	Similarity matrix B	Similarity matrix C
Prelude No. 1	−0.22	0.25	**0.52**	0.51
Prelude No. 5	−0.05	−0.11	0.72	**0.78**
Prelude No. 18	−0.06	0.73	0.50	**0.80**
Prelude No. 20	−0.08	0.12	0.55	**0.69**
Averages	−0.10	0.25	0.57	**0.70**

During the evaluation, Spearman's ρ was calculated between the *similarity matrix obtained from the experts* and the four *similarity matrices obtained from the recommender system*:

- Random generated matrix;
- Similarity matrix obtained by using Euclidean distance $(1 - ED)$—matrix A;
- Similarity matrix obtained by using Pearson's correlation coefficient—matrix B;
- Similarity matrix obtained by using Spearman's rank correlation coefficient—matrix C.

The obtained results of the evaluation are presented in Table 9 and pertain all analyzed compositions played in five different performances. For each composition, the bold font indicates the highest compliance with the experts' opinions. The values of the randomly generated matrix, which was chosen as the baseline for comparing our results, do not correlate with the experts' opinions (avg. $\rho = -0.10$, second column). The results obtained using Euclidean distance show slightly better compliance with the experts' opinions (avg. $\rho = 0.25$), but they are not too high (third column).

We see the positive values of Spearman's ρ for both of the other B and C matrices (from 0.50 to 0.80, fourth and fifth columns). They confirm a clear relation and compliance with the experts' opinions and the correlation matrices between the performances calculated by the recommender system. The results show that using correlations to find similarities between performances makes much more sense than Euclidean distance. We should note that the values for the ρ for matrix C (avg. $\rho = 0.70$) are even greater than the ρ for matrix B (avg. $\rho = 0.57$). This indicates that calculating correlations between performances using ranking made sense and significantly increased compliance with the experts' opinions.

7 Conclusions

In this study, a content-based music recommender system that uses emotion tracking was presented. The recommender system was limited to different performances of the same composition, i.e., similarities were found between recordings of different interpretations of the same musical material performed by different performers. Automatic detection of perceived emotions was used and the obtained values of arousal and valence, specifying placement on Russell's emotion plane, were used to chart the course of emotions over time.

The results obtained from the presented approach were evaluated using the opinions of music experts. Different metrics for similarity between the music items were used and the accuracy of the metrics was evaluated. The obtained results confirm that the detected values of emotions in music files can be used to recommend performances similar to those selected by the user and can be used to build a music recommendation system.

A music recommender system that helps to find similar performances or can arrange them from the most similar to the most different could be very useful for music lovers looking for different interpretations of the same composition. The question "Which performance of the same composition is similar or different?" is often asked during music competitions. Music students, educators, and musicologists studying the interpretation of compositions could also be interested in such a system.

Acknowledgements The work was supported by a grant from the Bialystok University of Technology and funded by the Ministry of Science and Higher Education in Poland.

References

1. Aggarwal, C.C.: Content-Based Recommender Systems, pp. 139–166. Springer International Publishing, Cham (2016). https://doi.org/10.1007/978-3-319-29659-3_4
2. Barrington, L., Oda, R., Lanckriet, G.R.G.: Smarter than genius? human evaluation of music recommender systems. In: K. Hirata, G. Tzanetakis, K. Yoshii (eds.) Proceedings of the 10th International Society for Music Information Retrieval Conference, ISMIR 2009, Kobe International Conference Center, Kobe, Japan, October 26-30, 2009, pp. 357–362. International Society for Music Information Retrieval (2009)
3. Bogdanov, D., Haro, M., Fuhrmann, F., Xambó, A., Gómez, E., Herrera, P.: Semantic audio content-based music recommendation and visualization based on user preference examples. Inf. Process. Manag. **49**, 13–33 (2013)
4. Bogdanov, D., Wack, N., Gómez, E., Gulati, S., Herrera, P., Mayor, O., Roma, G., Salamon, J., Zapata, J., Serra, X.: ESSENTIA: an audio analysis library for music information retrieval. In: Proceedings of the 14th International Society for Music Information Retrieval Conference, pp. 493–498 (2013)
5. Celma, O., Herrera, P.: A New Approach to Evaluating Novel Recommendations, pp. 179–186 (2008). https://doi.org/10.1145/1454008.1454038
6. Chen, P.Y., Popovich, P.M.: Correlation: Parametric and Nonparametric Measures. Sage, Thousand Oaks (California) (2002)
7. Dimitrova-Grekow, T., Klis, A., Igras-Cybulska, M.: Speech emotion recognition based on voice fundamental frequency. Arch. Acoust **44**(2) (2019)
8. Dixon, S., Widmer, G.: MATCH: a music alignment tool chest. In: ISMIR 2005, Proceedings of 6th International Conference on Music Information Retrieval, London, UK, 11-15 September 2005, pp. 492–497 (2005)
9. Grekow, J.: Music emotion maps in arousal-valence space. In: Computer Information Systems and Industrial Management: 15th IFIP TC8 International Conference, CISIM 2016, Vilnius, Lithuania, Proceedings, pp. 697–706. Springer International Publishing (2016)

10. Grekow, J.: Audio features dedicated to the detection of arousal and valence in music recordings. In: 2017 IEEE International Conference on INnovations in Intelligent SysTems and Applications (INISTA), pp. 40–44 (2017)
11. Grekow, J.: Musical performance analysis in terms of emotions it evokes. J. Intell. Inf. Syst. **51**(2), 415–437 (2018). https://doi.org/10.1007/s10844-018-0510-y
12. Kohavi, R., John, G.H.: Wrappers for feature subset selection. Artif. Intell. **97**(1–2), 273–324 (1997)
13. Kuo, F.F., Chiang, M.F., Shan, M.K., Lee, S.Y.: Emotion-based music recommendation by association discovery from film music. In: MULTIMEDIA '05 (2005)
14. Lu, C.C., Tseng, V.: A novel method for personalized music recommendation. Expert Syst. Appl. **36**, 10035–10044 (2009). https://doi.org/10.1016/j.eswa.2009.01.074
15. Quinlan, R.J.: Learning with continuous classes. In: 5th Australian Joint Conference on Artificial Intelligence, pp. 343–348. World Scientific, Singapore (1992)
16. Rabiner, L., Juang, B.H.: Fundamentals of Speech Recognition. Prentice-Hall Inc, Upper Saddle River, NJ, USA (1993)
17. Russell, J.A.: A circumplex model of affect. J. Personal. Soc. Psychol. **39**(6), 1161–1178 (1980)
18. Schedl, M., Knees, P., McFee, B., Bogdanov, D., Kaminskas, M.: Music Recommender Systems, pp. 453–492. Springer US, Boston, MA (2015). https://doi.org/10.1007/978-1-4899-7637-6_13
19. Schedl, M., Zamani, H., Chen, C.W., Deldjoo, Y., Elahi, M.: Current challenges and visions in music recommender systems research. Int. J. Multimed. Inf. Retr. **7**(2), 95–116 (2018). https://doi.org/10.1007/s13735-018-0154-2
20. Smola, A.J., Schölkopf, B.: A tutorial on support vector regression. Statist. Comput. **14**(3), 199–222 (2004)
21. Wang, Y., Witten, I.H.: Induction of model trees for predicting continuous classes. In: Poster papers of the 9th European Conference on Machine Learning. Springer (1997)
22. Witten, I.H., Frank, E., Hall, M.A., Pal, C.J.: Data Mining, Fourth Edition: Practical Machine Learning Tools and Techniques, 4th edn. Morgan Kaufmann Publishers Inc., San Francisco, CA, USA (2016)

Music and Healthcare Recommendation Systems

Mariusz Kleć and Alicja Wieczorkowska

Abstract This introductory chapter starts with an overview of healthcare recommender systems, supported by a comprehensive list of references. Next, the systems that recommend music for health purposes are briefly reviewed. Since the systems that recommend music explicitly for medical purposes are not commonly used yet, we focus on studies that explore the influence of music into human health in general. We also outline the inspirations for the future development of music recommendation systems used for medical purposes.

1 Introduction

Recommendation Systems (RS) help users to find various items, like books, movies, and other products from big repositories of data. In this survey, we start with describing recommendation systems used in healthcare, addressing various health problems. Next, the systems that recommend music for medical applications are also briefly reviewed. However, the publications that address music in the application for medicine are still rare. The theoretical and methodological basis of such systems is sought in music therapy. Therefore, we decided to reserve a significant place in this survey for research that examines the influence of music on human health in general [5, 10, 13, 26, 43].

We performed the literature review by searching the following databases: ACM Digital Library, IEEEexplore, ScienceDirect, and Google Scholar, which provides results from many other databases (see Table 1 and 2). We mainly focused on journal and conference papers published after 2016. The discussion of the outcomes of our search is presented in the next sections.

M. Kleć (✉) · A. Wieczorkowska
Polish-Japanese Academy of Informtion Technology, Koszykowa 86, 02-008 Warsaw, Poland
e-mail: mklec@pjwstk.edu.pl

A. Wieczorkowska
e-mail: alicja@poljap.edu.pl

Z. W. Ras et al. (eds.), *Recommender Systems for Medicine and Music*,
Studies in Computational Intelligence 946,
https://doi.org/10.1007/978-3-030-66450-3_12

Table 1 Literature review on Healthcare Recommender Systems where 77% of papers have been published after 2016

Keywords	ACM[1] (%)	IEEE[2] (%)	SD[3] (%)	Other[4] (%)	Literature
Surveys and reviews	0	40	0	60	[33, 37, 40, 42, 45]
Drug recommendation	0	25	0	75	[11, 30, 34, 38, 47]
Music recommendation for health	0	50	16	33	[1, 2, 16, 24, 39, 41]
Diagnoses, medical publication venue, medical videos, nutrition, and others	18%	45%	0%	36%	[3, 7, 8, 12, 17, 20, 22, 28, 36]

[1] ACM Digital Library
[2] IEEEexplore
[3] ScienceDirect
[4] Google Scholar

Table 2 Literature review on Music Therapy where 80% of papers have been published after 2016 year

Keywords	ACM[1] (%)	IEEE[2] (%)	SD[3] (%)	Other[4] (%)	Literature
Dementia and elderly care	20	0	20	60	[4, 6, 13, 43, 44]
Parkinson's, Alzheimer's and other diseases, stress and depressive disorders, palliative medicine	0%	0%	20%	80%	[6, 9, 10, 18, 19, 21, 25, 31, 32, 35, 46]
Others	66	0	0	33	[5, 26, 29]

[1] ACM Digital Library
[2] IEEEexplore
[3] ScienceDirect
[4] Google Scholar

2 Healthcare Recommendation Systems

Medicine is the domain where formal education is indispensable. Still, there exist many RS in health science, see [40, 42]. Such systems may recommend medications [7, 38, 40, 47], identify new targets for known drugs [30], or recommend healthcare-related videos [8]. Since patients often use social networks to understand their health condition, collaborative filtering is also applied in health recommender systems. In

[36], this approach is used, combined with big data analytics, using deep learning. Healthcare data are multi-structured data, including medical history, images, and prescriptions. These large amounts of data, processed together with social network activities of patients, may help healthcare professionals to treat patients better [3].

Healthcare RS may supply patients with additional information, helping them better understand their health status, in a layman-friendly way [45]. Such systems, apart from offering help to patients, also provide tools to assist doctors in the diagnosis of diseases [33, 37]. For example, the diagnosis of colon diseases is a big problem for specialists, because the symptoms may strongly resemble other diseases. The authors of [22] build classifying rules that help doctors to find symptoms which indicate a particular disease and exclude the others.

Besides helping doctors in diagnosis, RS can also assist in finding relevant scientific articles and collaborators. The system called Schosy recommends collaborators based on the authors' work, collaboration among the authors, Medical Subject Headings (MSH), terms and the productivity of relevant researchers [20]. Another medical RS helps researchers in choosing a biomedical publication venue [17].

Epilepsy. About 65 million patients have epilepsy globally. Chronic neurological syndromes are extremely hard to be definitively cured. However, approximately 70% of seizures can be under control by drugs. The authors of [11] propose a system that investigates epileptics' medical history to help doctors choose drugs. The authors of [34] solved the problem of complications associated with the inappropriate use of traditional herbal medicines. They apply ontology-based rules to provide the recommendations of traditional herbal medicines and their contraindications similar to a medical specialist.

Nutrition. Nutrition is essential for health. It is the primary determinant of major diseases such as diabetes, heart diseases, and obesity. However, current RSs are far from being mature enough to provide personalized food suggestion for daily usage. The exception is the RS described in [28], designed to propose local restaurant dishes that satisfy user needs. The system takes into account nutritional facts regarding products and recommends those that are healthiest according to the personalized health data of the user and the environmental context. Another personalized RS for optimized nutrition is introduced in [12]. It performs personalized grocery product filtering and recommendation. However, it is necessary to remember that such issues as conflicting nutritional theories and uncertainties regarding the users' nutritional state, and thus the personal health value of food items can lead to unreliable recommendations. These aspects need to be quantified and qualified in order to use a nutrition recommendation model in a food RS in a reliable way [28].

Activity-aware recommendations. Physical activity brings significant benefits to health, but many people exercise much less than it is recommended. Music can have a motivational effect and encourage people to exercise more or for a longer time. The authors of [16] propose a music RS motivating to exercise. The system is based on reinforcement learning. Activity-aware recommendations can also be based on signals captured from mobile and wearable devices [15]. For example, exercising movements can be captured using an accelerometer in a smartphone, and this information can be utilized to build activity-aware MRS, based on activity detection [23].

3 Systems for Recommending Music in Medicine

In this section, we would like to focus on systems that recommend music for therapeutic purpose or for supporting ongoing therapy [1, 16, 24, 39]. Regrettably, the publications in this field are still scarce, leaving many challenges and areas for further research. Despite the positive effect of music on health, we see a gap in music recommendation systems used explicitly in medicine. For example, tinnitus can be treated with music [1]. It is worth noting that music does not need to be selected, but it can also be generated. Automatic Music Generation (AMG) [27] can contribute to the creation of a new kind of systems. The example is ENDEL system,[1] which provides personalized sound environments to help the user to focus, relax, and sleep. Undoubtedly, such projects as Google Magenta[2] or AIVA[3] can inspire researchers for further investigations in connecting AMG with music RS used in medicine.

Music recommendation systems for stress relieving. Stress can be defined as the degree to which a person feels overwhelmed or unable to cope with, as a result of pressures that are unmanageable. The paper [39] presents an automatic stress-relieving music RS. The system uses a portable, wireless photoplethysmography module with a finger-type sensor, and interprets heartbeat signals from the sensor to calculate the stress index. The Sympathovagal Balance Index (SVI) is calculated from heart rate variability in order to assess the user's stress levels while listening to music. The results confirm that the system automatically recommends favourable music playlists to relieve stress for individuals, based on the SVI values.

We would like to also underline that using music as therapy is inexpensive and it constitutes highly enjoyable means of treatment.

4 The Influence of Music on Health

In this section, we present the results of our literature search (see Table 2). Music has become especially important in elderly care, for the benefits it has brought in the treatment of neurodegenerative diseases [4]. A music playing combined with user monitoring system can be beneficial in elderly care. For example, in [6], the authors describe the idea of such a cyber-physical system.

[1]https://endel.io/.

[2]https://research.google/teams/brain/magenta/.

[3]https://www.aiva.ai/.

Research shows that music can slow down heart rate, lower blood pressure and reduce levels of stress hormones [29]. The music can help patients to feel better and support ongoing therapy. The study in [46] determines the effect of music therapy on the spirituality of persons in an inpatient hospice unit. A spiritual well-being questionnaire was conducted before and after music therapy. Results indicate a statistically significant increase in spiritual well-being scores on music days. In recent years, music interventions have grown in popularity as a method of non-pharmacological treatment for persons with various types of diseases.

Heart diseases. According to WHO, cardiovascular diseases are the number one cause of death globally, taking an estimated 17.9 million lives each year. The work in [10] defines a conceptual framework to test the effectiveness of music listening on symptom burden and quality of life in Heart Failure (HF) patients. Music listening has been shown to improve outcomes in cardiovascular patients, but it has never been tested on HF patients. The authors conclude that listening to classical music is a feasible, noninvasive, safe, and inexpensive intervention, able to improve the quality of life in patients with HF in the home-care setting.

Cancer. According to the World Health Organization (WHO), cancer is the second leading cause of death globally, accounting for an estimated 9.6 million deaths, or one in six deaths, in 2018. The work in [31] examines adult cancer patients' views about music role before and after diagnosis. Results indicate that music helps the patients to remain connected with pre-illness identities, strengthens capacity for enduring treatment, ongoing survival, and even facing death. They conclude that the patient's preferred music should be available in diagnostic, treatment, and palliative settings, as it can promote endurance and life enrichment. Another research described in [9] proves improving the lifestyle of cancer patients by music therapy interventions. The results reported in [18] show a positive impact of music therapy on the stress levels, pain, and quality of life of the patients, family members and relatives in palliative medicine or in hospice care.

Ageing. Natural ageing processes make older patients more at risk of experiencing less favourable outcomes of treatment and complications after surgery. In this context, non-pharmaceutical interventions, such as music, may be preferable to medical interventions. Dementia in our ageing population needs developing treatments and activities that alleviate its symptoms. Music therapy influences the behaviour of older people with dementia. The work presented in [13] describes a clinically tested music therapy system that turned out to be useful for the elderly with mild cognitive impairment. Another study described in [43] assesses the effect of music on postoperative recovery in older patients with cancer. The research described in [44] reports a positive increase in participants' mood and socialization skills with carers when using music therapy in geriatric care.

Alzheimer's and Parkinson's diseases. Music also benefits patients treated for neurodegenerative diseases [4], such as Parkinson's disease (PD) or Alzheimer's disease (AD). The WHO states that AD is the most common form of dementia, with an estimated 50 million people living with the disease these days. Behavioural studies have shown that music can improve some cognitive functions in person with AD [25]. The PD, in turn, manifests itself in movement disorders, but it also influences perception, thoughts and emotions. One of the biggest problems for people with PD is the inability to spontaneously initiate movements. The movement can be interrupted, discontinuous, with many pauses. However, as described in [35], these interrupted actions give way to the peaceful rhythm of the music. Music can work as an external stimulus for those people, and control and regulate movement. Research shows the therapeutic potential of music in people with PD [19].

Autism. Music also has therapeutic potential in therapist's work with children with autism spectrum disorder, as investigated in [14]. The authors explore the use of music and its therapeutic potential in their work with autistic children, who have verbal skills. The musical interactions helped to create a shared experience between the child and therapist, and support the children's ability to regulate their emotions.

Sleep. Sleep deficiency may indicate chronic health problems, such as heart disease, kidney disease, high blood pressure, diabetes, stroke, obesity and depression. The article [6] addresses recent findings related to the potential of music to induce sleep in illness and wellness. The author also highlights the efficacy of music therapy as a potent and cost-effective intervention. Even healthy people suffer from sleep-related problems, which negatively influence their quality of life. The authors of [24] study the effect of pop music on both sleep and wake-up of young adults. Their analysis, involving carefully designed hardware and software, revealed types of musical features that are effective for fast sleep induction and wake-up. Based on these findings, they present scenarios of sleep music recommendation. Another system called HypnOS is designed for 'intelligent homes', aiming to improve the sleep quality of home residents [41]. The system monitors their sleep and provides personalized recommendations to overcome sleep-related issues by recommending, among others, music that helps the user to fall asleep.

Depression. Depression is a common mental disorder. According to WHO, more than 264 million people of all ages suffer from depression in the world. The results of music therapy described in [32] indicate gains in emotional fulfilment in patients with major depression or an acute phase of a schizophrenia spectrum disorder; the patients are becoming socially closer. Another music intervention described in [21] indicates positive results of short-term music therapy for arousal and attention regulation in patients with posttraumatic stress disorder. Participants of the experiment showed significant improvement on subscales of hyperarousal, mood and cognition, and attention.

All examples mentioned above highlight the importance of music in health, and they are inspiration for developing systems that support music therapists. Unfortunately, they are facing problems with handling new technologies due to complicated interfaces and the lack of training [26]. Therefore, helpful User Interfaces (UI) for music therapists are becoming an important aspect, explored in [5]. Taking into account little work on this topic, designing music RSs with user-oriented UI for music therapists seems to be a promising future research direction.

5 Summary

Medicine recommendation systems are becoming more popular, as they may help both physicians and patients. In this context, intuitive user interfaces, system explanation, and ease of use gain importance in medical applications. Still, the diversity of available digital data and increasing knowledge of their importance for health makes the development of effective health recommendation systems challenging.

A look at music recommendation systems used in medicine shows that there is a big room for further research on the development of personalized music recommendation systems for improving the health condition of their users. In this chapter, we reviewed the positive effect of music on human health, and how music can support treatment, as well as well-being.

We hope that the above review will contribute to new ideas for the development of personalized and context-aware music recommendation systems used in medicine.

References

1. Tinnitracks: Treat Tinnitus With Your Favorite Music! (06 Jul 2020). https://www.tinnitracks.com/en
2. Álvarez, P., Zarazaga-Soria, F., Baldassarri, S.: Mobile music recommendations for runners based on location and emotions: The dj-running system. Pervasive Mob. Comput. 101242 (2020)
3. Archenaa, J., Anita, E.M.: Health recommender system using big data analytics. J. Manag. Sci. Bus. Intell. 17–24 (2017)
4. Baird, A., Garrido, S., Tamplin, J.: Music and Dementia: From Cognition to Therapy. Oxford University Press (2019)
5. Baltaxe-Admony, L.B., Hope, T., Watanabe, K., Teodorescu, M., Kurniawan, S., Nishimura, T.: Exploring the creation of useful interfaces for music therapists. In: Proceedings of the Audio Mostly 2018 on Sound in Immersion and Emotion, pp. 1–7 (2018)
6. Bandini, S., Gasparini, F., Giltri, M.: Personalized music experience for the wellbeing of elderly people. In: International Conference on Internet Science, pp. 335–340. Springer (2019)
7. Bao, Y., Jiang, X.: An intelligent medicine recommender system framework. In: 2016 IEEE 11th Conference on Industrial Electronics and Applications (ICIEA), pp. 1383–1388. IEEE (2016)
8. Bocanegra, C.L.S., Ramos, J.L.S., Rizo, C., Civit, A., Fernandez-Luque, L.: Healthrecsys: a semantic content-based recommender system to complement health videos. BMC Med. Inf. Decis. Making **17**(1), 1–10 (2017)
9. Bradt, J., Potvin, N., Kesslick, A., Shim, M., Radl, D., Schriver, E., Gracely, E.J., Komarnicky-Kocher, L.T.: The impact of music therapy versus music medicine on psychological outcomes and pain in cancer patients: a mixed methods study. Support. Care Cancer **23**(5), 1261–1271 (2015)
10. Burrai, F., Sanna, G.D., Moccia, E., Morlando, F., Cosentino, E.R., Bui, V., Micheluzzi, V., Borghi, C., Parodi, G.: Beneficial effects of listening to classical music in patients with heart failure: a randomized controlled trial. J. Card. Fail. **26**(7), 541–549 (2020)
11. Chen, C., Zhang, L., Fan, X., Wang, Y., Xu, C., Liu, R.: A epilepsy drug recommendation system by implicit feedback and crossing recommendation. In: 2018 IEEE SmartWorld, Ubiquitous Intelligence & Computing, Advanced & Trusted Computing, Scalable Computing &

Communications, Cloud & Big Data Computing, Internet of People and Smart City Innovation (SmartWorld/SCALCOM/UIC/ATC/CBDCom/IOP/SCI), pp. 1134–1139. IEEE (2018)
12. Chen, C.H., Karvela, M., Sohbati, M., Shinawatra, T., Toumazou, C.: Person–personalized expert recommendation system for optimized nutrition. IEEE Trans. Biomed. Circ. Syst. **12**(1), 151–160 (2017)
13. Cheng, H.I., Alifa, R., Lee, H.: The effectiveness of music therapy system for the elderly with mild cognitive impairment. In: Proceedings of the 2019 7th International Conference on Information Technology: IoT and Smart City, pp. 445–448 (2019)
14. Epstein, S., Elefant, C., Thompson, G.: Music therapists' perceptions of the therapeutic potentials using music when working with verbal children on the autism spectrum: a qualitative analysis. J. Music Ther. **57**(1), 66–90 (2020). https://doi.org/10.1093/jmt/thz017
15. Erdeniz, S.P., Maglogiannis, I., Menychtas, A., Felfernig, A., Tran, T.: Recommender Systems for IoT Enabled m-Health Applications. In: Iliadis, L., Maglogiannis, I., Plagianakos, V. (eds.) 14th IFIP International Conference on Artificial Intelligence Applications and Innovations (AIAI), *Artificial Intelligence Applications and Innovations*, vol. AICT-520, pp. 227–237. Springer International Publishing, Rhodes, Greece (2018). https://doi.org/10.1007/978-3-319-92016-0_21. URL: https://hal.inria.fr/hal-01821320. Part 4: HEALTHIOT
16. Fang, J., Grunberg, D., Luit, S., Wang, Y.: Development of a music recommendation system for motivating exercise. In: 2017 International Conference on Orange Technologies (ICOT), pp. 83–86. IEEE (2017)
17. Feng, X., Zhang, H., Ren, Y., Shang, P., Zhu, Y., Liang, Y., Guan, R., Xu, D.: The deep learning-based recommender system "pubmender" for choosing a biomedical publication venue: Development and validation study. J. Med. Internet Res. **21**(5), e12957 (2019)
18. Gallagher, L.M., Lagman, R., Bates, D., Edsall, M., Eden, P., Janaitis, J., Rybicki, L.: Perceptions of family members of palliative medicine and hospice patients who experienced music therapy. Support. Care Cancer **25**(6), 1769–1778 (2017)
19. García-Casares, N., Martín-Colom, J.E., García-Arnés, J.A.: Music therapy in Parkinson's disease. J. Am. Med. Directors Assoc. **19**(12), 1054–1062 (2018)
20. Guerra, J., Quan, W., Li, K., Ahumada, L., Winston, F., Desai, B.: Scosy: A biomedical collaboration recommendation system. In: 2018 40th Annual International Conference of the IEEE Engineering in Medicine and Biology Society (EMBC), pp. 3987–3990. IEEE (2018)
21. Hakvoort, L., de Jong, S., van de Ree, M., Kok, T., Macfarlane, C., de Haan, H.: Music therapy to regulate arousal and attention in patients with substance use disorder and posttraumatic stress disorder: A feasibility study. J. Music Ther. **57**(3), 353–378 (2020)
22. Kasperczuk, A., Dardzińska, A., Daniluk, J.: Recommender system for diagnosis of colon diseases. In: 2018 International Conference BIOMDLORE, pp. 1–238. IEEE (2018)
23. Kim, H.G., Kim, G.Y., Kim, J.Y.: Music recommendation system using human activity recognition from accelerometer data. IEEE Trans. Consumer Electron. **65**(3), 349–358 (2019)
24. Lee, T., Moon, S.E., Baek, J., Lee, J.S., Kim, S.: Music for sleep and wake-up: an empirical study. IEEE Access **7**, 145816–145828 (2019)
25. Leggieri, M., Thaut, M.H., Fornazzari, L., Schweizer, T.A., Barfett, J., Munoz, D.G., Fischer, C.E.: Music intervention approaches for Alzheimer's disease: a review of the literature. Front. Neurosci. **13**, 132 (2019)
26. Li, Y.: Technologies and music therapy from the perspective of music therapists. In: Proceedings of the Fourth International Conference on Biological Information and Biomedical Engineering, pp. 1–5 (2020)
27. Louie, R., Coenen, A., Huang, C.Z., Terry, M., Cai, C.J.: Novice-ai music co-creation via ai-steering tools for deep generative models. In: Proceedings of the 2020 CHI Conference on Human Factors in Computing Systems, pp. 1–13 (2020)
28. Nag, N., Pandey, V., Jain, R.: Live personalized nutrition recommendation engine. In: Proceedings of the 2nd International Workshop on Multimedia for Personal Health and Health Care, pp. 61–68 (2017)
29. Norman, K.: Music as medicine. Lynchburg J. Med. Sci. **1**(3), 60 (2019)

30. Ozsoy, M.G., Özyer, T., Polat, F., Alhajj, R.: Realizing drug repositioning by adapting a recommendation system to handle the process. BMC Bioinform. **19**(1), 136 (2018)
31. O'Callaghan, C.C., McDermott, F., Michael, N., Daveson, B.A., Hudson, P.L., Zalcberg, J.R.: "A quiet still voice that just touches": music's relevance for adults living with life-threatening cancer diagnoses. Support. Care Cancer **22**(4), 1037–1047 (2014)
32. Paul, N., Lotter, C., van Staden, W.: Patient reflections on individual music therapy for a major depressive disorder or acute phase schizophrenia spectrum disorder. J. Music Ther. **57**(2), 168–192 (2020)
33. Pincay, J., Terán, L., Portmann, E.: Health recommender systems: a state-of-the-art review. In: 2019 Sixth International Conference on eDemocracy & eGovernment (ICEDEG), pp. 47–55. IEEE (2019)
34. Promkot, A.n., Arch-int, S., Arch-int, N.: The personalized traditional medicine recommendation system using ontology and rule inference approach. In: 2019 IEEE 4th International Conference on Computer and Communication Systems (ICCCS), pp. 96–104. IEEE (2019)
35. Sacks, O.: Muzykofilia: opowieści o muzyce i mózgu. Zysk i S-ka Wydawnictwo (2009)
36. Sahoo, A.K., Pradhan, C., Barik, R.K., Dubey, H.: Deepreco: deep learning based health recommender system using collaborative filtering. Computation **7**(2), 25 (2019)
37. Sezgin, E., Özkan, S.: A systematic literature review on health recommender systems. In: 2013 E-Health and Bioengineering Conference (EHB), pp. 1–4. IEEE (2013)
38. Shimada, K., Takada, H., Mitsuyama, S., Ban, H., Matsuo, H., Otake, H., Kunishima, H., Kanemitsu, K., Kaku, M.: Drug-recommendation system for patients with infectious diseases. In: AMIA Annual Symposium Proceedings, vol. 2005, p. 1112. American Medical Informatics Association (2005)
39. Shin, I.h., Cha, J., Cheon, G.W., Lee, C., Lee, S.Y., Yoon, H.J., Kim, H.C.: Automatic stress-relieving music recommendation system based on photoplethysmography-derived heart rate variability analysis. In: 2014 36th Annual International Conference of the IEEE Engineering in Medicine and Biology Society, pp. 6402–6405. IEEE (2014)
40. Stark, B., Knahl, C., Aydin, M., Elish, K.: A literature review on medicine recommender systems. Int. J. Adv. Comput. Sci. Appl. **10**(8), 6–13 (2019)
41. Tsolakou, E., Leonidis, A., Kouroumalis, V., Korozi, M., Antona, M., Stephanidis, C.: Hypnos: a sleep monitoring and recommendation system to improve sleep hygiene in intelligent homes. In: International Conference on Human Interaction and Emerging Technologies, pp. 433–439. Springer (2020)
42. Valdez, A.C., Ziefle, M., Verbert, K., Felfernig, A., Holzinger, A.: Recommender systems for health informatics: state-of-the-art and future perspectives. In: Machine Learning for Health Informatics, pp. 391–414. Springer (2016)
43. van der Wal-Huisman, H., Dons, K.S., Smilde, R., Heineman, E., van Leeuwen, B.L.: The effect of music on postoperative recovery in older patients: a systematic review. J. Geriatric Oncol. **9**(6), 550–559 (2018)
44. Wall, M., Duffy, A.: The effects of music therapy for older people with dementia. Br. J. Nurs. **19**(2), 108–113 (2010)
45. Wiesner, M., Pfeifer, D.: Health recommender systems: concepts, requirements, technical basics and challenges. Int. J. Environ. Res. Public Health **11**(3), 2580–2607 (2014)
46. Wlodarczyk, N.: The effect of music therapy on the spirituality of persons in an in-patient hospice unit as measured by self-report. J. Music Ther. **44**(2), 113–122 (2007)
47. Zhang, Y., Zhang, D., Hassan, M.M., Alamri, A., Peng, L.: Cadre: cloud-assisted drug recommendation service for online pharmacies. Mob. Netw. Appl. **20**(3), 348–355 (2015)

Emotion-Based Music Recommender System for Tinnitus Patients (EMOTIN)

Katarzyna A. Tarnowska

Abstract The chapter presents a personalized recommender system (RS) for tinnitus therapy, called EMOTIN. It is based on the automatic indexing of music by emotions. A framework and an algorithm for emotion-based music recommendations for tinnitus patients are proposed. The contribution is expected to be novel, as nobody yet proposed a music RS specifically to target negative emotions associated with tinnitus. The chapter is organized as follows. First, the medical problem of tinnitus, a common but non-curable hearing disorder, is presented. An overview of existing therapies, based on tinnitus retraining and music interventions, is provided. The background information includes work done previously in this research, including RECTIN (Recommender for Tinnitus) system and its prototype GUI-based version—eTRT (electronic Tinnitus Retraining Therapy). Next, the methods used to enhance an existing prototype by adding the music recommendation functionality are presented. The high-level overview of the content-based approach for music recommendation is described. A formal definition of the music recommendation is given and a recommender algorithm based on neighborhood approach and similarity metrics is described in detail. The methods to build a user profile are proposed, including user input data and a dimensional model of emotions. For item content analysis, an approach based on music emotion recognition and audio notching is outlined. The preliminary results on music item content analysis include datasets preparation, audio feature extraction, and testing regression models for music emotion recognition. Discussion includes future directions for this research, including full implementation of the system and evaluating the system's recommendations with tinnitus patients.

K. A. Tarnowska (✉)
San Jose State University, One Washington Square, San Jose, CA, USA
e-mail: katarzyna.tarnowska@sjsu.edu

Z. W. Ras et al. (eds.), *Recommender Systems for Medicine and Music*,
Studies in Computational Intelligence 946,
https://doi.org/10.1007/978-3-030-66450-3_13

1 Introduction

This section provides an introduction to the medical problem of tinnitus, as well as management therapies based on retraining and music-based interventions, which the proposed recommender system attempts to support.

1.1 Tinnitus

Tinnitus, known as "ringing in the ears", remains an enigma from the medical point of view [25]. Tinnitus is highly prevalent, estimated to affect 15% of the general population, with 2–3% having clinically significant tinnitus [3]. Tinnitus's effect on life can range from mild or low to severe. Despite its prevalence and debilitating effect on a significant portion of the population, there is still no known drug to treat tinnitus. The current methods are based on the management of symptoms. In this research, we focus on two such therapies: (1) tinnitus retraining therapy (TRT), which is a combination of sound therapy and counseling; (2) music therapy, which involves listening to tailored "notched" music.

1.2 Tinnitus Retraining Therapy

TRT has been developed by Dr. Jastreboff in the late '80s based on studies on animal models and the neurophysiological model of tinnitus [13]. It has been clinically practiced for over 25 years [14]. Both clinical trials and practice confirm the efficacy of the therapy with about 80% of patients being successfully helped to manage their tinnitus. The main goal of the therapy is the habituation of the symptoms achieved through retraining negative feedback loops between the auditory system, where tinnitus signal occurs, and cortical and subcortical areas of the brain, where the signal is detected and perceived. Additional counseling aims at retraining negative emotions developed due to the prolonged perception of tinnitus, physiologically, by retraining negative loops between brain and nervous system—limbic and autonomic nervous systems. The clinical protocol involves initial diagnosis into one of five categories of a hearing problem, and subsequent treatment protocol with sound instruments and individual counseling. The therapy must be highly personalized and spans up to 18 months to achieve habituation. It is relatively a niche therapy with scarce clinical expertise and experience in its delivery. It is not offered as a standard of care for tinnitus, but only by specialized clinics.

1.3 Music Therapy

Music therapy is the clinical and evidence-based use of music interventions to accomplish individualized goals within a therapeutic relationship [2]. It is provided by a music therapist, who works with a patient on an individualized treatment plan that manages the psychological and emotional aspects of tinnitus. Similar, as in TRT, the goal is the habituation of symptoms. It is based on a mindfulness approach that involves music-based exercises to practice acknowledgment and acceptance of symptoms. Music therapy can support sound therapy treatment, but the scope of music therapy practice also extends to psychosocial and mental health. Music therapy provides a "productive distraction" that aims at shifting cognitive focus from the irritating stimulus to a more productive stimulus. The goal to achieve acceptance implies a state of acknowledgment of sound perception without resistance. Acceptance and acknowledgment help reduce negative emotions, such as anger, frustration, resentment, anxiety, and physical tension. The treatment involves music recommendations, particularly preferred music, which offers a pleasant and enjoyable stimulus to assist the shift to a more productive cognitive focus. The Heidelberg Model is a protocol that combines sound therapy with counseling and psychological approaches [4, 12]. This model combines both acoustic and psychotherapeutic techniques. As developed in Europe, it is less known in the United States. There is still a small number of music therapists with advanced education and training who focus on research in music therapy for hearing disorders.

2 Background

This section provides background information on previous research, including the prototype of a clinical decision support system for tinnitus. It also provides mathematical foundations of the system, including the theory of decision rules and action rules. The section concludes with preliminary results on diagnostics and recommendations for TRT.

2.1 RECTIN—Recommender for Tinnitus

In [26] a recommender system for diagnosis and treatment of tinnitus (RECTIN) was proposed. A *recommender system* (RS) is a piece of software that aims at recommending *items* of particular interest to the *users*. RS technology has been used mainly in business-to-consumer setting and deployed mainly within e-commerce websites. Novel applications of RS emerge, such as in medicine or business-to-business setting [26, 27]. In the medical domain, the *users* would be patients or medical professionals, and *recommendable items* would be a piece of medical information, such as

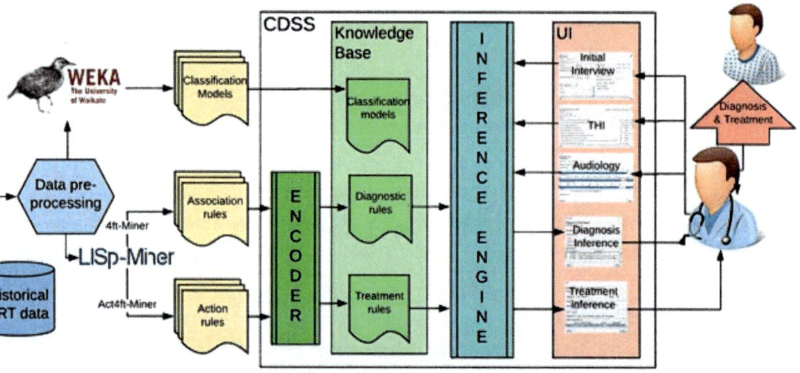

Fig. 1 The architecture of the knowledge-based Clinical Decision Support System (CDSS) for Tinnitus, called RECTIN ("Recommender for Tinnitus"). The historical TRT data constitutes a source for the knowledge base, from which classification models, association rules, and action rules are mined. The system provides knowledge-inferred recommendations for diagnosis and treatment to a physician through a Java-based user interface

diagnosis suggestion or treatment recommendation. The system proposed in [26] is data-driven and produces recommendations based on decision (classification) rules for diagnosis and action rules for the treatment adjustments (see Fig. 1). These rules were extracted in a series of data mining experiments and preceded by data cleansing and transformation [28].

2.1.1 Decision Rules for Diagnosis

Definition 1 A *decision rule* is a rule r in the form $(\phi \Rightarrow \delta)$, where ϕ is called *antecedent* (or assumption), and δ is called *descendant* (or thesis).
Each rule is characterized by *support* and *confidence*. *Support* $sup(\phi \Rightarrow \delta) = sup(\phi \wedge \delta)$ is defined as the number of tuples supporting ϕ and δ. *Confidence* is defined as $conf(\phi \Rightarrow \delta) = \frac{sup(\phi \wedge \delta)}{sup(\phi)}$.

Sample decision rules, extracted from tinnitus clinical datasets using LISp-Miner 4ft-Miner module [23], are presented in Table 1. These rules are interpreted as follows:

Table 1 Examples of discovered decision rules for the predicted category of a hearing problem based on the interview and audiometry input data

A sample diagnostic decision rule	Confidence
$H_{pr}(< 0; 0.5)) \wedge HL_{pr}(< 0; 0.5)) \wedge T_{pr}(< 6; 8)) \Rightarrow Category(1)$	85%
$L_2 \geq 50 \wedge R_6 \leq 75 \Rightarrow Category(2)$	87%

- *If* hyperacusis H_{pr} and hearing loss HL_{pr} indicated as not problematic, but tinnitus T_{pr} as a problem—*then* a patient is diagnosed into Category 1 with 85% confidence.
- *If* audiometric values of L_2 (audiogram at 2 kHz for the left ear) is greater or equal to 50 and R_6 (audiogram at 6 kHz for the right ear) is less or equal to 75, *then* a patient is categorized into Category 2 with 87% confidence.

2.1.2 Action Rules for the Treatment

The concept of an action rule was first proposed by Ras and Wieczorkowska in 2000 [19], and since then, its application was proposed, among others, for business, medicine, and music indexing [19, 20, 27, 30]. Action rules are especially promising in the field of medical data, as a doctor can examine the effect of treatment decisions on a patient's improved state. This technique is also particularly useful for building knowledge-based recommender systems.

Definition 2 *Action rule r* is a term $[(\omega) \wedge (\alpha \rightarrow \beta) \Rightarrow (\theta \rightarrow \psi)]$, where $(\omega \wedge \alpha) \Rightarrow \theta$ and $(\omega \wedge \beta) \Rightarrow \psi$ are classification rules, ω is a conjunction of stable attribute values, $(\alpha \rightarrow \beta)$ shows changes in flexible attribute values, and $(\theta \rightarrow \psi)$ shows the desired effect of the action.

Sample action rules extracted with LISP-Miner's Act4ft-Miner package [23] are presented in Table 2. These rules are interpreted as follows:

- *If* tinnitus was induced by other medical condition (*OMTI*), and as a side effect of taking medications (T_{side}), *then* changing the sound generator model GH hard (GHH) to the Viennatone model (V) at the first visit and changing the follow-up contact to the telephone-based (T) will improve a patient with 82% confidence.
- *If* the current treatment involves sound generator *SG*, *then* changing the mixing point for the right ear Mix_{RSL} from $< 11; 12)$ to $< 9; 10)$ will improve a patient's state with 100% confidence.

2.2 eTRT—Electronic Tinnitus Retraining Therapy

eTRT is a GUI-based prototype implementation of a clinical decision support system for tinnitus diagnosis and therapy [9], which follows the design of RECTIN system.

Table 2 Examples of discovered action rules for recommending treatment in TRT

A sample treatment action rule	Conf.
$T_{side}(yes) \wedge OMTI(yes) \wedge (Ins_{vis(01)} GHH \rightarrow V) \wedge FU(0 \rightarrow T) \Rightarrow Ch(better)$	82%
$Ins(SG) \wedge (Mix_{RSL}(< 11; 12) \rightarrow < 9; 10)) \Rightarrow Ch(better)$	100%

It is a three-tier application that supports clinicians who diagnose and treat tinnitus patients using the TRT method. The system utilizes a user-friendly graphical interface to enter patient- and visit-related data and to display the system's inference of diagnosis and effective treatment options (see Fig. 2). The rule engine was implemented using the Java Expert System Shell (JESS) framework. The system utilizes a pattern-matching algorithm to provide a diagnosis for a new patient based on a pre-coded set of *decision rules*. These decision rules encoded into the system were extracted from clinical datasets in previous work [28]. Each decision rule assigns a TRT category based on characteristics of a patient, such as initial interview and

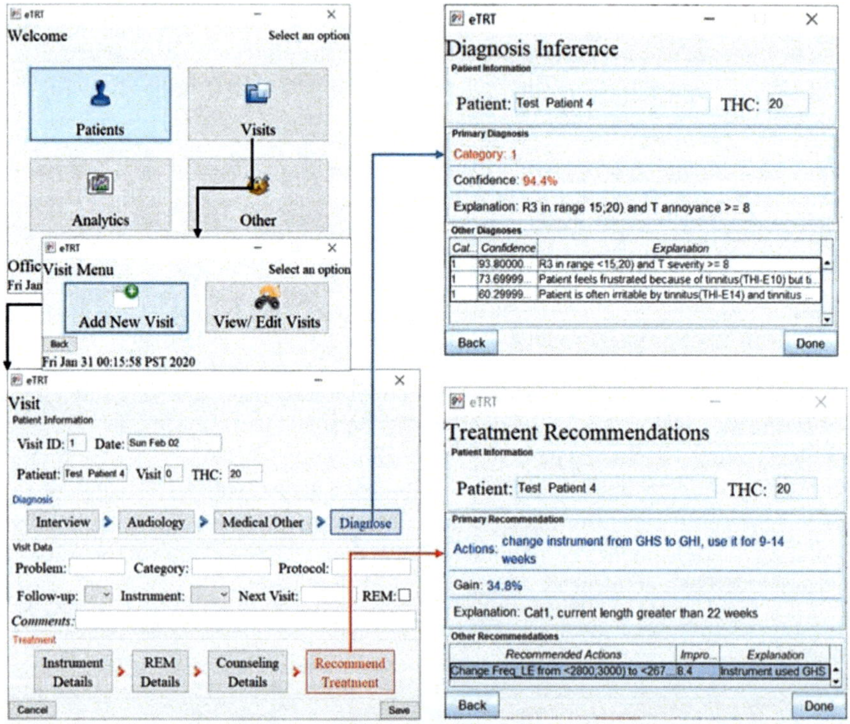

Fig. 2 eTRT—implementation of the GUI-based clinical decision support system for tinnitus diagnosis and therapy [9]. A sample workflow depicts adding new visit data and generating a corresponding inference of a diagnosis and treatment recommendations personalized for a patient

audiometry. The treatment recommendations are inferred from *action rules* extracted from clinical datasets first and encoded into the knowledge base next.

Preliminary results on evaluating the eTRT system in terms of accuracy and explainability are presented in Tables 3 and 4 on the chosen patient cases.

Table 3 eTRT evaluation results on predicting diagnosis by the system on the chosen patient test cases—actual category versus category predicted by the system, characterized by the confidence and explanation

Test case	Actual	Prediction	Conf.	Explanation
1: male, 38, noise exposure	Cat 4	Cat 4	66.7%	LSD <= 100, L4 < 10, and LL3 < 75
2: male, 49, ear surgery	Cat 3	Cat 3	100%	LL3 in < 85; 91), Hyper. Annoy >=8, H Eff on Lif >=8, and H Sev >=7.5
3: female, 77, hearing loss	Cat 2	Cat 2	96.2%	LR8 >= 999, R6 >= 75, and T_{sv} >= 8
4: male, 53, stress	Cat 1	Cat 1	94.4%	LL3 in < 15; 20) and Tin. annoy. >= 8
5: male, 36, car accident	Cat 0	Cat 1	60.3%	Patient often irritable by tinnitus (E14) and tinnitus makes him anxious (E22)

Table 4 eTRT evaluation results on recommending treatment actions, characterized by an expected improvement gain in percentage points and explanation(s) for the patients' test cases

Test case	Recommended action(s)	Gain	Explanation
1	Change instrument from GHH to GHS	41 pp	A male whose tinnitus was induced by noise
4	Change instrument from GHS to GHI, use it for 9–14 weeks	34.8 pp	Cat1, instr. duration greater than 22 weeks
5	Change Freq LE from < 2800; 3000) to < 2670; 2800) in REM	8.4 pp	Instrument used GHS

3 Methods

The method section presents an approach used for music recommendation in EMOTIN. The content-based approach is described, together with methods for user profiling and item content analysis. The RS neighborhood-based algorithm is proposed with the similarity metrics, such as Euclidean distance and cosine similarity. User profiling utilizes a dimensional model of emotions and content analysis uses regression models for emotion recognition in music items.

3.1 Music Recommendations

This work aims at augmenting the previous work on RECTIN and eTRT implementation by adding the music recommendation module (see Fig. 3). Currently, the system supports the clinical delivery of tinnitus retraining therapy. Adding personalized music recommendations for tinnitus patients will additionally support music therapy for tinnitus. The pleasant sound enrichment with recommended music items will augment sound therapy used in TRT. The system will recommend music pieces to the patient according to their preferences and personalized to their tinnitus acoustic characteristics. The goal of the music recommender system incorporated into eTRT is to present a ranked list of *items*, in this case, music pieces (see Fig. 4).

The ranking is generated by applying prediction algorithms, based on the *content* of the music pieces, the *user's* profile, preferences, and constraints. Here, the user is the patient, and the data for music recommendations is collected implicitly with clinical tinnitus data, as well as explicitly with music preferences questionnaire (see Fig. 5). The goal of the built-in music recommender is to assist the physician in delivering music therapy without directly consulting music therapists. The user profile is represented by both *personal health records* and music preferences collected in eTRT. When supplied with facts about the new patient, the music recommender system computes a set of potentially relevant music *items* of interest to the target user (tinnitus patient). Such an RS will address the insufficient number of both TRT specialists as well as music therapists, which is a niche specialty. The recommendations generated based on the patient's examination and questionnaires will be presented to the physician, and next the physician will present and consult the choices with the patient.

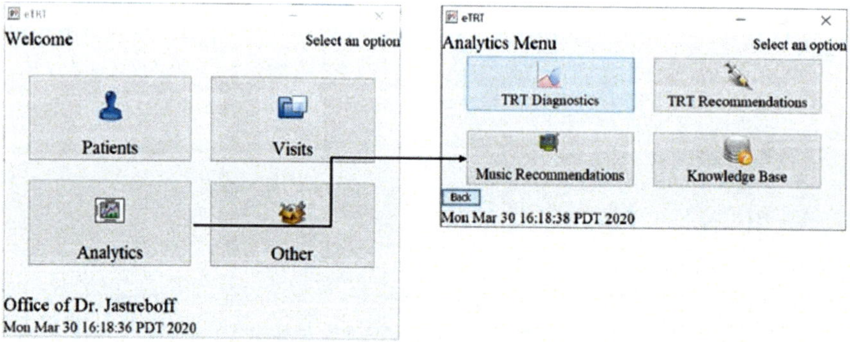

Fig. 3 eTRT system expanded with the music recommendations option in the analytics menu

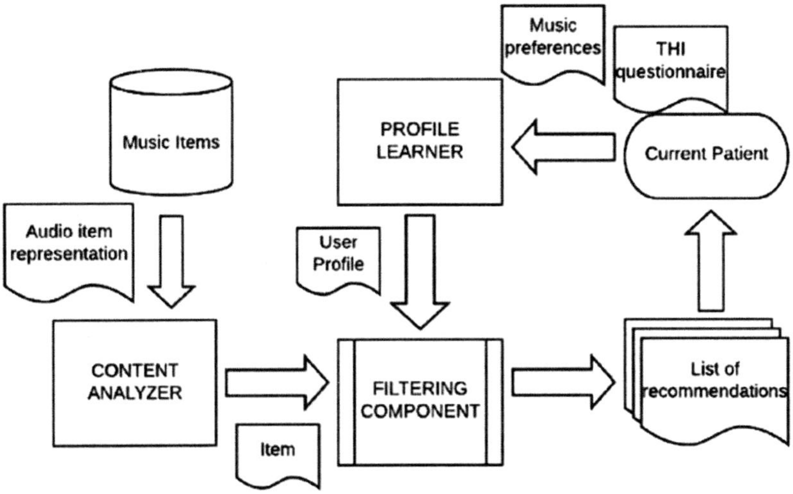

Fig. 4 High-level architecture of a content-based music recommender system for tinnitus patients

3.1.1 Content-Based Approach

The content-based approach for building recommender systems stems from the concepts such as information retrieval and is suitable for music recommendation problem. In this approach, discrimination between relevant and irrelevant items is based on exploiting information derived from the items' contents. In the considered problem area, the content of a music piece is understood as acoustic characteristics that translate into an emotion carried by the music piece. The derived emotional content of a music piece is then matched against the patient profile, described by their emotional state and music preferences. The system will also learn to recommend items similar to those that the user liked in the past. In this work, it is proposed to build a hybrid recommender system for music that integrates content and emotion-based filtering.

3.2 Music Therapy Protocol

Music therapy takes place in sessions for either individuals or small groups. The first step in the protocol is the therapist conducting an initial assessment with the goal of understanding the individual needs and aims related to their health and well-being. The patient's individualized goals are explored to tailor the use of music-based interventions. This includes a review of musical preferences, likes, and dislikes. Certain features, such as rhythm or tempo can be customized. For patients with tinnitus, the focus can be on intensity (loudness), melody, and pitch to facilitate relaxation, dampen general anxiety, and/or help with sleep disturbances. It may also be beneficial to filter or mask certain sound frequencies that match the patient's tinnitus.

3.2.1 Music Preferences

Music preferences are elicited explicitly by using a form for choosing the preferred music genres and artists (see Fig. 5). The set of genres to choose from is fixed in the system (i.e. blues, electronic, rock). Favorite artists can be searched from the database of artists of the available music pieces.

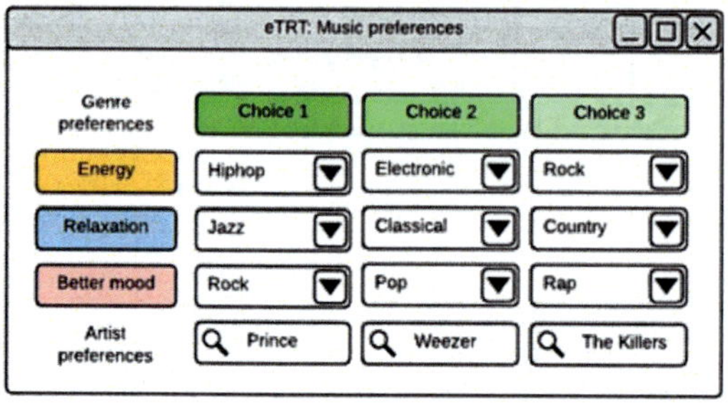

Fig. 5 Design of the screen for entering the user's music preferences. This includes 3 choices of the preferred genre for improving arousal (energy), lowering arousal (relaxation), improving mood (increased valence), and preferred artist. The choices are used as constraints in the music recommender filtering algorithm

3.3 *Detecting Affective States*

Affective states of the recommender system's users can be detected in two ways: explicitly or implicitly [29]. The self-report SAM (Self-Assessment Manikin) tool was proposed in [7] to elicit the emotional state of a patient. In [15, 16] Emotion Indexing Questionnaire was developed to gather initial data about users and their music preferences. In this research, it is proposed to use standard questionnaires for tinnitus to derive the emotional state of a patient. Tinnitus Handicap Inventory (THI) consists of 25 questions divided into functional, control, and emotional sections. All questions from the emotional section, 2 questions from functional, and 1 question from control were selected for building the emotional "profile" of a patient (see Table 5). Each question is answered with no/sometimes/yes by a patient. The categorical answers are translated to numerical scores of 0/2/4, correspondingly, and used to calculate the total score of THI, which in turn determines the severity of tinnitus.

Table 5 Selected questions from the Tinnitus Handicap Inventory (THI) used to detect negative emotions associated with tinnitus. The table shows arbitrary mappings between THI questions and emotions. Names for emotions were defined by the Sherer dimensional model [22]. The table also shows their corresponding values of arousal and valence (in the 0–9 scale)

THI code	THI question	Emotion (Sherer)	Arousal	Valence
E-3	Tinnitus make you angry?	Angry	7.2	−1
F-4	Tinnitus make you confused?	Confused	6.29	6.14
C-5	Because of your tinnitus, do you feel desperate?	Desperate	−4.6	−7.3
E-6	Do you complain a great deal about your tinnitus?	Discontented	3	−6
E-10	Tinnitus make you feel frustrated?	Frustrated	3.5	−5.4
E-14	Tinnitus make you often irritable?	Annoyed	6	−4
E-16	Tinnitus make you upset?	Sad	−3.6	−7.4
E-17	Tinnitus has caused stress on your relationships with family and friends?	Distressed	5.1	−6.4
F-20	Tinnitus make you often feel tired?	Tired	−9	−0.15
E-21	Tinnitus make you feel depressed?	Depressed	−4.2	−7.4
E-22	Tinnitus make you feel anxious?	Anxious	−7.3	−6.6
E-25	Does your tinnitus make you feel insecure?	Insecure	−7.8	−7.6

3.4 *Emotion Model*

An assumption for emotion representation is that emotion can be considered as a set of continuous quantities and mapped into a set of real numbers. The dimensional emotions model describes each emotion as a point in a continuous multidimensional space. Each dimension represents a quality of the emotion, and the most popular model uses valence and arousal as dimensions [21]. Emotion terms are described as silent to energetic along the arousal dimension and negative to positive along the valence dimension (see Fig. 6).

3.4.1 User Profiling

The patient's profile is represented by their *current* and *desired* emotional state. The *current* emotional state is expressed as a set of valence-arousal points on a 2D plane (see Fig. 7) derived from the THI questionnaire and the mapping proposed in Table 5. To match patient data with music pieces that address their emotional state, first, the representation of the patient profile must be developed. It is proposed to map the emotional state of a patient, as detected by THI to a standard dimensional model of emotion, such as the ones proposed in [21, 22].

The patient's current emotional state (*CES*) is a vector of points (v_n, a_n), where each point represents the n-th emotion E_n, as elicited from THI questions.

$$\mathbf{CES} = [w_1, w_2, \ldots, w_n]^T \cdot [(v_1, a_1), (v_2, a_2), \ldots, (v_n, a_n)] \quad (1)$$

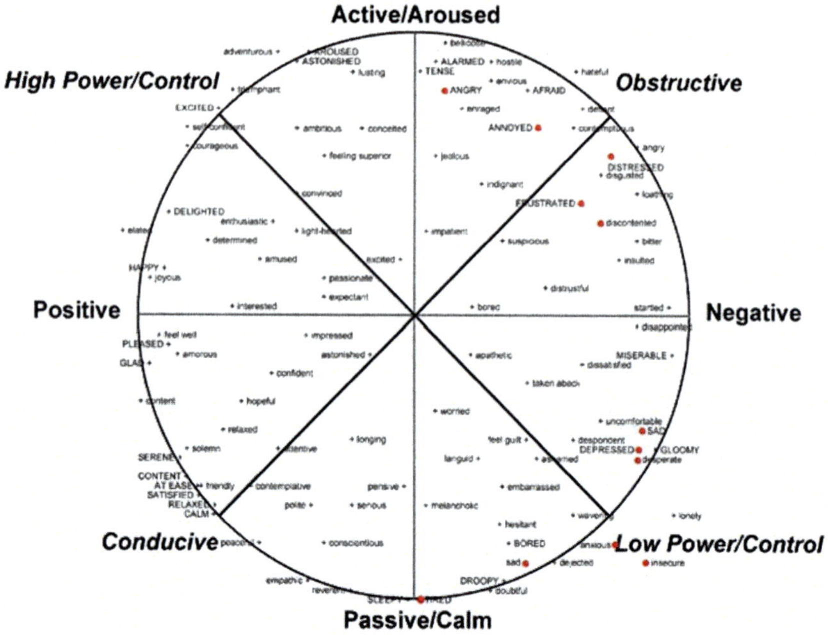

Fig. 6 Two-dimensional valence-arousal (V-A) Sherer model [22] is used to annotate THI questions by emotions. Highlighted in red are negative emotions associated with tinnitus as mapped from the THI questionnaire

Fig. 7 A sample current emotional state CES of a patient (named points in blue) derived from THI questions depicted in the V-A space. The corresponding desired state of emotions DES consists of points opposite to CES in the V-A space (points A-J)

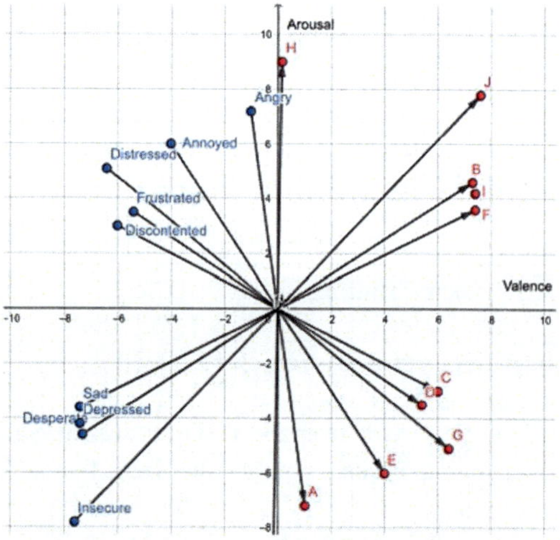

where v_n is the valence coordinate of E_n in the V-A emotion model and a_n is the arousal coordinate. Additionally, each point is assigned weight w_n: {0; 0.5; 1} depending on whether the question was answered as *no*, *sometimes*, or *yes*.

The patient's desired emotional state (*DES*) is derived as the opposite of the current emotional state:

$$\mathbf{DES} = -\mathbf{CES}, \tag{2}$$

that is the goal is to change each emotion to its counterpart in the dimensional space (see Fig. 7 for a sample transformation). For example, if the current emotional state includes emotion E_1 with $(-6, 7)$ coordinates in V-A space, the desired emotion would be $-E_1$, that is, emotion identified by coordinates $(6, -7)$.

3.5 Music Emotion Recognition

The goal of this step is to map each music piece from the song database into the same V-A space, as used for the representation of the patient's emotional state. That is, each music piece M_k can be assigned a certain emotion. Since manual annotation is not feasible for a large database of songs, the proposed approach is to use the prediction model. The regression-based model will predict the valence v_k and arousal a_k value of a music piece M_k. Since the values of arousal and valence are real values (as opposed to discrete values), emotion recognition in music can be handled as a regression machine learning problem. To train the model, a song dataset annotated with arousal and valence values was used [1]. The prediction model is built from audio features extracted with the pyAudioAnalysis library [11, 18]. The process of the music emotion recognition adapted for this work is depicted in Fig. 8.

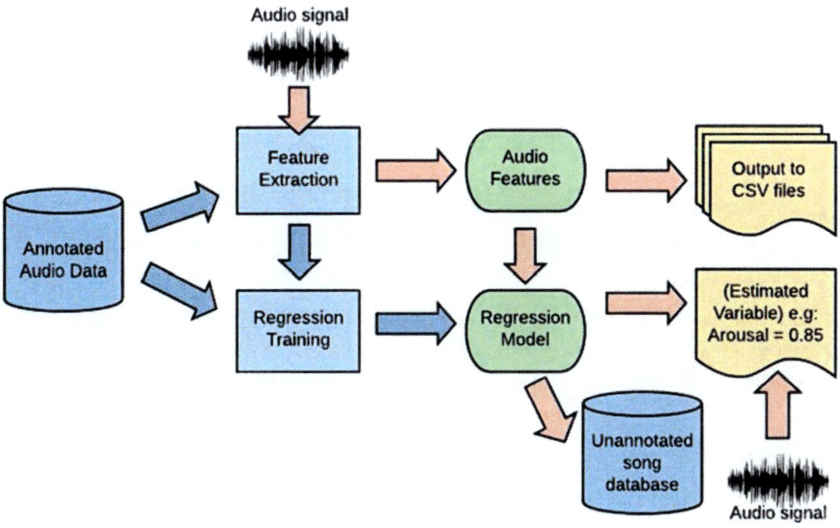

Fig. 8 The process of music emotion recognition adopted for the EMOTIN recommender system

3.5.1 Dataset

In experiments, the dataset created by Soleymani (DEAM: MediEval Database for Emotional Analysis in Music) was used [1, 24]. It contains more than 1800 songs and corresponding annotations of the valence and the arousal values. The dataset is intended to detect emotions that are expressed by the music and musicians from the content. The annotated songs are royalty-free and were obtained from several sources: freemusicarchive.org (FMA), jemando.com, and the medleyDB dataset [6, 8, 10]. The songs' excerpts shortened to 45 seconds include relevant annotations, such as arousal, valence, and averages for a sampling rate 2 Hz.

3.5.2 Audio Feature Extraction

The first step in music emotion recognition is to represent each music item, given in the form of an audio signal, as a set of audio features. These numerical features, such as energy, spectral centroid, chroma vector, describe the physics of sound. Converting music representation to numerical format allows for applying machine learning algorithms to train models that will predict the values of arousal/valence of new (unannotated) music items in the database. pyAudioAnalysis library was adopted to extract a total of 34 audio features per each music item (45 s) or per 500 ms frame [11, 18]. It is an open-source library written in Python, which offers a wide range of procedures for audio analysis, including feature extraction and music classification. The implemented procedure for data pre-processing and feature extraction consists of the following steps:

1. Converting song files in the database from *mp3* to *wav* format;
2. Converting from *stereo* to *mono* signal;
3. Audio feature extraction:
    a. Short-term feature extraction using a sampling window of 500 ms and no overlapping. This results in extracting a vector of 34 short-term features for each of 90 frames per song.
    b. Mid-term feature extraction using a sampling window of 2 s, and long-term averaging mid-term features resulting in one vector of mean feature values per song.
4. Merging individual per-song datasets into a single dataset with song-frame features (variant 1) or song-level mean features (variant 2);
5. Merging audio feature datasets with the corresponding annotations of the valence and arousal values provided by the DEAM dataset.

The resulting dataset from variant 1 (short-term feature extraction) consists of 97,732 song-frame instances, while per-song audio features dataset (variant 2) consists of 1,630 instances.

3.6 *Audio Notching*

The previous studies indicate that listening to spectrally "notched" music leads to an innovative tinnitus treatment strategy aimed at reducing tinnitus loudness [17]. The researchers attempted to reduce the loudness of patients' tinnitus by exposing them to the music of their choice that was modified, or "notched", to contain no energy in the same frequency range as the patient's tinnitus. In the proposed music recommender system EMOTIN, the music items suggested by the system in the ranking process will be optionally "notched" to further increase the effectiveness of music therapy on tinnitus patients. This will be implemented programmatically with a digital notch filter that will remove a frequency band corresponding to the tinnitus frequency from the music energy spectrum. The tinnitus frequency is a measure collected with standard eTRT procedure which includes audiology assessment of tinnitus pitch match. The studies show that removing from the auditory input a range of frequencies around the tinnitus frequency can cause long-term depression of auditory neurons corresponding to the tinnitus frequency [17].

3.7 *Emotion-Based Music Recommender Model*

3.7.1 The Formal Definition of a Problem

In our problem domain, we define a set of *users* (tinnitus patients) as U, and a set of music *items* available from a free music database as I. We define a utility function $F : U \rightarrow I$ that computes the utility value $f(u, i)$ of item i to the user u. We define music recommendation for tinnitus patients formally as a *top-N recommendation problem*. Within this work, we propose a *neighborhood-based* approach to recommending music. Neighborhood-based methods are intuitive and relatively simple to implement. They also provide a concise and intuitive justification for the computed predictions. Another strong point of neighborhood-based systems is their efficiency. The user profile (emotional state and music preferences) is used to recommend music items to a user u, by suggesting items whose feature vector $\mathbf{x_i}$ is the most similar to the profile vector $\mathbf{x_u}$, using similarity measures, such as *Euclidean distance* and *cosine similarity*.

3.7.2 Correlation-Based Similarity

The similarity measure plays an important role in the neighborhood-based recommendations, as it has an impact on both: accuracy and performance. A common measure of similarity between two objects a and b is the *cosine similarity* which computes cosine angle between two vectors $\mathbf{x_a}$ and $\mathbf{x_b}$ that represent these objects in space:

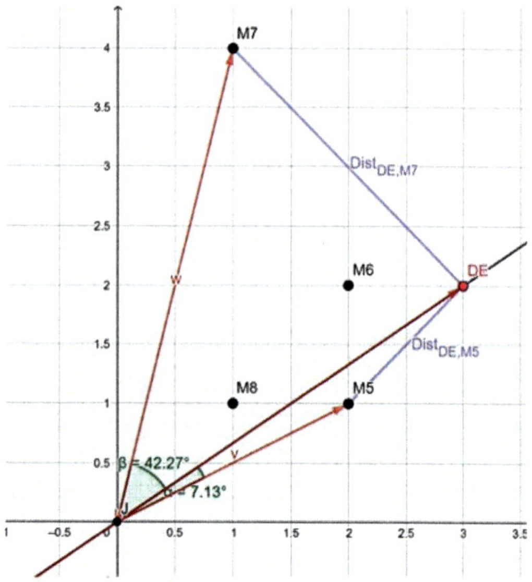

Fig. 9 Illustration of neighborhood-based recommendation using cosine similarity (green) and Euclidean distance (purple) between desired emotion DE and two music items—$M5$ and $M7$. The cosine of an angle between vectors represented by the patient's emotion and the music item determines the similarity in space, while Euclidean distance measures the absolute distance between two points. Both metrics are used to determine the utility of the music recommendation

$$cos(\mathbf{x_a}, \mathbf{x_b}) = \frac{\mathbf{x}_a^T \mathbf{x}_b}{||\mathbf{x}_a|| ||\mathbf{x}_b||}. \tag{3}$$

The *Euclidean distance* is the simplest and the most common measure of distance. The distance between two data objects a and b is measured as follows:

$$d(a, b) = \sqrt{\sum_{i=1}^{n} (a_i - b_i)^2} \tag{4}$$

where n is the number of dimensions (attributes) and a_i and b_i are the ith attributes (components) of data objects a and b, respectively. The two measures used in neighborhood-based recommendations are presented in Fig. 9 for a sample user's emotion (DE) and music items (M5 and M7).

3.7.3 Neighborhood Selection

The number of nearest neighbors to select and criteria used for this selection can have a significant impact on the quality of recommendations. The selection of neighbors used in this system is based on pre-filtering criteria and choosing the best candidates per prediction. In a recommender system that involves a large database of songs, possibly in millions, it is important to perform pre-filtering. The pre-filtering step that only keeps a subset of music items will reduce computational requirements for calculating similarity measures between each pair of a patient's emotion and a music item. Here, it is proposed to apply pre-filtering based on the user's preferences for the music genre. The recommendation algorithm also applies ranking based on the user's preferences for artists.

3.8 Recommendation Algorithm

The pseudocode of the music recommendation algorithm for the current user u is given in Algorithm 1 and illustrated in Fig. 10. First, the patient fills out the Tinnitus Handicap Inventory (THI) as a part of a standard visit process. The system computes the current emotional state (CES) of a patient as a vector of points using the 2D-emotional model (line 3 in the algorithm). The weights are considered to scale the vectors, depending on whether the patient answered "yes", "sometimes", or "no" to a question. Then, CES is used to calculate the desired emotional state DES (line 4) as the vector of the points opposite to the current emotions in 2D space (see Fig. 7). Next, we consider each desired emotion (DE_i) at a time. First, a preliminary pre-filtering is applied based on genre preferences of the current user u (line 6). The set of all music items MIS is reduced to include only these genres preferred by the user to improve their mood, increase energy, or relaxation accordingly to the desired change. After pre-filtering based on the genre, the algorithm prioritizes two subsets of music items in the dimensional space (see Fig. 10). The prioritized subset consists of music items with values of valence and arousal better that the current DE (depicted as an area in brown in Fig. 10). If this item set is found to be empty, then the secondly

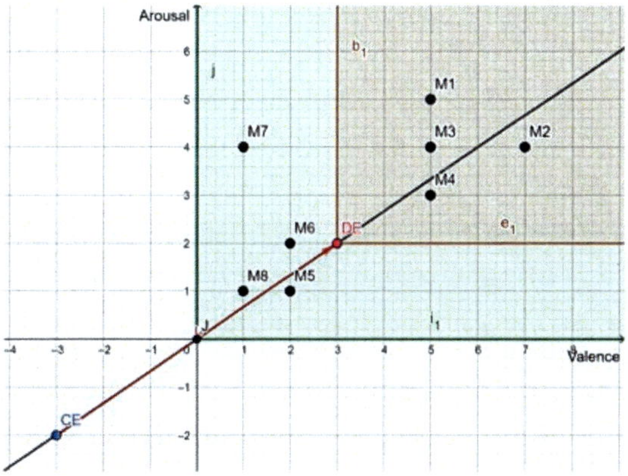

Fig. 10 Illustration of an emotion-based music recommendation in EMOTIN. The starting point is the current emotion (CE) and the goal is to convert it into the polar positive desired emotion (DE). The algorithm considers music items with valence and arousal values closest to the line connecting CE and DE. The algorithm applies priority for items "above" DE (here: $M1$, $M2$, $M3$, $M4$ in the "brown" area). Secondly, it considers items above (0, 0) and "below" DE (here: $M4$, $M5$, $M6$, $M7$ in the "green" area)

prioritized subset consists of music items with values of valence and arousal better than the point (0, 0)—depicted as the green area in Fig. 10. Next, for each music item MI_i in the subset, the cosine similarity metric is calculated between the current DE_i and MI_i (line 12). The same way, we compute Euclidean distance between the emotion point DE_i and music item MI_i (line 13). After processing all music items from the considered set, a corresponding rank is assigned to MI_i based on the cosine similarity value (line 17) and another rank based on distance (line 18). Based on these two rank values the average rank is computed (line 19). The average rank and user's preferences for the artist are considered to return the top music recommendation set (line 21).

Algorithm 1 Music recommendation algorithm in EMOTIN

1: u = current user
2: MIS (musicItemSet) = entire music database
3: Compute CES (current emotional state) of u from THI questionnaire
4: Compute DES (desired emotional state) of u from CES
5: **for** `each` DE_i `in DES` **do**
6:     MIS = `doFiltering(genre)`
7:     MIS = `Subset1`
8:     **if** MIS is empty **then**
9:         MIS = `Subset2`
10:     **end if**
11:     **for** `each` MI_j `in MIS` **do**
12:         $ComputeCosSim(DE_i, MI_j)$
13:         $ComputeDist(DE_i, MI_j)$
14:     **end for**
15: **end for**
16: **for** `each` MI_j `in MIS` **do**
17:     $AssignRankCos(MI_j, cosSim)$
18:     $AssignRankDist(MI_j, dist)$
19:     $AssignAvgGlobalRank(MI_j, RankCos, RankDist)$
20: **end for**
21: **return** $TopMusicItems(AvgGlobalRank, artistPrefer)$

4 Results

This section discusses the preliminary results of this work in the following aspects:

- Audio feature selection for valence and arousal.
- Regression models for classifying emotions (estimating the values of valence and arousal) in music items.

The experiments on emotion recognition in songs were performed on two types of the dataset (see Sect. 3.5.2). The first dataset (frame-level) combines feature extraction for each song-frame in the dataset. The annotations available at a frame-level were used. The same sampling rate was used in feature extraction as in the data annotations (the window size of 500 ms). For 45 s audio excerpts, it resulted in 90 frames per song. The second dataset used annotations at song-level, and audio features were extracted using averaging mid-term features (see Sect. 3.5.2 for the details). The song-level dataset is annotated on a 0–9 scale, and the frame-level dataset is annotated on a 0–1 scale for the valence and arousal.

4.1 Audio Feature Selection for Music Emotion Recognition

The first experiment included feature selection using WEKA. Correlation analysis was used to reduce the dataset dimensionality for further training of the regression model. The features most correlated to valence and arousal (based on the correlation rank metric) include: mel frequency cepstral coefficients (MFCC), spectral centroid, spectral spread, spectral entropy, zero-crossing rate (ZCR), and energy (see Table 6 for details). This experiment reduced the dimensionality of the regression model from 34 to 6 most correlated audio variables.

4.2 Regression Models for Music Emotion Recognition

In the context of music emotion recognition, where the emotion annotations are provided not as discrete classes, but rather real-valued measurements, the machine

Table 6 Audio feature selection for datasets annotated at the frame- (on 15,000 instances) and song-level (1,565 instances), with the corresponding correlation rank

Dataset	Rank	Arousal	Correlation	Valence	Correlation
Frame-level	#1	MFCC 1	0.62	MFCC 1	0.44
	#2	Spectral centroid	0.55	Spectral centroid	0.42
	#3	ZCR	0.48	Spectral spread	0.34
	#4	Spectral entropy	0.47	ZCR	0.33
	#5	Spectral spread	0.39	Spectral entropy	0.30
	#6	Energy	0.38	MFCC 3	0.22
Song-level	#1	MFCC 1	0.57	Spectral centroid	0.42
	#2	Spectral centroid	0.55	Spectral spread	0.40
	#3	Spectral entropy	0.51	ZCR	0.32
	#4	ZCR	0.50	MFCC 1	0.29
	#5	Spectral spread	0.47	Spectral entropy	0.29
	#6	Energy	0.42	MFCC 3	0.28

learning problem, here, is considered a regression problem. The trained regression model will be used to estimate the value of an unknown variable (here, valence and arousal) to an unknown sample (in our case audio signal). The model is built from the datasets that represent mappings from audio features to real-valued variables.

4.2.1 Regression Results in WEKA

WEKA was used, first to perform feature selection (based on correlation analysis), and then build a regression model from feature-reduced datasets. After feature selection, the experiments were conducted in training regression models for valence and arousal. Regression models tested in WEKA include linear regression, additive regression (meta-classifier), and linear nearest neighbor search (IBk in WEKA). The metrics used to assess the performance of the regression models included:

- The correlation coefficient (CC)—a measure of how closely the observation points conform to the regression model.
- Mean absolute error (MAE)—the sum of the squared differences between the predicted value and the actual value.
- Root mean squared error (RMSE)—the square root of MSE, measures how close the model's predictions are to the actual target values.

Table 7 compares the results for different types of datasets (frame- and song-level) and for different algorithms, using tenfold cross-validation as a method of testing. Linear regression was the best-performing model for song-level datasets, and additive regression for frame-level datasets. Valence was estimated more precisely than arousal for both types of datasets.

4.2.2 Regression Results in Python

Additionally, machine learning (ML) algorithms implemented in Python scikit-learn library were used. This ML library is incorporated into the pyAudioAnalysis library to facilitate audio classification and regression. The library supports SVM regression in order to map audio features to supervised variables. The library also provides a random forest algorithm for regression models. The regression training functionality includes a parameter tuning procedure, where cross-validation is performed to find an optimal mean square error (MSE). Experiments on regression models using the pyAudioAnalysis library were conducted on datasets without dimensionality reduction. The different variants of regression models (support vector machine with different kernels and random forest) were tested using tenfold cross-validation splitting the dataset randomly in ratio 9:1 (90% instances used for training and 10% used for testing). Finally, the 10 error estimates are averaged to yield an overall error estimate. The following metrics were collected:

- Mean squared error (MSE)—primarily used to evaluate the regression model.

Table 7 Different regression models tested for arousal and valence with the frame- and song-level annotated and dimensionally reduced datasets. The metrics include correlation coefficient (CC), mean absolute error (MAE), and root mean squared error (RMSE)

Dataset	Label	Algorithm	CC	MAE	RMSE
Song-level	Arousal	**Linear regression**	0.7	0.73	**0.94**
		Additive Regression	0.68	0.75	0.96
		kNN	0.5	0.99	1.23
	Valence	**Linear regression**	0.46	0.72	**0.92**
		Additive regression	0.44	0.73	0.94
		kNN	0.25	1.0	1.27
Frame-level	Arousal	Linear regression	0.59	0.18	0.232
		Additive regression	0.61	0.18	**0.229**
		kNN	0.5	0.21	0.29
	Valence	Linear regression	0.37	0.18	0.218
		Additive regression	0.38	0.17	**0.217**
		kNN	0.34	0.19	0.27

- Mean squared error on the training dataset (T-MSE) to provide the level of "overfitting".
- "Baseline" MSE (RMSE)—the MSE achieved when the unknown variable is always set equal to the average value of the training set.

Figure 11 and Table 8 present the details on parameter tuning and regression.

SVM Linear performed better on song-level datasets and random forest on frame-level datasets. Valence was more precisely estimated than arousal for all tested cases. Once different algorithms have been trained and compared and the optimal regression model is chosen, pyAudioAnalysis function will be used to estimate the regression

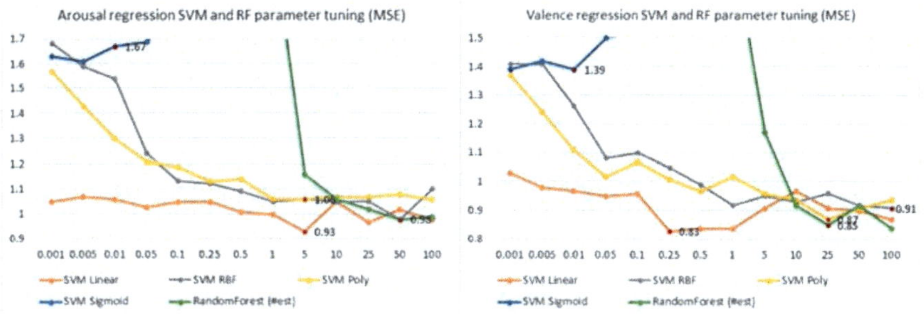

Fig. 11 Parameter tuning results—finding the optimal parameter value (c-parameter) for SVM regression models with different kernels and random forest (number of estimators). The charts present the optimal parameter value for each algorithm that minimizes MSE tested on the song-level dataset

Table 8 Different regression models tested for arousal and valence with the frame- and song-level annotated datasets in Python. The metrics include a mean squared error (MSE), MSE on training data (T-MSE), and "baseline" MSE (RMSE)

Dataset	Label	Algorithm	MSE	T-MSE	RMSE
Song-level	Arousal	Random forest, n = 50	0.95	0.29	1.64
		SVM Linear, c = 5	**0.93**	0.76	1.61
	Valence	Random forest, n = 100	0.84	0.28	1.37
		SVM Linear, c = 0.25	**0.83**	0.75	1.37
Frame-level	Arousal	**Random forest**, n = 50	**0.034**	0.05	0.08
		SVM Linear, c = 5	0.049	0.17	0.08
	Valence	**Random forest**, n = 50	**0.033**	0.05	0.06
		SVM Linear, c = 5	0.047	0.17	0.06

variable for an unknown audio file. The open-source music database of unannotated songs, such as the one in [5] will be used for testing in the future.

4.2.3 Regression Results in RapidMiner

RapidMiner software was used to test additional algorithms for regression. RapidMiner allows for running several algorithms at a time and produces comparative results. The following algorithms were compared for regression models: generalized linear model, deep learning, decision tree, random forest, gradient boosted trees, and support vector machine. Additionally, an automatic feature selection was used for each model. Table 9 presents the number of selected features and regression metrics for each algorithm.

The models were compared using root mean square error (RMSE), the relative error (%), squared error, and correlation. In all tested cases, the deep learning model outperformed other algorithms in all these metrics. The models built on frame-level were characterized with much higher relative error than models built on the song-level feature datasets. Valence value was estimated better than arousal on the song-level datasets, but on the frame-level datasets arousal was estimated better than valence.

5 Discussion

Within this work, a framework for emotion-based music recommender system, called EMOTIN, was presented. The preliminary results included testing regression models for music emotion recognition (MER). Further experiments will be conducted to improve the accuracy of MER with the goal of providing more accurate music recommendations. The future work on EMOTIN includes the implementation of the presented system, including music RS input and output screens, and recommenda-

Table 9 Comparison of regression models tested in Rapid Miner for the song- and frame-level datasets using optimal feature selection

Dataset	Label	Algorithm	No of features	RMSE	Relative error	Squared error	Correlation
Song-level	Arousal	Generalized linear model	9	1.066	16.2%	1.14	0.526
		Deep learning	13	**1.049**	16.0%	1.106	0.557
		Decision tree	1	1.178	18.1%	1.39	0.427
		Random forest	11	1.069	16.2%	1.146	0.547
		Gradient boosted trees	15	1.086	16.2%	1.182	0.533
		Support vector machine	2	1.154	16.9%	1.334	0.465
	Valence	Generalized linear model	13	1.009	14.9%	1.022	0.537
		Deep learning	16	**0.986**	14.7%	0.976	0.573
		Decision tree	1	1.106	16.1%	1.225	0.389
		Random forest	8	0.99	14.5%	0.985	0.554
		Gradient boosted trees	16	1.019	14.8%	1.043	0.53
		Support vector machine	5	0.987	15.1%	0.979	0.579
Frame-level	Arousal	Generalized linear model	29	0.223	67.0%	0.05	0.631
		Deep learning	15	**0.209**	63.9%	0.044	0.685
		Decision tree	10	0.23	69.6%	0.053	0.598
		Random forest	6	0.224	69.1%	0.05	0.633
		Gradient boosted trees	7	0.225	67.4%	0.051	0.621
		Support vector machine	5	0.229	67.3%	0.052	0.605
	Valence	Generalized linear model	34	0.216	78.7%	0.047	0.404
		Deep learning	24	**0.204**	76.1%	0.042	0.502
		Decision tree	1	0.227	82.8%	0.051	0.275
		Random forest	2	0.22	80.0%	0.048	0.343
		Gradient boosted trees	6	0.214	78.0%	0.046	0.41
		Support vector machine	6	0.229	80.9%	0.052	0.267

tion algorithm. Next, the goal will be to evaluate the prototype with clinical experts and tinnitus patients. Once sufficient feedback data is gathered, the system will be expanded with the learning-from-user-feedback functionality. The end result of this interdisciplinary research is expected to provide better and more personalized healthcare for tinnitus patients based on retraining negative emotions with sound therapy, counseling, and music interventions.

References

1. Aljanaki, A., Yang, Y. H., Soleymani, M.: Developing a benchmark for emotional analysis of music. PLoS ONE **12**(3) (2017)
2. American Music Therapy Association: What is Music Therapy? https://www.musictherapy.org (2019)
3. American Tinnitus Association: Understanding the Facts. www.ata.org/understanding-facts (2020)
4. Argstatter, H., Grapp, M., Hutter, E., Plinkert, P., Bolay, H.V.: Long-term effects of the "Heidelberg Model of Music Therapy" in patients with chronic tinnitus. Int. J. Clin. Exp. Med. **5**(4), 273–288 (2012)
5. Bertin-Mahieux, T., Ellis, D.P.W., Whitman, B., Lamere, P.: The million song dataset. In: Proceedings of the 12th International Conference on Music Information Retrieval (ISMIR 2011)
6. Bittner, R., Salamon, J., Tierney, M., Mauch, M., Cannam, C., Bello, J.P.: MedleyDB: a multitrack dataset for annotation- intensive MIR research, In: Proceedings of the 15th International Conference on Music Information Retrieval (ISMIR 2014)
7. Bradley, M.M., Lang, P.J.: Measuring emotion: the self-assessment manikin and the semantic differential. J. Behav. Ther. Exp. Pychiatry **25**(1), 49–59 (1994)
8. Defferrard, M., Benzi, K., Vandergheynst, P., Bresson, X.: FMA: a dataset for music analysis. In: 18th International Society for Music Information Retrieval Conference (2017)
9. Dispoto, B., Tarnowska, K.: A clinical decision support system for tinnitus diagnosis and therapy. In: Poster Session Presented at: 32nd Annual CSU Biotechnology Symposium, Santa Clara, CA (2020)
10. Free Music Archive. http://freemusicarchive.org (2020)
11. Giannakopoulos, T.: pyAudioAnalysis: an open-source Python library for audio signal analysis. PloS ONE. **10**(12) (2015)
12. Grapp, M., Hutter, E., Argstatter, H., Plinkert, P.K., Bolay, H.V.: Music therapy as an early intervention to prevent chronification of tinnitus. Int. J. Clin. Exp. Med. **6**(7), 589–593 (2013)
13. Jastreboff, P.J., Hazell, J.W.P.: Tinnitus Retraining Therapy: Implementing the Neurophysiological Model. Cambridge University Press, Cambridge (2004)
14. Jastreboff, P.J.: 25 years of tinnitus retraining therapy. HNO **63**(4), 307–311 (2015)
15. Kohli, D., Ras, Z.W., Thompson, P.L., Jastreboff, P.J., Wieczorkowska, A.: From music to emotions and tinnitus treatment, initial study. In: Foundations of Intelligent Systems, Proceedings of ISMIS 2012 Symposium, LNAI, vol. 7661, pp. 244–253. Springer (2012)
16. Mostafavi, A.C., Ras, Z.W., Wieczorkowska, A.: From personalized to hierarchically structured classifiers for retrieving music by Mood. In: Post-Proceedings of NFMCP 2013, ECML/PKDD Workshop, Prague, Czech Republic, LNAI, vol. 8399, pp. 231–245. Springer (2014)
17. Okamoto, H., Stracke, H., Stoll, W., Pantev, C.: Listening to tailor-made notched music reduces tinnitus loudness and tinnitus-related auditory cortex activity. Proc. Natl. Acad. Sci. **107**(3), 1207–1210 (2010)
18. pyAudioAnalysis. https://github.com/tyiannak/pyAudioAnalysis (2020)
19. Ras, Z.W., Wieczorkowska, A.: Action-rules: how to increase profit of a company. In: Principles of Data Mining and Knowledge Discovery, pp. 587–592. Springer (2000)
20. Ras, Z. W., Wieczorkowska, A.: Advances in Music Information Retrieval. Studies in Computational Intelligence. Springer (2010)
21. Russell, J.A.: A circumplex model of affect. J. Personal. Soc. Psychol. **39**(6), 1161–1178 (1980)
22. Scherer, K.R.: What are emotions? And how can they be measured? Soc. Sci. Inf. **44**(4), 695–729 (2005)
23. Simunek, M.: LISp-Miner control language description of scripting language implementation. J. Syst. Integr. **5**(2), 28–44 (2014)
24. Soleymani, M., Caro, M.N., Schmidt, E.M., Sha, C., Yang, Y.: 1000 songs for emotional analysis of music. In: Proceedings of the 2nd ACM International Workshop on Crowdsourcing for Multimedia, pp. 1–6 . ACM (2013)

25. Swain, S.K., Nayak, S., Ravan, J.R., Sahu, M.C.: Tinnitus and its current treatment—still an enigma in medicine. J. Formos Med. Assoc. **115**(3), 139–144 (2016)
26. Tarnowska, K.A., Ras, Z.W., Jastreboff, P.J.: Decision support system for diagnosis and treatment of hearing disorders. The case of Tinnitus. Studies in Computational Intelligence, vol. 685. Springer, International (2017)
27. Tarnowska, K., Ras, Z.W., Daniel, L.: Recommender System for Improving Customer Loyalty. Studies in Big Data, vol. 55. Springer, International (2020)
28. Tarnowska, K.A., Ras, Z.W., Jastreboff P.J.: Mining for actionable knowledge in tinnitus datasets. In: Thriving Rough Sets, pp. 367–395, Springer, International (2017)
29. Tkalcic, M., Kosir, A., Tasic, J.: Affective recommender systems: the role of emotions in recommender systems. In: A Felfernig et al. (eds.) Joint Proceedings of the RecSys 2011 Workshop on Human Decision Making in Recommender Systems (Decisions@RecSys '11) and User-centric Evaluation of Recommender Systems and their Interfaces-2 (UCERSTI 2) Affiliated with the 5th ACM Conference on Recommender, pp. 9–13 (2011)
30. Wasyluk, H., Ras, Z.W., Wyrzykowska, E.: Application of action rules to HEPAR clinical decision support system. Exp. Clin. Hepatol. **4**(2), 46–48 (2008)

A Model of Typhlo Music Therapy in Educational and Rehabilitation Work with Visually Impaired Persons

Pawel Cylulko and Joanna Gladyszewska-Cylulko

Abstract The aim of this paper is to present the specifics of a support intervention for visually impaired persons, carried out according to the author's model of typhlo music therapy. The model is based mainly on the sightless approach to experiencing music, the healing potential of music and, above all, the rehabilitative and therapeutic dimension of the human–music relationship. As a result, the fundamental feature which distinguishes the proposed method from other models of support interventions is primarily the tactile and auditory nature of the measures, programmes, session structures and therapy session scenarios used. Consequently, the rehabilitation and therapeutic activities do not require the participants to use unimpaired visual perception and forms of behaviour requiring a fully functional visual analyser. This model plays an important role in stimulating the individual development of persons with a disability, improving the impaired body functions and in optimal adaptation to everyday functioning without sight or with serious visual impairment. The model was developed in the early 1990s and it was later modified, improved and evaluated in the Department of Music Therapy at the Karol Lipinski Academy of Music in Wroclaw and in the Maria Grzegorzewska Lower Silesian Special Educational Centre for Blind and Visually Impaired Children in Wroclaw (Poland) over the last thirty years. The authors of the article, professionals in such disciplines as clinical psychology, music therapy, music education and special education, share their thoughts, observations, experiences and conclusions based on their many years of work. They attempt, among other things, to standardise the basic terms, concepts and definitions in the field of music therapy for visually impaired persons by relating them to the paradigms of special education.

P. Cylulko (✉)
Karol Lipinski Academy of Music in Wroclaw, Wroclaw, Poland
e-mail: pawel.cylulko@amkl.edu.pl

J. Gladyszewska-Cylulko
Institute of Pedagogy, University of Wroclaw, Wroclaw, Poland
e-mail: joanna.gladyszewska-cylulko@uwr.edu.pl

Z. W. Ras et al. (eds.), *Recommender Systems for Medicine and Music*,
Studies in Computational Intelligence 946,
https://doi.org/10.1007/978-3-030-66450-3_14

1 Introduction

Persons with permanent visual impairment form a complex and diverse population in terms of type, degree and extent of disability. This population comprises children, teenagers and adults who are, generally speaking, fully or almost fully blind or partially sighted. There are also persons with additional developmental deficits and chronic diseases within this group. Fully or almost fully blind persons orient themselves in the surrounding space, move around, monitor their own and other people's behaviour, communicate and obtain information in a sightless manner, i.e. mainly through touch and hearing, but also through smell and taste. Partially sighted persons mainly use their residual sight, followed by hearing, touch, smell and taste. The functioning of both of these groups of people usually progresses in a specific, unique and characteristic way for each group. The main and fundamental reason for this state of affairs is, aside from fully or significantly impaired visual perception, the secondary effects of the disability, and improper conditions of development, rehabilitation and education. These factors generate, to varying degrees and extents, psychophysiological, emotional and social problems, which in turn may transform into difficulties, limitations, deficiencies and setbacks in the everyday lives of these persons [18, 23, 27]. All these adverse factors often require support intervention from the dedicated associations, institutions and specialists, including such professionals as doctors, psychologists, educators, speech therapists and music therapists.

In the context of working with visually impaired persons, music therapy intervention is often perceived as an unorthodox and innovative healing, educational, rehabilitation or therapeutic approach. On the one hand, it is met with great commitment and dedication on the part of music therapists and family members of persons with disabilities. On the other hand, it is met with misunderstanding, disbelief, scepticism, lack of knowledge or even resistance. Both in theory and practice, this type of art therapy is often considered to be of secondary importance. This may be due to such factors as attachment to traditional forms of rehabilitation through teaching these persons to handle everyday activities, orientation and locomotion in space and the Braille alphabet. In addition, there are prejudices and stereotypes about the innate and extraordinary musical talents of such persons [22].

When analysing publications in the field of music therapy, it can be noticed that they very rarely discuss matters concerning the therapeutic effect of music on visually impaired persons. Even if papers are published on the subject, they usually cover general, superficial issues and often do not fully convey the essence of the artistic and healing impact of music. Most often, these publications are of a popular or popular science nature. This can be evidenced by the lack of theoretical foundations (references to the paradigms of such disciplines as medicine, pedagogy and psychology), substantive instruction (presentation of therapeutic approaches, methods and techniques used in the professional clinical practice of music therapy), and above all, failure to relate theoretical knowledge and practical experience to the abstract, asemantic and amorphous nature of the art of music (professional discussion of forms of musical activity in terms of their artistic and aesthetic dimension). For example, according to certain publications, music therapy for children with visual impairment is the integration of musical structures with educational methods in order to eliminate inappropriate behaviour and stimulate their individual development [26]. Others focus on the amateur musical activity of children or their musical education. In those publications, the problems of music education, special education, rehabilitation and music therapy are often discussed synonymously as a single issue. Thus, there is definitely a shortage of scientific papers which explore and describe, in a professional manner, i.e. methodically, the sightless character of music therapy activities carried out with persons with visual impairment in and through music.

2 Music—The Most Accessible of All the Fine Arts

Every person, including the visually impaired, from the first moments of their life has a creative potential, shows great interest in music and their musicality is almost innate [17]. For them, music is the closest, the most accessible and the most communicative of all the fine arts, as it is perceived directly through the auditory analyser [15]. By making music, the person becomes completely free and fully independent in the field of music, as visual impairment does not prevent them from experiencing this form of art [12]. This allows them to compete on an equal footing with able-bodied persons, and in certain situations achieve even better results [1, 10, 13, 14]. Through music, they can discover their perceptive, creative and imitative potential, and thereby fully experience the intuitiveness, creativity and agency behind their artistic activity [11]. It can be argued that music, on the one hand, evokes emotions and the desire to express them and, on the other hand, provides a sense of security [20]. These positive experiences can be transferred from the sphere of the healing effects of music to the daily functioning of a person with a disability and thus, despite the disability, they can gain a sense of their aptitudes and abilities, not only musical but also motor, verbal and vocal. This contributes to the fact that these individuals can experience their autonomy, subjectivity and dignity to a fuller extent and thus influence their quality of life [28]. However, very often, due to the serious secondary effects of visual impairment, frequent additional dysfunctions and developmental deficits as well as improper conditions of the educational environment, the contact of visually impaired persons with music is still significantly hampered. For instance, for many of them, practising music using a properly trained voice, professional musical instruments and in the full artistic and aesthetic dimension is virtually impossible. In order to remedy this situation, some specialists propose, on the one hand, music therapy interventions, and on the other, simple percussion instruments, such as drums, maracas, tambourines, claves, cymbals or Orff instruments as the most appropriate form of contact with music and the most suitable musical instruments for this group.

3 The Concept of Typhlo Music Therapy

Until the mid-1990s, neither theoretical knowledge nor practical experience in the field of music therapy for the visually impaired had been consolidated under a single coherent theoretical and practical system developed as a complete model of support intervention. Among other things, there was no exhaustive definition of music therapy for this population or the right term allowing for its precise definition. Neither in the academic literature nor in the practical experience of professionals were there any complete and fully developed models for educational, rehabilitation or therapeutic procedures using the art of music in working with visually impaired persons.

The model presented in this paper has been developed and modified for thirty years in terms of its theoretical foundations, methodology for carrying out practical activities, and with a view to teaching candidates for the profession of music therapist. It is based on the Polish Scientific Concept of Music Therapy developed by the progenitor of the Polish and Wroclaw school of music therapy, Prof. Tadeusz Natanson, PhD, which orders that, generally speaking, music therapy activities be carried out according to the paradigm of the humanistic and objective concept of disability while maintaining the balance between theoretical knowledge and practical experience [9, 19]. Due to its theoretical and practical assumptions, the concept is embedded in the subjective, social dimension of music, special education and music therapy. It also refers to the idea of humanistic psychology, focusing on the visually impaired person and their individual experience. Under this model, particular importance is attached to their individuality, autonomy and self-determination, and thus to their personal experience, creativity and musical activity. This humanistic and, at the same time, holistic approach to the visually impaired person provides optimal conditions for the full development of their personality. Such a holistic approach to the visually impaired person is indicative of the healing nature of the rehabilitation and therapeutic actions aimed towards them, and directs these actions mainly towards the positive potential inherent in the person. As a result, their creative abilities necessary to overcome the effects of visual impairment and thus to achieve a new quality of life are activated.

The model of typhlo music therapy, through the system of specific assumptions, terms, concepts, definitions and the relations between them, serves to explore theoretical, practical and research problems arising in the area of music therapy for the visually impaired. The mental construct contained within it allows us to discern the unique health situation of persons with disabilities in terms of the aetiology of visual impairment, its secondary effects and accompanying diseases. This model is based on the author's own concept of music therapy for visually impaired persons, in which the author's own definition of music therapy for the visually impaired has been adopted [4, 5, 7, 8]. Along with the term typhlo music therapy, it was first presented in 1995 in Poland at an international scientific conference on special education [3]. Then both the definition and the term were presented as part of an academic presentation at the 8th World Congress of Music Therapy held in 1996 at the Hamburg University of Music and Theatre (Germany) [2]. The development of the definition, the introduction of the term and the emergence of typhlo music therapy as a separate subdiscipline of music therapy mainly resulted from the specific perception and functioning of visually impaired persons, the unique place of music in their lives, and the specific functions, goals and measures used in typhlo music therapy interactions.

The term "typhlo music therapy" is derived from three Greek words: typhl?s—blind; mousiké—musical works, the art of composing from sounds or reproducing them using musical instruments; therape?a—treatment, medical activity aimed at restoring people's health, mental and physical fitness by means of medicines and medical procedures. For the purposes of this model, the definition of typhlo music therapy is as follows: typhlo music therapy (TMT) is a form of support intervention aimed at persons with visual impairment, using multiple forms of music and other acoustic (non-musical) phenomena in order to stimulate, develop, correct, compensate and improve the impaired body functions and optimally adapt such persons to active participation in various areas and domains of life, in particular social life. This definition allows us to determine within the adopted model how the process of treatment with music should proceed, who should participate in it, how the measures should be applied, and how to design and implement the typhlo music therapeutic programme.

Typhlo music therapy is mainly based on a sightless intervention aimed towards visually impaired persons, i.e. a tactile and auditory approach both to the art of music and to therapy. This specific basis guarantees the uniqueness of the TMT model and its originality, which fundamentally distinguishes it from other therapeutic, educational and rehabilitation procedures. Although the sightless aspect is a true hallmark of this model, it is not its main defining feature, but rather a fundamental feature distinguishing the model from other therapeutic options used. This effect is mainly accompanied by the sightless interaction between the therapist and the patient, developing as a result of auditory, tactile and kinaesthetic, olfactory and even taste sensations. It is mainly a sound and musical interpersonal relationship where the typhlo music therapist, assisting the patient in their development, offers them friendly, emotional and dynamic support through music as well as therapeutic intervention [21]. Instead of visual sensations, the therapist offers the patient new experiences enriched with auditory and tactile sensations. This way, the patient perceives themselves, their problems and the surrounding reality in a new and different way, providing them with a sense of security, intimacy, community and interpersonal bonds within the framework of therapeutic interventions using music [16, 25].

4 Typhlo Music Therapeutic Procedure

Typhlo music therapy implemented according to the described model can and should be used in working with children, teenagers and adults, including those with additional diseases and developmental deficits, i.e. patients (clients) in various life, social and cultural situations. The condition for participation in typhlo music therapy sessions is having permanent visual impairment, manifesting a variety of physical, psychomotor, mental, emotional and social problems, difficulties and irregularities hindering everyday functioning, not always resulting from the visual impairment itself or from its secondary effects. In order for the therapeutic intervention to generate the expected results, the person with a disability should be taught to consciously take advantage of the health benefits of the art of music and music therapy from the earliest months of their life. This type of activity, generally speaking, can be referred to as preparation for music therapy [6]. It can take place, for example, in a child's home, crèche, kindergarten, school (at various educational levels), hospital, rehabilitation, education, recreation, or sports centre and at the workplace. A serious contraindication for the use of therapy according to the discussed model may be inadequate space, furniture, equipment and lighting of the office, as for the participants of therapy sessions all this significantly hampers spatial orientation and locomotion, distorts the perception of human speech and various acoustic phenomena as well as music created "live" or played from recordings, and above all, it may result in a feeling of fatigue, agitation, confusion and danger. The same applies to the quality, quantity and variety of the musical instruments used and the electronic equipment that reproduces and records sound and video. Other unacceptable items in the studio include steps, pillars, protruding objects, sharp edges, rolling carpets, slippery floor or walls that are too bright or too dark. All this can fundamentally hinder or even prevent interventions using the TMT model.

Typhlo music therapy may perform various functions in the life, treatment, education and rehabilitation of visually impaired persons, including diagnostic, developmental, physiotherapeutic, psychotherapeutic, healing, educational, integrative (community), recreational and play, aesthetic and adaptive functions. The main objective of this type of assistance is to support the individual development of visually impaired persons, to improve their impaired functions and to cultivate their mutual cooperation. Other equally important goals and objectives include, among others:

- inspiring cognitive, motor, intellectual and social activity;
- stimulation of the senses: auditory, tactile, kinaesthetic and motor, and visual (for partially sighted persons);
- correcting abnormal posture and reducing blindisms;
- improving motor functions (mainly locomotion and manipulation);
- improving orientation in one's own body and in space;
- improving speech, mental dispositions (thinking, attention, remembering etc.);
- reducing fear and anxiety;
- channelling and sublimation of aggression;
- reducing excessive psychophysical and emotional tension;
- stimulation and modification of expression (motor, speech, vocal, artistic, musical, etc.);
- encouraging self-acceptance, embracing of one's disability, illness and its consequences;
- overcoming reluctance to tackle difficulties, limitations and obstacles;
- increasing self-esteem, independence and resourcefulness;
- building confidence in oneself, one's potential and capabilities;

- modifying abnormal social behaviour;
- teaching how to establish and maintain interpersonal relations and cooperate in a social group;
- improving mood and well-being;
- providing pleasure, joy and a sense of satisfaction.

In order to achieve the set therapeutic goals and objectives in the most effective way possible, it was necessary to develop an appropriate arrangement of the TMT model's components, which are therapeutic, artistic and logistical in nature. In order for them to be suitable for working with visually impaired persons, they are optimally adapted to their specific perception and functioning in everyday life. Both the individual components, as well as their arrangements and the dynamic interrelationships between them, provide the model with structure, coherence and internal stability, and thus ensure the substantive correctness, effectiveness and efficiency of the intervention. The key components of the TMT model include, among others:

- the term and concept of "typhlo music therapy";
- the therapeutic functions, goals and objectives;
- the measures used in the support intervention (sound and music material, therapeutic techniques, aids etc.);
- the intervention programme (individual and group);
- the conditions and methods of carrying out the therapeutic process;
- the structure of the therapy session;
- early initiation of typhlo music therapy;
- the active participation of the patient's family members in the intervention.

The substantive, organisational and musical assumptions adopted in the TMT model for its components, in a fundamental way, involve the various stages of intervention in the area of music therapy for visually impaired persons. They include, among others:

- carrying out promotional, preventive and educational activities in the patient's environment, e.g. through talks, demonstrations, publications;
- preliminary diagnosis, i.e. making an initial diagnosis concerning the patient's functioning and their immediate family environment, as the therapy progresses, including formulating partial diagnoses;
- construction, modification and verification of the tools necessary for diagnostic activities;
- formulation of indications and contraindications for the use of the therapy, its course;
- specification of the goals and objectives of the therapeutic intervention;
- planning the therapeutic measures to be used;
- implementing the typhlo music therapy programme (individual and group);
- secondary diagnosis, including modification of the predetermined intervention programme and patient progress;
- carrying out further therapeutic treatment;

- evaluation, consulting the patient, their family and other specialists on the effectiveness and efficiency of the TMT model.

Since the structure of the components and the step-by-step approach adopted within the typhlo music therapy model serve to achieve better stability, predictability and thus the safety of the intervention when working with visually impaired persons, they should not be omitted nor replaced by other procedures.

5 Acoustic Material

The main means of therapy applied in each model, approach and method of music therapy is the art of music and its individual components such as melodics, metrorhythmics, agogics, dynamics, articulation, timbre, phrasing and a range of musical instruments. In a typhlo music therapeutic intervention, various non-musical acoustic materials are used to the same extent as music, and sometimes even more frequently and to a greater extent. It can include, on the one hand, music (songs, ballads, instrumental, vocal, and vocal-instrumental pieces, accompaniments, dances, soundtracks, music videos, etc.) and non-musical sound phenomena (e.g. single sounds, noises, murmurs, rustling, rumbling, crackling, knocking and gurgling) and silence. This material, programmed so as to meet the expectations, capabilities and preferences of patients and the therapeutic goals set, is essential for the success of the TMT model by providing its participants with:

- emotional and aesthetic sensations (by experiencing the beauty of art and single sounds);
- cognitive information (supporting the identification of sounds emitted by objects and various acoustic phenomena);
- orientation cues (making it easier to get acquainted with one's own body, space and the possibilities of moving around in it);
- control data (helping to check practical activities—performing movements, everyday activities etc.);
- communicative signals (facilitating the establishment and maintenance of interpersonal relations and communication with other people).

In terms of effective support for the development and functioning of persons with disabilities, all this information and these experiences are very important, and sometimes even fundamental. When used improperly during a therapeutic intervention, they may result in unnecessary chaos and confusion in the interpretation of the patients' surroundings by means of hearing. In clinical practice, this means that, on the one hand, the acoustic space must not be enriched by too many auditory stimuli and their excessive intensity and, on the other hand, it must not be impoverished by too few stimuli and their insufficient power and range of influence. Thus, under certain conditions, the acoustic space accompanying typhlo music therapy sessions may be a source of too bland or too intense, and sometimes even overwhelming, auditory stimuli. In both cases, it may hinder the proper course of TMT intervention. In other words, the sound environment must be clear and understandable to all patients (children in particular) at all times, as it is only accessible for them by hearing (and to a limited extent).

When discussing the therapeutic significance of the patient's acoustic space, it is worth mentioning silence as a fundamental acoustic, linguistic, musical and therapeutic phenomenon. Due to the compensatory role of hearing in the lives of persons with disabilities, it is a very important means of therapy used under the TMT model, as well as musical and non-musical sounds. Most often, silence is not even mentioned in the literature on the subject—as a very important, in certain situations even essential, means of therapy. It can communicate that which neither verbal nor musical means can express, convey or portray. Since the auditory analyser of a visually impaired person is always in a state of constant vigilance and operation, in their everyday life such persons often lack room for the silence to "resonate", and sometimes even the permission or opportunity for it to occur. This may be caused by constant "scanning" of the audiosphere and searching for various sensations and auditory information, compensating in a partial and limited way for the lack, or significant impairment, of visual sensations.

6 Music Therapy Sessions

Implementation of the TMT model in clinical practice requires the creation of an intervention programme that does not require the patient's visual perception and that is based on the sightless use of therapeutic measures, i.e. acoustic material, therapeutic techniques, forms of musical activity, methods of implementation, props, office equipment, scenarios and therapeutic session structures. When working with fully blind and visually impaired persons, this approach gives priority to modes of action based mainly on tactile, kinaesthetic and auditory impressions, and secondly, on olfactory and taste ones. In the case of the partially sighted, there are also activities that stimulate damaged sight. The typhlo music therapist modifies the standard means of music therapy, adapting them to larger sizes, diverse shapes, clearer surface textures, different elasticity of materials, enlarged print, contrasting background, more intense colours, flavours, smells and vibrations, and designs completely new measures based on the activities carried out [16, 24]. The use of sightless means of therapy under the TMT model requires that they be used in accordance with the principle of demonstration, consisting of e.g. verbal instruction and the patient "examining" using touch, smell and sometimes also taste. This procedure leads to the elimination from the intervention of those methods of therapy whose success is dependent on direct, unimpaired visual cognition. In practice, this requires the specialist to be able to shift from the music therapy methods based on sight to methods based only on auditory, tactile and kinaesthetic, olfactory and taste sensations and information. Thus, the sightless approach to music, its healing potential and the rehabilitative and therapeutic dimension of the human–music relationship could be referred to as typhlological.

The basic method of typhlo music therapy intervention is musical and sound interaction with the use of gestures, motions, verbalisation, vocalisation, simple musical instruments, dancing and psychodrama. This results in sightless therapeutic situations which arise through the use of specific methods referred to as therapeutic techniques, which differ in terms of the type of musical activity, the use of sound, body and the degree of difficulty. Based on the criterion of the main objectives of these techniques, five main groups can be distinguished:

- activation and compensation techniques (tactile exercises, listening exercises, exercises improving the sense of rhythm, singing songs, making music with gestures, making music with everyday objects, making music on instruments made by hand, making music on simple percussion instruments, practising natural forms of locomotion, movements imitating everyday activities, music and movement games, dancing, etc.);
- imagination and projection techniques (listening to music, artistic interpretation of music, etc.);
- creative techniques (verbal improvisations, vocal improvisations, musical and movement improvisations, mimic exercises etc.);
- intrapersonal and interpersonal techniques (improvisation on children's percussion instruments, pantomime, psychodrama, role-playing staging a song, therapeutic conversations etc.);
- relaxation techniques with a musical background (breathing exercises, relaxation massage, Schultz autogenic training, Jacobson's progressive relaxation technique, etc.).

Intervention situations constructed using single therapeutic techniques or various compilations thereof create typhlo music therapy sessions carried out according to the TMT model. Such sessions, due to difficulties in adaptation of persons with disabilities to numerous and diverse changes, situations, events and circumstances occurring in time and space, should be conducted according to a strictly defined organisational and therapeutic plan, if possible fixed and unchanging from the beginning until the end of the series of meetings. The plan allows patients to anticipate the successive stages of therapeutic activities, and thus offers them a greater sense of security. Therefore, a single session under the model should consist of three main phases: (1) initial; (2) proper and (3) final.

Each of them is a set of exercises and games. The first phase includes introductory activities and serves to build mutual trust between all the participants and the therapist, and to activate their psychomotor functions, improving their concentration. This stage puts the group members in the mood of the music therapy session and motivates them to play and create. This phase may include, for example: getting to know the typhlo music therapy office, its furniture and equipment, the therapist greeting the whole group and each patient individually and all the participants greeting each other, breathing exercises, rhythmic exercises, verbal improvisations, singing songs, making music with gestures, making music with everyday objects, making music on instruments made by hand, practising natural forms of locomotion and movements that imitate everyday activities.

The second (proper) phase is the main part of the therapeutic session. Its objective is to stimulate and develop the dynamics of the group, foster the patients' acceptance of themselves and their disabilities as well as their sense of their own value, uniqueness and exceptionality, improve functioning in the therapeutic group and enable assimilation of specific skills (e.g. proper communication, tolerance, empathy, orientation and movement in space). This part of the meeting may involve, for example: listening exercises, tactile exercises, vocal improvisations, improvisations on children's percussion instruments or Orff instruments, music and movement improvisations, music and movement games, elements of dancing, pantomime, psychodrama, listening to music and artistic interpretations of music.

The third phase includes the final activities and is aimed at reacting to psychophysical and emotional tensions, calming down or relaxing of the TMT session participants, and thus ending the session and saying goodbye to all participants and the therapist. These activities may include, for example: relaxing massage, Schultz autogenic training, Jacobson's progressive relaxation technique, therapeutic conversations, summing up the meeting and saying goodbye to the participants, leaving the therapy room and finding yourself outside it.

The proposed division of the TMT session into three phases serves the purpose of accomplishing the established goals and objectives more efficiently, as well as achieving better structuring, predictability, stability and safety of the music therapy activities. For these reasons, no phase should be omitted or replaced by another. However, it is possible, depending on the individual needs, capabilities, limitations and expectations of individual patients and therapeutic groups participating in the session, to modify and expand this plan according to the needs and progress of therapeutic activities.

7 Conclusions

Over time, the model of typhlo music therapy (TMT) has been constantly developed, modified, improved and thus shaped to fit the current definitions of disability, the conceptualisation of the place of the person with a disability in modern society, and the requirements and paradigms of music therapy and related disciplines such as medicine, special education, rehabilitation and music education. In clinical practice, this type of therapeutic intervention allows for positive diagnosis, correct planning of therapeutic action, the optimal music therapy approach tailored to the individuality and uniqueness of the visually impaired person, and thus respect for their full dignity, subjectivity and autonomy. It should be added that, along with the theoretical assumptions of the model, the practical approach to the visually impaired person, their participation in music therapy, their process of creating music and its result in the form of musical works have also changed over the past years from a more objective approach towards a fully subjective one. It seems that the ongoing evolution of the TMT model guarantees respect for the autonomy, uniqueness, creativity and artistic works of persons with disabilities.

Certainly, this paper is not in a position to exhaustively discuss the complex issue concerning the specifics of typhlo music therapy and the related intervention procedures under the proposed model. Despite the many difficulties in its implementation in facilities for visually impaired persons, it can be expected that over time both their immediate family members and specialists will approach the subject with increasing interest, understanding and trust. We believe that the model of typhlo music therapy presented in this paper will inspire various specialists to use it in their everyday work with visually impaired persons, to modify and improve it by seeking newer, more effective and more efficient methods of music therapy, and to carry out empirical research based on this approach.

8 Notes on the Authors

Pawel Cylulko, Ph.D., DSc—Master of Music Therapy, Master of Music Education, is acting Head of the Department of Music Therapy and the Rector's Representative for Persons with Disabilities of the Karol Lipinski Academy of Music in Wroclaw. President of the Board of the Polish Music Therapists Association for almost 10 years, he is currently the President of the National Music Therapy Council and the founder of the quarterly academic journal "Muzykoterapia Polska" [Polish Music Therapy]. He is the author of numerous publications in the field of music therapy, including three monographs and research papers. His main areas of interest include the rehabilitation and education of children with disabilities using the therapeutic benefits of music, and teaching the new generation of music therapists.

Joanna Gladyszewska-Cylulko—Doctor of Humanities in the field of pedagogy, clinical psychologist, music therapy teacher for blind and visually impaired persons, assistant professor at the Institute of Pedagogy of the University of Wroclaw. The author of numerous academic publications, including two monographs and research papers. She presents her experiences at national, international and foreign academic conferences. Her areas of scientific interest are focused on the education and rehabilitation of persons with visual impairment, in particular on the use of the art of music in their diagnosis and rehabilitation.

Acknowledgements The authors are grateful to Aileen Benedict from the CS Department at the University of North Carolina at Charlotte for formatting this paper into the required format.

References

1. Antović, M., Bennett, A., Turner, M.: Running in circles or moving along lines: conceptualization of musical elements in sighted and blind children. Musicae Sci. **17**(2), 229–245 (2013)
2. Cylulko, P.: Consequences of music therapy in the rehabilitation of the blind and visually impaired. In: Book of Abstracts. VIII World Congress of Music Therapy, II Congress of the World Federation of Music Therapy, p. 187 (1996)

3. Cylulko, P.: Tyflomuzykoterapia jako forma stymulacji rozwoju malych dzieci [typhlo music therapy as a form of stimulating the development of small children]. In: G. Walczak (ed.). Problemy wczesnej rehabilitacji niewidomych i slabowidzacych dzieci [Problems in early rehabilitation of blind and visually impaired children] pp. 71–79 (1996)
4. Cylulko, P.: Muzykoterapia w rehabilitacji ruchowej dzieci niewidomych i słabowidzących [Motor therapy in the rehabilitation of blind and visually impaired children] (1998)
5. Cylulko, P.: Muzykoterapia niewidomych i słabowidzących dzieci [music therapy for blind and visually impaired children. a methodological guide]. Zeszyty Tyflologiczne **16**, 1–112 (1999)
6. Cylulko, P.: Therapy and upbringing of visually impaired children by the use of music. In: M. samoraj (ed.) Essays on Education through Art Time Passing and Time Enduring, pp. 256–260 (2002)
7. Cylulko, P.: Tyflomuzykoterapia dzieci: teoria i praktyka muzykoterapii dzieci z niepełnosprawnością wzrokową [Typhlo music therapy for children. The theory and practice of music therapy for children with visual impairment]. Wydawn. Akademii Muzycznej im. Karola Lipińskiego we Wrocławiu (2004)
8. Cylulko, P.: A pediatric typhlo music therapy model. In: P. Cylulko, J. Gladyszewska-Cylulko (eds.). Wroclaw Music Therapy Models, pp. 41–60 (2016)
9. Cylulko P.G.C.J.: Polska naukowa koncepcja muzykoterapii - w trzydziestolecie wydania ksiazki Tadeusza Natansona wstep do nauki o muzykoterapii [the polish scientific concept of music therapy - on the thirtieth anniversary of the publication of tadeusz natanson's book introduction to the science of music therapy]. in: A. granat-janki (ed.). Tadeusz Natanson. Kompozytor, uczony, pedagog [Composer, Scholar, Pedagogue] pp. 173–184 (2010)
10. Darrow, A.A., Novak, J.: The effect of vision and hearing loss on listeners' perception of referential meaning in music. J. Music Ther. **44**(1), 57–73 (2007)
11. Dauber, M.: What is essential is invisible to the eye: A music therapy tale of a young woman with visual impairment. Approaches: Music Therapy & Special Music Education, Special Issue pp. 20–29 (2011)
12. Decker-Voigt, H.: Musiktherapeutische hilfen für die begleitung von blinden und sehbehinderten. Musiktherapeutische Umschau **15**(2), 135–142 (1994)
13. Eitan, Z., Ornoy, E., Granot, R.Y.: Listening in the dark: congenital and early blindness and cross-domain mappings in music. Psychomusicol. Music Mind Brain **22**(1), 33 (2012)
14. Flowers, P.J., Wang, C.H.: Matching verbal description to music excerpt: The use of language by blind and sighted children. J. Res. Music Educ. **50**(3), 202–214 (2002)
15. Hamilton, R.H., Pascual-Leone, A., Schlaug, G.: Absolute pitch in blind musicians. Neuro Report **15**(5), 803–806 (2004)
16. Lam, R.C., Wang, C.: Integrating blind and sighted through music. Music Educ. J. **68**(8), 44–45 (1982)
17. Malloch, S.N.: Mothers and infants and communicative musicality. Musicae Sci. **3**(1_suppl), 29–57 (1999)
18. Miedziak, A.I., Perski, T., Andrews, P., Donoso, L.A.: Stargardt's macular dystrophy–a patient's perspective. Optometry (St. Louis, Mo.) **71**(3), 165–176 (2000)
19. Natanson T, Wstep do nauki o muzykoterapii [An introduction to the science of music therapy], 1979, Wroclaw-Warsaw-Kraków-Gdansk: The National Ossolinski Institute
20. Nordoff, P., Robbins, C., Bryndal, A., Masiak, E.: Terapia muzyką w pracy z dziećmi niepełnosprawnymi: historia, metoda i praktyka [Music therapy in working with children with disabilities. History, method and practice]. Oficyna Wydawnicza "Impuls" (2008)
21. Pavlicevic, M.: Dynamic interplay in clinical improvisation. J. Br. Music Ther. **4**(2), 5–9 (1990)
22. Pfammatter, X.: Music as a leisure-time occupation for the blind (1988)
23. Preisler, G.M.: A descriptive study of blind children in nurseries with sighted children. Child Care Heal. Dev. **19**(5), 295–315 (1993)
24. Rummel, M.: Ein bad in vibrationen, das klavier in der musiktherapie mit taubblinden. Musiktherapeutische Umschau **13**(2), 109–111
25. Sobey, K.: Out of sight—out of mind? reflections on a blind young woman's use of music therapy. J. Br. Music Ther. **7**(2), 5–11 (1993)

26. Steele, A.L., Crawford, C.: Music therapy for the visually impaired. Educ. Vis. Handicap. **14**(2), 56–62 (1982)
27. Tröster, H., Brambring, M.: Early motor development in blind infants. J. Appl. Dev. Psychol. **14**(1), 83–106 (1993)
28. Wolf, F.: Music therapy with the blind. J. Br. Music Ther. **9**(3), 28–30 (1978)